THERAPEUTIC ENDOSCOPY IN GASTROINTESTINAL SURGERY

RAPHAEL S. CHUNG, M.D., F.A.C.S.

Professor of Surgery, State University of New York
Health Science Center at Syracuse
Director, Surgical Endoscopy Service
Attending Surgeon, State University Hospital
Veterans Administration Medical Center
and Crouse Irving Memorial Hospital
Syracuse, New York

With illustrations prepared by David Factor, M.S.

CHURCHILL LIVINGSTONE
New York, Edinburgh, London, Melbourne 1987

Library of Congress Cataloging-in-Publication Data

Chung, Raphael S.
    Therapeutic endoscopy in gastrointestinal surgery.

    Includes bibliographies and index.
    1. Gastrointestinal system—Surgery.   2. Endoscopic
surgery.   I. Title.   [DNLM: 1. Endoscopy.
2. Gastrointestinal Diseases—surgery.   WI 100 C559t]
RD540.C48   1987   617'.43   86–32692
ISBN 0–443–08394–0

Distributed in the United Kingdom by Churchill Livingstone, Robert
Stevenson House, 1–3 Baxter's Place, Leith Walk, Edinburgh EH1 3AF,
and by associated companies, branches, and representatives throughout
the world.

Accurate indications, adverse reactions, and dosage schedules for drugs
are provided in this book, but it is possible that they may change. The
reader is urged to review the package information data of the
manufacturers of the medications mentioned.

Copy Editor: Julia Muiño
Production Designer: Gloria Brown
Production Supervisor: Jane Grochowski

Printed in the United States of America

First published in 1987

Therapeutic Endoscopy: Its Role in Gastrointestinal Surgery

THE NATURE OF THERAPEUTIC ENDOSCOPY

As the lumen of the gastrointestinal (GI) tract becomes readily accessible to the endoscope, the logical concept of treating luminal lesions by a luminal approach becomes practical. The inherent advantage of such a direct approach is obvious; it eliminates much of the surgical trauma, as it does not require an incision. Indeed, the open surgical approach, in comparison, can only be considered indirect, as luminal lesions are approached from the serosal aspect. The therapeutic importance of endoscopic procedures is such that in a few instances they have acquired the stature of surgical operations. Several surgical operations are no longer (or should no longer be) performed because the equivalent endoscopic procedures have been so successful, with markedly reduced morbidity.

Endoscopic operations, however, have different skill requirements. As an example, consider the open operation of colonic polypectomy. The colon is first exposed by laparotomy, and then the polyp by colotomy. A large variety of surgical instruments, plenty of room for the operator, and the use of assistants tend to make the task

simple. By contrast, the endoscopic procedure is performed by insertion of the endoscope into the colon via the anus. The exposure is restricted, and there is little room to maneuver. The choice of instrument is strictly limited. Even more different is the way the operation is done: The endoscopic polypectomy is done by ''remote control.'' It demands much patience, a high degree of hand–eye coordination, and considerable resourcefulness and ingenuity, even more so than does the equivalent open operation. In some ways endoscopic procedures are more difficult to do, and much more difficult to do well, than the corresponding open operations. If the outcome of operative surgery is dependent on technical skill and judgment, it is even more so in therapeutic endoscopy. The obvious advantages of the endoscopic approach more than make up for the disadvantages: No anesthesia is required and recovery is always rapid, as there are no incisions to heal. Indeed, the relative noninvasiveness of therapeutic endoscopy is so attractive that many overlook the fact that it is also more skill dependent, sometimes more difficult, and less effective in many instances than operative surgery. The price of diminished invasiveness is increased demand of manual dexterity and a higher failure rate. As surgeons know only too well, increased technical complexity is also attended by increased technique-related complications. Therapeutic endoscopy is by no means complication free; many of the complications are life threatening and require treatment with operative surgery. Even though operative surgery is often resorted to after therapeutic endoscopy has failed, it does not necessarily mean that therapeutic endoscopy must always be attempted at all. An illustrative example is esophageal myotomy versus brusque dilation ("blunt myotomy") in the treatment of achalasia. In a center where consistently good results are obtained from myotomy, a strong case can be made for offering the operative treatment for all good-risk patients without first attempting brusque dilation.

THE RATIONALE OF THERAPEUTIC ENDOSCOPY

There are only a limited number of mechanical manipulations with which the endoscopist can treat lesions of the GI tract using the luminal approach. Each of these is the subject of a different chapter. The indications for these procedures fall into three broad categories. First, endoscopic treatment can only be done when the pathology is primarily intraluminal, readily lending itself to mechanical manipulation, such as excision of polyps, dilation of strictures, disimpaction and retrieval of foreign bodies, cautery of a discrete bleeding vessel, and division of the intraluminal part of the sphincter of Oddi. Any intraluminal lesions that, when finally confronted on the operating table, would cause the surgeon to exclaim: "What a pity we have to operate for this," is probably suitable for endoscopic treatment, provided it is within reach of the endoscope. The second broad indication is when and where operative surgery would be hazardous. The endoscopic approach makes more sense in patients considered to be poor operative risks because of systemic disease. Similarly, where the operations are known to be technically difficult and hazardous, such as

in reoperations in the porta hepatis, a luminal route avoiding bloody, tedious, and dangerous dissection should be given a first try. The third indication is for conditions in which the results of operative surgery are known to be poor, such as resection of esophageal stricture or advanced carcinoma of the esophagus.

Despite these broad considerations, the selection of operative surgery versus therapeutic endoscopy is not always clear cut in any individual patient, especially since objective data from controlled clinical trials are difficult to come by. Most decisions are quite subjective, so it is important for the clinician to have a realistic idea of the risks and results of both therapeutic endoscopy and operative surgery in order to make an intelligent, albeit still subjective, choice. It would be ideal for the care of the patient for the therapeutic endoscopist to work hand in hand with the surgeon in an integrated unit attended by gastroenterologists/endoscopists and surgeons. There are only a few of such units in this country, but I believe it will be the trend for the future.

THE PRACTICE OF THERAPEUTIC ENDOSCOPY

Just as in operative surgery, there are certain general requirements for success in therapeutic endoscopy. First and foremost is preparation, including mental preparation of the endoscopist. It is important that therapeutic endoscopy not be scheduled as a minor event, sandwiched between major commitments. Therapeutic endoscopy demands much more time and resourcefulness than diagnostic endoscopy of the same region of the GI tract. Particularly when the procedure is done on a new patient, events have a way of taking an unexpected turn, more often than not for the worse. What the endoscopist does not need under these circumstances is the added pressure of running out of time. Patience and perseverance are essential qualities; they are the only help available to the beleaguered endoscopist during a difficult procedure. Preplanning may need to be elaborate, including careful study of the radiographs and obtaining all relevant measurements. Special instruments and accessories must be at hand. A dry run may be necessary if the instrument has been improvised or has not been used before. When fluoroscopy is considered desirable and the endoscopy suite is not equipped with a fluoroscope, some advance arrangement must be made rather than making do without. The patient too must be adequately prepared. Sedation does not supersede clear explanation of the procedure to allay fear of the unknown. Voluntary cooperation is a sine qua non for operations done under local anesthesia—a well-known surgical truism. If the patient is unable to cooperate, the procedure should be performed under general anesthesia, unless there is some absolute contraindication, an infrequent event. An example is performing sclerotherapy in the intoxicated alcoholic bleeding from esophageal varices: The risk of a general anesthetic is well worth taking in exchange for a controlled airway, a nonthrashing patient, and a calm working environment. There are few data on the risks of instrumental injury in an uncooperative patient, but most experienced endoscopists show a healthy respect by avoiding such encounters. Numerous examples demonstrate that forethought significantly reduces risks. For procedures in the colon, not only is a well-prepared colon essential for a good examination, but it would eliminate the hazard of explosion when cautery is used, as well as minimize mortality and morbidity in the event of a perforation. For procedures in a biliary tract that has been the focus of chronic sepsis, administration of prophylactic systemic antibiotics covering the appropriate spectrum reduces the risks of septicemia. As with operative surgery, or for that matter any clinical undertaking, good judgment is an absolute requirement. It often makes the difference between consistent success and a practice strewn with disasters. Enthusiasm must be tempered with caution; procedures must never be attempted for the sake of technical bravura. Overconfidence in one's technical ability is the basis of untold tales of woe.

Much has been spent by the endoscope manufacturers in advertising for the "therapeutic endoscope." What is a therapeutic endoscope? A simplistic view is that it is a fiberoptic endoscope in which the biopsy channel has been renamed the "instrument channel." The therapeutic endoscope had its real beginning as the result of tinkering by a few endoscopists who were not content merely to insert biopsy forceps down the channel. In order to keep the power of suction intact while the channel is being occupied with an instrument, the channel is made as large as possible. Some therapeutic endoscopes have two channels at the expense of light supply. Light bundles are either smaller or, as in many models, only one bundle instead of two provides the illumination. This is not always a desirable trade-off, as a single bundle illumination may cast a shadow and may take some getting used to. Others have built-in forceps-elevators or a forward-firing water jet. Special modifications are required for laser work, including a built-in filter in the eyepiece for ocular safety and a heat-resistant coat for the tip section. Therapeutic endoscopes are convenient but not essential; for the endoscopist engaged in a substantial volume of therapeutic work, however, investment in such an endoscope is well worthwhile.

Holding great potential for therapeutic endoscopy, particularly for procedures done in a sterile field, is the videoendoscope. When the view is displayed on a high-resolution color monitor, the operator is freed from the eyepiece, a great fatigue factor in endoscopic procedures. In a sterile field (e.g., in choledochoscopy), both the hands and endoscope are secure from contamination by the face and mask of the operator. The assistant can coordinate in intricate maneuvers without the need for verbal communication. Furthermore, the resolution is three to four times as good as the fiberoptic endoscope, and even better resolution is possible in the future. The resolution of the fiberoptic instruments is governed by the size of the individual fiber, which has already attained the smallest size possible, since smaller fibers will not transmit the wavelength of the entire visible spectrum. Even a miniature TV camera attachment installed on the conventional fiberoptic endoscope can provide many of the above advantages and is highly popular with therapeutic endoscopists.

The field of therapeutic endoscopy is exciting and rapidly expanding; application of the existing modalities is limited only by the ingenuity of the endoscopist. The introduction of new technologies will spur new applications. Guided by interdisciplinary cooperative effort, new applications may find their proper role in the existing therapeutic armamentarium. It is safe to predict that as a result of advances in therapeutic endoscopy and the integration of new skills into the practice of GI surgery, the treatment of GI diseases will be more cost effective and the patients better served.

2

Management of Upper Gastrointestinal Bleeding: The Role of Diagnostic and Therapeutic Endoscopy

THE NATURAL HISTORY OF UPPER GASTROINTESTINAL BLEEDING: RATIONALE OF THERAPEUTIC ENDOSCOPY

The natural history of upper gastrointestinal (GI) bleeding has been well studied.[2,4,48,64–66] An overall mortality of 10 percent is expected in all admissions carrying this diagnosis, a figure that has remained virtually unchanged over the past four decades. The proportion of older patients (over age 60) with this diagnosis, however, has steadily risen, from 30 percent in series collected 40 years ago to 60 percent in series of this decade. Of all patients admitted for bleeding, in 80 percent bleeding stops spontaneously within 48 hours; for this group the mortality is less than 3 percent. For those with continued bleeding, or bleeding recurring in the same hospitalization, the mortality is 20 percent. Emergency surgery for continued bleeding carries a mortality of more than 15 percent.[2,4,20,59] In addition, mortality is adversely affected by prognostic factors such as massive bleeding, old age, coexisting systemic diseases, and certain conditions carrying increased risk of rebleeding, such as esophageal varices, giant duodenal ulcers, and ulcers with exposed vessels. Massive bleeding has been variously defined, but most studies agree that hypotension at presentation is a valid index of severity. It is also commonly accepted that bleeding at a rate requiring more than 1 unit of blood replacement every 6 to 8 hours is called massive. Massive bleeders are more apt to be found actively bleeding at emergency endoscopy, and the mortality of actively and massively bleeding patients is many times higher.[2,25,48]

The contribution of endoscopy in diagnosis is nowhere more evident than in GI hemorrhage. There is little controversy that diagnostic accuracy has been much enhanced with timely endoscopy, especially for upper GI hemorrhage.[14,33,65] It therefore seems somewhat puzzling that almost all controlled studies showed that, despite the use of emergency endoscopy which resulted in earlier and more accurate diagnosis, there has been no demonstrable improvement in survival of these patients.[19,21,27,40,54,62] Emergency diagnostic endoscopy has been defined, for the purpose of these studies, as a procedure performed either when the patient was actively bleeding or within the following 12 hours. If the results of these studies are somewhat surprising, it is because of the common assumption that better diagnosis would automatically lead to better survival, without consideration of the patient's condition or the treatment rendered. In Peterson's series,[54] for example, a standardized antacid treatment was given to all study patients irrespective of the findings at endoscopy, including variceal bleeding. It is clear that the outcome cannot be improved by an early diagnosis if the information is not appropriately used. Another reason that outcome may not benefit from earlier and more accurate diagnosis is the nature of the disease. For example, the patient with inoperable cancer who presents with bleeding is unlikely to be affected by any current therapy, or the poor-risk patient correctly diagnosed to be bleeding from a peptic ulcer and referred for surgery as a last resort is still a poor risk irrespective of how early the bleeding source has been identified. As Conn[13] pointed out, one must not blame the diagnostic technique for the inadequacy of the therapy. It may well be that those patients who died would not have survived an operation; therefore, early diagnosis made little difference, a mortality described as inevitable by Avery-Jones.[4] The therapeutic nihilists argue that, on the face of these controlled studies, it is pointless to do emergency endoscopy. If the mortality of upper GI hemorrhage is to improve, however, the mortality of this high-risk subgroup must be reduced. It is for this subgroup of patients that therapeutic endoscopy holds the greatest potential. New techniques introduced by recent advances in technology have put a number of therapeutic options at the disposal of the endoscopist. Early results of many techniques show considerable promise. If such results are obtainable communitywide, and not just confined to specialized centers, therapeutic endoscopy may well hold the key to an overall improvement in mortality in GI hemorrhage in the years to come. Various endoscopic measures may be applied to the bleeding

lesions without an open operation, avoiding the major metabolic disturbances due to anesthesia, surgery, and, not infrequently, sepsis, as well as the attendant morbidity and mortality. Since the vast majority of GI hemorrhage stops spontaneously, the efficacy of therapeutic endoscopy can only be assessed with well-conducted controlled trials.

A major therapeutic impact of endoscopic diagnosis in GI hemorrhage has been the introduction of the concept of stigmata of recent bleeding. There are no equivalent signs in radiology. It has been clearly shown that patients with these stigmata are at increased risk of continued or recurrent bleeding; clinically, these stigmata are important prognosticators of impending bleeding.[23,29,67,79] The importance of these signs, such as the visible vessel sign, has recently been evaluated prospectively by Wara,[79] who found that, of 52 patients who had visible vessels, less than one-third rebled massively. By itself, the sign is not as predictive as earlier investigators thought; when combined with other endoscopic data such as oozing, an overlying clot, or location within a gastric or duodenal ulcer, however, the predictive value is enhanced.[79] Swain et al.[75] showed a much higher rate of rebleeding in those with visible vessel; as much as 58 percent did. Moreover, these investigators demonstrated the pathologic nature of the visible vessels in resected gastric ulcers[75]: an exposed vessel running across the ulcer bed, with a pinpoint lateral opening 0.1 to 1.8 mm in diameter. More than 80 percent of these vessels have histologic changes of arteritis, and one-half of them have aneurysmal dilatation. Other workers found the size or height of the clot to be important as well: The higher the clot, the more likely the rebleeding. When small, the clot can be whitish, probably equivalent to the platelet–fibrin plug seen in esophageal varices (Chapter 3). Arterial sputting seen during endoscopy constitutes irrefutable evidence that the source of bleeding has been found, but it is also another important prognostic factor: 80 percent of these patients have continued or recurrent bleeding. Continuous oozing is said to have a lesser chance of rebleeding, although

at 0.5 MHz. At this range, tissue membrane potentials are not affected, as the direction of voltage alternates too quickly for discharge to occur. Even so, current does flow through tissue (in alternating directions), and the resistance to the flow of current results in heat. The waveform, or how the RF voltage varies over time, is important in determining the tissue effect of the spark. A spark is generated when the power is turned on and the electrode is brought close to the tissue but not in contact with it. In cutting mode, a simple sine waveform causes high current density in the tissue and results in cleavage with no hemostasis (Fig. 2-1A). During cutting, the cells are struck by numerous tiny ''lightning bolts'' and, as the water content vaporizes, they burst and the tissue is cleanly separated. In coagulation, the waveform of the spark is that of rapid intermittent bursts of a family of spikes (Fig. 2-1B). Such sparks do not carry a high current density to the tissue, vaporization does not occur; and there is no cutting, but tissue is coagulated through denaturation of protein. A blend of both effects, that is, hemostatic coagulation with less than clean cutting, is a combination of both waveforms (Fig. 2-1C). When

the electrode is in direct contact with the tissue, sparks are not formed; either waveform will result in desiccation. In this phenomenon, continuous steam formation limits the tissue temperature to the boiling point, so the desiccated tissue is soft. Softened tissue facilitates mechanical cutting, a fact put to good use in polypectomy.

Fulguration is spark gap-induced coagulation. The electrode does not make physical contact with the tissue, so there is no sticking of the electrode to the coagulum. Unlike desiccation, fulguration can heat tissue to far higher temperatures, causing the formation of a firm coagulum. Even in the presence of a thin layer of flowing blood, good-quality fulguration can coagulate a bleeding arteriole of up to 1.5-mm diameter. However, unpredictable depth of tissue damage makes this a hazardous modality.

THE POWER CONTROL

Power in electrosurgery is defined as the heat energy (joules) delivered to the patient. Watts are joules delivered per second. Theoretically, the output of electrosurgical units should be calibrated in watts; operators can then specify watts used in performing certain operations, such as fulguration of a 1-mm arteriole. Unfortunately, tissue resistance varies in real-life situations. When the electrode is in contact with the tissue, the resistance varies with the area of contact and the amount of moisture in contiguity. Also, as coagulation proceeds, tissue resistance increases. When the electrode is not in contact with the tissue and sparking results, energy is dissipated to the electrode, to the flash, as well as to the tissue. All these variables in resistance affect the current output, so there is no simple way of knowing that the watts dialed in are actually delivered. All power settings are therefore calibrated in an arbitrary scale. A special analogue computer, however, has been used to record the total electrical energy delivered in experimental work, but this is too cumbersome for clinical use. From the practical

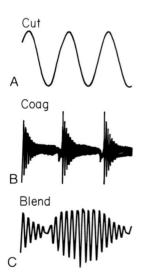

Fig. 2-1 Waveforms in different modes of electrocautery. (A) Cutting. (B) Coagulation. (C) Blended A and B not-so-clean cutting with moderate coagulation.

point of view, when electrosurgery is performed, the power should be dialed from zero upward until the first visible effect is detected, hence the use of an arbitrary scale in the power setting of most electrosurgical units.

CURRENT FLOW PATHWAYS

A monopolar electrode allows the current to flow from the electrode to the tissue and to return to the unit by the patient plate, which provides a large area of contact. Failure of contact of the grounding plate causes the current to ground through small areas of contact such as the ECG electrodes, causing burns. Many new electrosurgical units provide a ground fault or warning signals when such breaks in the circuit are detected. In addition, stray currents of low frequency (''noise'') may develop, which may be harmful to the patient or the endoscopist if not grounded properly. A bipolar electrode has an active electrode through which the current enters the tissue, as well as an adjacent electrode to return the current back to the unit, dispensing with the patient plate. The current thus passes only through the tissue between the two electrodes, thereby eliminating hazards of stray currents, ground faults, and excessive tissue damage. By the same token, however, bipolar electrodes are less effective: They do not spark, and they operate only when in contact with tissue (desiccation).

The endoscope must be grounded (connecting the S-cord), even when it is completely insulated, because the insulated instrument may serve as a capacitor when alternating RF current passes down an electrode that has been inserted through it. If not grounded, current is stored in the endoscope, which may cause shocks or even burns to the patient and to the eyes and hands of the endoscopist when it escapes through a small area of contact.

Visual check of these pathways is essential to ensure electrical safety of electrosurgery before use. The patient plate should be of the disposable type that adheres to the patient, commonly used in the operating room, so that changing the patient's position will not interrupt the contact. The endoscope must not have bare metallic parts exposed, and the eyepiece and buttons must have a rubber or plastic cover. The insulation coat of the electrode must be intact at all times.

FUNCTIONS OF ACTIVE ELECTRODES

Within limits imposed by the design of the power generator, the larger the electrode in contact with the tissue, the lower the resistance, hence the larger the current delivered. Current density is the same, however, as is the desiccation effect. As the temperature in the water in the cells approaches the boiling point, further temperature rise is temporarily halted as steam is formed. When the tissue dries up, conductivity is lost and the electrical resistance rises. Current flow drops and heating decreases. If the power setting has been selected appropriately, completion of desiccation turns off the current automatically. In such cases, the depth of penetration of necrosis is roughly equal to the width of the electrode. The temperature of the electrode is dependent not only on size, but also on material. A relatively poor heat conductor such as stainless steel (compared, for example, with silver) can attain very high temperatures; such electrodes produce an effect similar to the branding iron, such as the heater probe. Hot electrodes are likely to stick to tissue as a result of desiccation of tissue in immediate contact with it. Electrodes designed specifically for desiccation use are either water or air cooled (e.g., with a central lumen for either irrigation or aspiration) or are made with silver or gold. Wire electrodes, such as those used in polypectomy snares and sphincterotome loops, cut better when made with fine wire (0.3 mm), but if the wire cuts mechanically through the tissue before the electrical current is passed, bleeding may result. Thicker wire (0.6 mm) usually results in better hemostasis.

Clinical Applications

MONOPOLAR ELECTROCOAGULATION

This is the most common mode of electrosurgery employed in general surgery; and most surgeons are familiar with the tissue effects of cutting, coagulating, and blended waveforms. The major concern in the use of this mode of electrosurgery is that the depth of tissue injury is unpredictable: It depends on many variables such as the power, duration of current flow, tissue resistance, electrode size and shape, area of contact with the mucosa, and pressure of application of the electrode, to name just a few. Thus Blackwood and Silvis[5] showed that in the canine intestine, the ball-tipped electrode produced a depth of tissue necrosis roughly the diameter of the ball. Papp et al.[51] showed that the pressure and duration of electrode application are important, and not the diameter. Using a computer to monitor the total energy delivered by an electrosurgical generator, Piercy et al.[56] showed that even when pressure of application was standardized, hemostatically effective monopolar electrocoagulation produced an unpredictable depth of necrosis. Protell et al.[58] treated 71 acute experimentally induced bleeding gastric ulcers with monopolar electrocoagulation using a mean of 11 (0.6-second duration) applications of 22 joules each. Hemostasis was obtained in all cases, but evidence of full-thickness damage to the gastric wall was found in 44 percent in follow-up histologic studies performed up to 28 days later. The extent of tissue necrosis did not correlate with the number of electrode applications, joules per application, or total joules per ulcer treated.

Despite this reservation, clinical application of monopolar electrocoagulation in uncontrolled studies has repeatedly confirmed its efficacy. No complications were reported by Gaisford,[24] Volpicelli et al.,[77] Papp,[52] and Sugawa et al.[68] in substantial experience. A 1.8 percent incidence of perforation was reported in a survey of European endoscopists, who also confirmed the high success rate for hemostasis.[78]

MONOPOLAR ELECTROFULGURATION

When the current is turned on before the tissue comes into contact with the electrode, a spark occurs after the power reaches a certain threshold. Coagulating waveform current thus delivered constitutes fulguration. Studying this modality in dogs, Dennis et al.[16] found it effective in causing hemostasis, but the depth of injury was again unpredictable. A 30 percent incidence of full-thickness injury was reported. The use of CO_2 or a mixture of CO_2 and argon to enhance ionization and spark formation did not reduce the incidence of deep injury. Since this technique is no more effective than monopolar electrocoagulation but appears to cause deeper injury, it has not been used clinically. Most surgeons' experience with fulguration in operative surgery supports this view—more tissue destruction yet marginally more effective than coagulation for hemostasis.

BIPOLAR ELECTROCOAGULATION

A bipolar electrode has two active electrodes in close proximity to each other, both in contact with tissue during use. The electric current returns to the generator via one of the electrodes; thus the pathway is more localized than monopolar electrocoagulation. Experimentally, Moore observed two full-thickness injuries in a series of 87 gastric ulcers treated with bipolar electrocoagulation. Using the analogue computer to deliver a predetermined amount of energy for bipolar electrocoagulation, and also controlling the pressure of application, Protell et al.[58] showed that bipolar electrocoagulation was effective in controlling bleeding from experimental ulcer models, but a 25 percent incidence of full-thickness injuries was observed. Comparison with monopolar electrocoagulation[58] confirmed that the bipolar mode is less likely to cause deep injury.

A multipolar electrode (Fig. 2-2) has been marketed by ACMI (BICAP endoscopic electrocoagulation system) for clinical use. The tech-

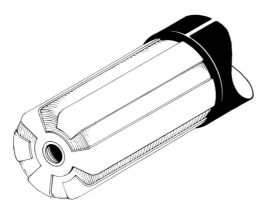

Fig. 2-2 Details of the tip of the BICAP multipolar electrode (ACMI).

nique is similar to monopolar coagulation, but the patient plate is not essential. The central lumen may be used to aspirate blood or smoke produced during cautery or for irrigation to cool the electrode and keep the field clear.

Photocoagulation

LASER PHYSICS

By applying an external electromagnetic force to the atoms, they may be stimulated to emit energy, as shown by Planck's equation of the quantum theory of light:

$$Ep = hc/l$$

where Ep is the energy per photon, h is Planck's constant, c is the speed of light, and l is the wavelength. When the electromagnetic energy has a frequency of oscillation equal to that which the atom would have in spontaneous emission, stimulated emission is induced. This emission is an energy or light of a specific wavelength (monochromatic), highly focusable (coherent), known as laser, an acronym for light amplification by stimulated emission of radiation.

Figure 2-3 shows how commonly used medical lasers are produced. The lasing material (source of lasers) is either a gas or solid com-

pound. For gases such as argon or CO_2, an electric field can be applied to a glass cylinder containing the gas to increase their energy to induce light formation (electrical discharge-pumped); the light is collected by totally reflecting mirrors and is allowed to escape through partially transmitting mirrors (Fig. 2-3). For solids such as the neodymium-doped yttrium aluminum garnet (Nd:YAG) crystal, an intense light source, such as the xenon arc lamp, can be used as the means of excitation (optically pumped). The lasers produced are named after the source, and each has a unique wavelength characteristic of the molecule. All lasers are capable of being highly focused and totally transmitted, the single most useful characteristic that distinguishes lasers from ordinary light.

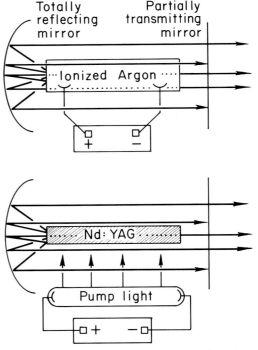

Fig. 2-3 Diagram of two types of medical laser sources. (A) Electrical discharge pumped (e.g., argon, CO_2). Electrical energy is used to energize the gas element contained in a glass tube to produce laser. (B) Optically pumped (e.g., Nd:YAG). Strong light is used to stimulate laser emission from a rod of the crystal used for laser source.

LASER BIOLOGY

The absorption of the laser by the tissues is dependent on its wavelength. The CO_2 laser is readily absorbed by water, causing a rise in temperature. Since water is present in all tissues, the energy is dissipated early, accounting for shallow penetration. The argon laser is absorbed by the hemoglobin (Hb) molecule and not by water; therefore it heats tissues only when blood is present. In the gastric mucosa, the argon laser penetrates typically to a depth of 1 mm. The Nd:YAG laser is not significantly absorbed by water, and only partially by blood; it therefore penetrates deeper into tissues. In the stomach Nd:YAG can penetrate a depth of 4 mm. In doing so, however, it affects a cone-shaped amount of tissue in its pathway due to the generation of ''scatter.''

Figure 2-4 shows the effect of thermal transfer in lasers to tissues. Unlike heat transfer by heater probe or electrocautery, penetration by laser is instantaneous. The final amount of tissue damage, however, is altered by thermal conduction and is wider and deeper than the initial penetration. A certain amount of scattering by fibrous

tissue tends also to fan out the path of destruction. If the tissue is well perfused with blood, vascular cooling may render a protecting effect. A well-known cause of failure to reach coagulating temperature is the remarkable heat-sink phenomenon attributable to conduction by an underlying artery with high flow rate. The effect of heat on the cells depends on the temperature attained. Protein denaturation (thermal coagulation) occurs at 50° to 80°C, but at 100°C water evaporation occurs and the temperature will not rise further until evaporation has been complete. Thereafter the temperature rise will continue with heat transfer until a carbon residue is formed. Almost instantaneous evaporation of tissue water by deep penetrating lasers, such as the Nd:YAG, imparts a dramatic visual effect: An instant crater is created accompanied by a slight explosion due to rapid steam formation. This can be disastrous if applied to a vessel wall; instead of hemostasis, an injudicial direct hit of the vessel wall may create a larger hole, hence more bleeding (see technique).

The main limiting factor in attaining hemostasis is the diameter of the bleeding vessel. The upper limit for the Nd:YAG laser is about 3 mm, and for the argon laser about 1 mm; although experts may quibble somewhat about the figures. In histologic studies, the immediate effect of laser photocoagulation is dehydration and shrinkage of the vessel, which is also compressed by the shrinkage of the surrounding tissue. The endothelial lining appears swollen in freshly coagulated specimens, with the lumen packed with red cells. Higher energy density and longer exposure to the laser result in disruption of the continuity of the vessel without coagulation of the contents, accounting for the clinical observation of exacerbation of bleeding.

Because of the focusing function of the lens of the human eye, laser entrance into the eye can cause serious damage. A beam incident on the eye is focused on the retina as a concentrated area of high energy and can cause permanent thermal and mechanical damage, a principle put to good use in the ophthalmologic practice of photocoagulation of microaneurysms of retinal vessels. Reflected scattered laser light may be

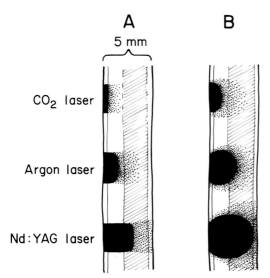

A **B**

5 mm

CO_2 laser

Argon laser

Nd:YAG laser

Fig. 2-4 Tissue penetration by lasers. Final damage (B) is always greater than which is immediately apparent (A) due to the delayed effect of scatter. The deeper the penetration, the wider the scatter.

focused on the retina too, but the effect is much less, as the light is no longer well collimated or as focusable, carrying only a small fraction of the energy of the original beam. Nevertheless, reflected laser from shiny mucosal surfaces may cause significant retinal damage if no filter has been installed in the eyepiece of the endoscope.

Clinical Applications

The commonly used lasers for therapeutic endoscopy are the argon and the Nd:YAG lasers; both are conducted by fiberoptics. The argon laser is a good coagulator used widely in ophthalmology and gastroenterology; the Nd:YAG laser is also a coagulator, but it finds important application for tumor ablation as well. In therapeutic endoscopy, the laser waveguide, made of a quartz fiber coated with glass of a lower refractive index for total internal refraction, is used to conduct the laser to the tissues. The waveguide fiber itself is housed in a slightly larger sheath, which permits ancillary installations such as a coaxial jet of CO_2 gas and aiming light to facilitate accurate photocoagulation. The aiming light provides a preview of the spot size of the laser on the mucosa, especially important for the Nd:YAG laser, which is invisible to the human eye. The coaxial jet of gas tends to expose the bleeding vessel under a layer of blood, but it also decreases the risk of blood coming into contact with the tip of the fiber, causing carbon deposits and even burning of the fiber.

The dose of energy delivered is governed by power output and duration of application, but obviously the amount of tissue over which the energy is spread determines the local result. All laser machines provide precise controls for presetting time of application and power output, and most compute total energy delivered automatically as well. It is up to the endoscopist to control the area (hence the volume) of the tissue receiving the energy. This is done primarily by regulating the spot size. Spot size is influenced by divergence angle (the angle of spread made by the laser as it emanates from the tip

of the waveguide) and the tip-to-target distance. The angle of divergence is usually between 4 and 16 degrees: By adjusting the distance of the tip to the mucosa, a suitable spot size can be attained. The typical useful spot size is 1.5 to 4 mm diameter, depending on the lesion to be treated. For an angle of divergence of 14 degrees, a 1-cm distance from the mucosa gives a spot size of 2.5 mm, a commonly used spot size for treating bleeding. It is not very meaningful in describing clinical laser treatment simply to state energy density, that is, joules per square centimeter (joules/cm^2) delivered, since thermal conduction, scattering due to differing amounts of fibrous tissue, and vascular cooling due to differing rates of tissue perfusion are uncontrollable biologic variables. Instead, the power density, that is, watts/square centimeter (watts/cm^2), duration of application, spot size, and the kind of laser used should be specified for a more finite description.

A clinical laser is an expensive, often bulky, apparatus. It requires a high-voltage electrical outlet (like x-ray machines), plumbing connections (faucet and drain for water cooling), precautions for ophthalmic safety, and a working environment in which other patients and personnel are excluded and where biohazard warning signs can be clearly posted as required by law. In many hospitals these requirements make the laser unsuitable for use by the bedside of critically ill patients, who require intensive monitoring and are often best treated in a special care unit. By contrast, electrocoagulation units are portable, do not require special biohazard posting regulations, and can easily be brought to the patient's bedside. Admittedly there are a good many advantages in the use of laser for hemostasis, not the least of which is the ease of use and efficacy, but the hurdles posed by logistics make it a much less attractive tool for emergency work.

The recent development of an artificial sapphire crystal free of air bubbles permitted delivery of the Nd:YAG laser to tissue by contact (contact irradiation), eliminating a number of disadvantages of the noncontact laser.[15] A laser scalpel, for example, is made of a sapphire crys-

Electrocoagulation

Electrocoagulation is described for the most common application, namely, treating a discrete bleeding point in a gastric ulcer. The equipment required consists of an insulated endoscope with a wide channel, either a monopolar coagulator probe with a central lumen for suction or a bipolar probe as found in the BICAP (ACMI), and an electrosurgical generator with a foot switch. The current flow pathway is visually checked, the patient plate is securely fastened and skin contact ensured with generous application of ECG electrode jelly, and the S cord is connected grounding the endoscope to the generator ground terminal.

The stomach is cleansed by preliminary irrigation. Endoscopy is performed and the bleeder identified; the position of the patient is changed, if necessary, to shift a pool of blood for exposure of the underlying mucosa. There are many different techniques, all effective in the hands of their proponents.

For monopolar coagulation, the author prefers applying the electrode directly to the bleeding spot as accurately as possible, using barely enough pressure for tissue contact. The mucosa should not be dimpled excessively by the electrode during coagulation. Many electrodes come with interchangeable tips; in the author's practice, a medium-size spherical tip (2.5-mm diameter) works well; it can be used more effectively than the finer tips for direct tamponade of the bleeding vessel before application of current as a test of accuracy. Once pressure is shown to decrease bleeding, the pressure is released. The power setting on coagulation is set low in the dial (e.g., 1 to 2) and the foot switch is activated. The assistant then slowly turns up the power and stops as soon as the effect of electrocoagulation is observed. The first signs are tiny bubbles and steam or faint smoke coming from the site of contact. A whitish round spot almost immediately follows, indicating completion of the coagulation process. The bursts should be between 0.5 and 2 seconds. Gaisford[24] uses a Valleylab SSE-2 with the power setting on 5 to 7 of the dial. Irrigation of saline via the central lumen of the electrode

throughout the entire process of coagulation not only keeps the view clear but also cools it to prevent it from sticking to the eschar.[73] Repeat application to the adjacent site is only needed if oozing is continuing. Smoke should be cleared by aspirating through the endoscope. Hemostasis has been achieved if no bleeding occurs under observation for 5 to 10 minutes. Matek et al.[46] used a similar way of applying the electrode, except that distilled water was continuously instilled down the central lumen of the electrode at the rate of 20 to 40 ml/min during the entire process of coagulation. The probe, called the electrohydrothermal (EHT) probe, is easily made from an existing coagulation probe. The hemostatic energy required is less than that needed for other techniques, the visibility is enhanced by the jet stream, and, most importantly, sticking to either the tissues or eschar has been completely avoided. They use a Martin Elecktrotom 170RF at a power setting of 6 to 8. Swain et al.[73] similarly demonstrated the superiority of the ''liquid'' over the dry monopolar electrode. Saline was pumped down the central lumen of the liquid electrode at 0.5 ml/sec. Papp[52] used a different technique, encircling the bleeding vessel 2 to 3 mm away from it applying 4 to 5 spots each of 2 to 2.5 seconds until the bleeding stops, employing a Cameron-Miller electrocoagulation unit with a power setting of 5. The practice is based on the theory that electrocoagulation causes coaptation in the muscular and submucosal layers and thus tamponades the vessel, whereas direct application may destroy the vessel causing more bleeding. Surgeons who operate with electrocoagulation every day find this hard to reconcile with their practice, since failure to stop bleeding from small vessels with the electrocautery on the operating table is almost invariably caused by lack of accuracy. It is true that direct hit of the vessel may cause more bleeding, but this occurs under certain circumstances: too much current, too large a vessel, and on very thin-walled vessels lacking tissue support. A classic example is the larger omental vein, where electrocautery almost always creates more bleeding, as the unsupported thin-walled vein bleeds from the larger hole created by a direct hit. The novice must remember that accuracy is crucial in monopolar coagulation, as the therapeutic range is smaller than with other modalities such as bipolar coagulation.

For bipolar electrocoagulation much the same technique is used. The BICAP probe is also shaped like a catheter with a central lumen except that the tip has three pairs of bipolar electrodes (six elements) arranged like the spokes of a wheel, with the active elements extending from the tip up the sides of the probe. It comes in 2.3- and 3.3-mm sizes. Chances are that lateral or tip contact with any part of the probe suffices for bipolar electrocoagulation. To use it, accurate aiming is important: Ideally, the current is passed on one side of the vessel and is conducted away from the other side, an ideal situation in which the vessel is straddled by two electrodes, not always achievable in practice. A Medi-Tech bipolar electrode works similarly: It consists of two steel wire loops 2 mm apart embedded in an insulated sheath, with current flowing between the tissue contacting the two loops. However, bipolar action is confined only to using the tip end-on.

Infrequently a spurting artery is seen protruding into the lumen, a perfect setting for using the monopolar hemostatic coagulating forceps.[70] It looks like a pair of ordinary biopsy forceps except that the cups are replaced with flat electrodes. The arteriole is grasped between the electrodes and coagulated with minimal tissue damage. A bipolar hemostatic coagulating forceps can be constructed very similarly, except that one of the electrodes conducts current back to the ground, rather than exiting from the patient plate. A similar principle has been used in the construction of a bipolar polypectomy snare (see Chapter 8).

The Heater Probe

The heater probe, also a catheter instrument, handles rather differently. First, it acts rather slowly as compared with all other modalities. Since its temperature is limited to 250°C, it does not produce an effect like electrocoagula-

tion. It has a rounded tip, and irrigation ports are situated away from the very end, so that the probe can be apposed to the target without disabling the irrigation. It comes with a jet irrigation system, similar to a WaterPik. The tips are rather large, 3.2 or 2.4 mm, and are coated with nonstick material such as Teflon. When the lesion is actively oozing or spurting, the unactivated probe is used to press directly at the bleeding site with moderate pressure to decrease bleeding so that as much blood can be removed as possible (Fig. 2-8). When tamponade is successful, blood clears in a few moments with irrigation. Several continuous pulses of 30 joules are applied to provide a thermal seal for the tamponaded vessel. Each 30-joule pulse takes about 8 seconds to deliver with current machines, although a faster probe is being developed. By pressing circumferentially a little away from the vessel, it is possible to find a quadrant that effectively decreases bleeding, indicating that the vessel courses directly underneath the probe. Energy is then switched on to effect a thermal seal.[40,57] When the lesion presents as a visible vessel, or an adherent blood clot, the vessel or the clot can be directly touched and the probe turned on to deliver the required energy. There are other less obvious advantages: Depth of coagulation can be varied not only by duration of pulses but also by the amount of pressure applied. No smoke is produced, and no suction venting is necessary. It costs about as much as an expensive electrocautery machine. Johnston et al.[38] recently compared the efficacy and safety of the heater probe with the Nd:YAG laser and found the probe to be superior in both qualities.

Laser Photocoagulation

The techniques are not standardized, although there is some broad agreement that Argon laser and Nd:YAG lasers are used differently.

ARGON LASER. Since the argon laser, a bluish-green light, is absorbed by blood pigment, the bleeding lesion must be exposed first;

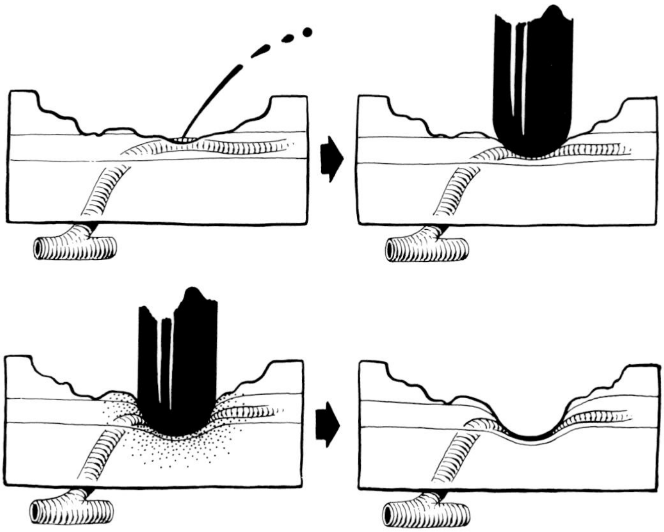

Fig. 2-8 Heater probe is initially used to tamponade the bleeding vessel to gain a clear view. When heat is switched on, a thermal seal is effected. (Adapted from Johnston JH: Endoscopic thermal treatment of upper gastrointestinal bleeding. Endoscopy Review 2:21, 1985)

otherwise the flowing stream will act as a heat sink, preventing the tissue from reaching the necessary coagulation temperature. This is achieved by blowing the blood away by a coaxial jet of CO_2 built into the waveguide. Most guides have a continuous background flow to keep the tip from being fouled by blood, switchable to a stronger jet (7 to 8 L/min) whenever needed, for example, just prior to photocoagulation. Venting is essential to prevent excessive distention, which has been shown to predispose to full-thickness injury, probably because of marked thinning of the distended wall. Venting is achieved either by using a double-channeled endoscope, a separate indwelling nasogastric tube, or a recyling system provided by some laser waveguides. Guidelines to the safe use of the argon laser have been published by Johnston et al.[37] based on systematic experimental studies. Using waveguides incorporating a 0.2- or 0.4-mm quartz fiber with an angle of divergence of 8 degrees, a power setting of 8 to 10 watts at a treatment distance (distance of tip of guide to target) of 1 to 3 cm is recommended; the target should be irradiated en face as much as possible. The treatment distance is vitally critical. With too close a treatment distance, such as a few millimeters, a spot size of 1.1 mm or smaller will result, and tissue erosion

and vaporization effect will be observed, highly likely to cause more bleeding and even perforation. At the recommended treatment distance of 1 to 3 cm, the spot size will be 1.8 to 3.2 mm in diameter and effective hemostasis is obtained, yet relatively free from risk of perforation, provided the stomach is not markedly distended. The spot size is so much easier to judge than treatment distance during actual clinical use. In these experiments using a spot size of 2 to 3 mm and a power setting of 10 watts, pulses of 15- to 20-second duration were required for hemostasis at the bleeding edges of the mucosal defect created by an "ulcer maker," modified from a suctional biopsy capsule, in dog stomachs without full-thickness coagulation injury. At lower power settings, such as 6 to 8 watts, a mean of 33 seconds of application was required in the same model. A power setting or 4 watts or less was ineffective. Bleeding vessels up to 1.5 mm can be coagulated with this laser.

The clinical practice is based on experimental work. The aiming light, usually the same blue-green argon laser but at only 0.1 percent of full power, is first used to adjust the treatment distance (judged by spot size) and to direct the beam squarely at the bleeding vessel. When the 2-mm blue-green disk of light comes to rest on the bleeder, the switch is activated for a burst of 2 to 3 seconds, watching for the effect of coagulation (Fig. 2-9). If the first two or three bursts result in no effect or only slightly diminished bleeding, more bursts are given and for longer duration. However, if after many bursts in quick succession totaling close to 30 seconds and bleeding still is ongoing, it is wise to reassess rather than continue blasting away. Often edema that ensues during the following minutes helps stop the bleeding, but the major decision the endoscopist has to make is when to recognize a failure and resort to something else. There are no experimental data to guide the clinician as to what to do next: Can electrocoagulation or sclerosant injection be safely used to supplement partially or totally unsuccessful argon photocoagulation? Should the Nd:YAG laser be used instead? Few have the luxury of having both systems right at hand. The endoscopist who has ever had to make this unpleasant decision but once is likely to develop a lasting unfavorable impression of the argon laser.

THE Nd:YAG LASER. The Nd:YAG laser handles quite differently from the argon laser. Although the waveguide is similar, this laser has much more penetration and demands an altogether different touch. The pattern of energy dissipation in the tissue has a conical shape due to greater ''scatter'' (Fig. 2-4). Not only is the tissue in the direct path of the beam affected, but the scatter brings the effect sideways for a small distance. Bleeding vessels are coagulated best by the scatter, as the direct hit may cause vaporization, creating a larger hole in the vessel. When a visible stream of blood is flowing, the heat delivered to the vessel is conducted away by the stream, the heat-sink effect, and the coagulation effect on the vessel is minimized. Coagulation of the tissue surrounding the vessel also serves to compress on the feeding vessel, and the scatter eventually coagulates it. Therefore the Nd:YAG is best used by shooting next to the vessel rather than directly at it. For hemostatic work, a power setting of 60 to 70 watts is recommended. A jet of CO_2 is not essential but is helpful for better visibility. The treatment distance should be about 2 cm; and working with a waveguide that has an angle of divergence of 8 to 10 degrees, that translates to a spot size of 2 to 3 mm. In the esophagus and duodenum, where short treatment distances may have to be used, the power setting or the duration of the pulse (or both), must be reduced. Since the Nd:YAG laser is invisible, an aiming light (usually a red beam of He Ne) is used. The coagulation effect is obvious and instantaneous on short bursts, typically 0.5 seconds, and a rimming or ringing technique should be used to get the bleeding vessel to coagulate (Fig. 2-10). This technique consists of shooting rapid short bursts around the bleeding target, 1 mm or so away, to surround it with three to four coagulating hits. Vaporization in the form of visible cavitation must be avoided; when that happens, it is usually because the spot size is too small, that is, the tip of the waveguide is too close to the target. Hemorrhage from high pressure sources such as arterial bleeding or portal hypertensive venous bleeding may be more difficult to stop. The options are to increase

Direct   Ring

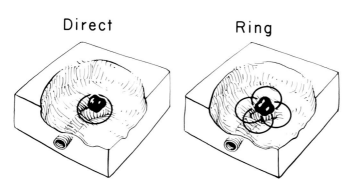

Fig. 2-9 The argon laser is usually (not always) used for on-target direct irradiation (direct). The Nd:YAG laser is best applied by shooting next to the vessel—the ringing or rimming technique (ring).

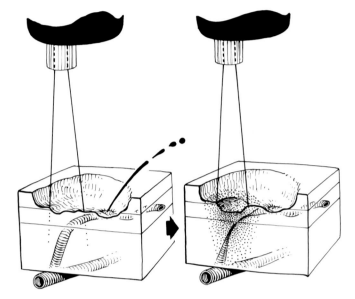

Fig. 2-10 Using the scatter of the Nd:YAG laser to effect coagulation of a vessel by shooting next to it.

the power setting to 80 to 90 watts, longer bursts to 1 to 2 seconds, and shorter intervals between bursts to maximize buildup of heat. As in the use of the argon laser, if the bleeding continues after these measures, and after a total of 8 to 10 pulses of 0.5 to 1 seconds at 80 watts have been given, it is important not to panic and keep delivering larger and larger doses of energy. An interval of waiting works wonders at such times. Both tissue swelling and vessel spasm take time to reach their height. One may take this time to double-check the equipment to make sure everything is as it should be.

Clinicians used to the relatively slow argon laser tend to look on the Nd:YAG laser as too dangerous, but that is because one needs to develop a different touch to handle it. Dixon[17] showed, in the dog model, that a reasonable margin of safety exists in that the duration of bursts that results in perforation is three times that for hemostasis. Vessels up to 3 mm in diameter can be coagulated with this laser.

The contact Nd:YAG laser probe handles quite like the monopolar electrode. A power setting of 8 to 16 watts is sufficient for coagulation of most bleeders, using a sapphire crystal tip of 1-mm diameter. At present there is insufficient experience to formulate guidelines for

widespread endoscopic practice, although open surgical use is already very successful (Joffe SN, personal communication).

INJECTION OF SCLEROSANTS. The tissue necrosis effect of absolute alcohol has long been known; now it is mainly used clinically for permanent nerve block. Recently it has been used successfully to stop peptic ulcer bleeding in Japan.[3] It has also been studied in the animal model for its efficacy as a sclerosant for gastric hemorrhage and has been found to be safe and effective.[69] Sugawa and co-workers[69,70] have a substantial experience with the clinical application and their technique is as follows:

A tuberculin syringe containing 1 ml of 98 percent ethanol is mounted on a sclerotherapy flexible injector, which has a 25-gauge, 4-mm retractable needle. After identification of the bleeding vessel, the needle is inserted directly into the base of the ulcer for a depth of 2 to 3 mm and injection of 0.1 to 0.2 ml of alcohol is given (Fig. 2-11); if the first injection does not result in hemostasis, it can be repeated by sequential injections in adjacent areas until a maximum dose of 0.8 ml has been given. Blanching and swelling may occur, but the hemostatic effect is immediate. According to Su-

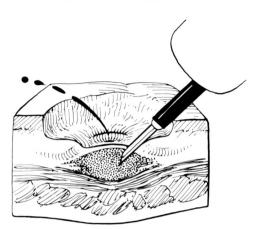

Fig. 2-11 Injection of ethanol for hemostasis: direct injection into base of ulcer, 2 to 3 mm deep, using 0.2 ml for each injection. One to four injections usually suffice.

gawa, brisk bleeding can be stopped in this way. Recurrent hemorrhage (within 72 hours) was encountered in 4 out of a total of 58 patients in his experience. He has reported no other complications (see Results).

This low-tech method is attractive because of the extreme simplicity, low cost, general availability, and absence of special training requirements. Confirmation of Sugawa's favorable results is pending. Increase in size of the ulcer due to the tissue necrotizing effect alone should not be an objection, since all other effective modalities (lasers, heater probe, electrocoagulation) also increase the size of the ulcer. There have been reports of other sclerosants such as hypertonic sodium chloride, but the efficacy and safety remain unproven.

SUMMARY OF TECHNIQUES

Different lesions require somewhat different technique. Also, some modalities may be more suitable than others for certain lesions. It is often difficult to get to an optimal position to treat lesions in the duodenal bulb, but most gastric and esophageal lesions are open to a number of options. In this author's practice, monopolar electrocoagulation has been used

most extensively purely because of familiarity. It is likely that the contact laser probe may eventually displace the monopolar electrode but probably may never replace it. For the spurting arteriole, this author prefers the contact method of the monopolar electrocoagulation with the ball-tipped electrode, compressing the artery first with the cold electrode. While water is being irrigated, pressure is released and electric current passed, using medium power and watching for the whitening effect. Hemostasis usually results after a 2-second application. An identical technique is used with the heater probe, except that pressure is continually applied to effect a coaptive seal. However, a much longer period (15-second application to deliver 300 joules) is necessary for sealing of the vessel. For the ulcer with a sentinel clot with or without oozing underneath it, the monopolar electrode is applied directly through the clot to touch the vessel and pass current as for a spurting artery. A visible vessel without bleeding or a clot is treated in the same way. A raised or protruding vessel, bleeding or not bleeding, is grasped with the monopolar coagulating forceps and current passed. For diffuse slow oozing, low-current monopolar electrocoagulation without pressure is applied to the area of oozing repeatedly until all oozing stops. For angiodysplasia lesions, bleeding or nonbleeding, the hot biopsy forceps are used to perform piecemeal removal of the entire area supplemented by electrocoagulation with either the closed forceps or the ball-tipped electrode. This author would have used the argon laser for these routinely if he had an argon laser machine at his disposal. The alcohol injection technique as recommended by Sugawa was used recently; it was successful in obtaining permanent hemostasis for arterial spurting in two cases and in one case of oozing under a sentinel clot.

POSTTREATMENT MANAGEMENT

The patient should be monitored for continuing hemorrhage with vital signs and serial hematocrit determinations. Most endoscopists would dispense with the nasogastric tube, as it can be a factor in provoking hemorrhage; if it is used, however, it should not be put to suction, but test irrigated hourly, making no effort to retrieve the entire amount of irrigant. Cimetidine and intensive antacid treatment is justified if the patient is suffering from a bleeding peptic ulcer, but also if ulcers have been created due to the therapy. There is no role for vasopressin infusion in this author's opinion; the bleeding has either stopped or it has not and, if it has not, the sooner the clinician knows about it the better.

Rebleeding is usually an indication for surgery but, depending on the severity, time of occurrence after the first treatment, accessibility of the lesion, and the general medical condition of the patient, repeat therapeutic endoscopy may also be considered. The morbidity is somewhat increased, since the area treated is usually in the phase of softening and also because an additional depth of necrosis would be created. Against this must be balanced the considerable advantage that the endoscopist knows exactly what to look for and the appropriate modality to use. In any case, if the patient is not a prohibitive operative risk, surgery should not be delayed.

Even if the patient appears to have no bleeding and is free from symptoms of abdominal pain, delayed perforation still has to be watched for in the first 48 to 72 hours. An upright chest radiograph should be taken routinely on the second or third day to look for pneumoperitoneum.

In this author's practice, all patients in whom the extent of damage due to the therapeutic effort is not certain are reendoscoped. Examination on the fifth or sixth day usually shows a larger ulcer with a clean base or a small whitish area if no ulcer has existed before. The previously visible vessel may no longer be visible, but if it is, the patient is endoscoped again within 2 weeks and the vessel recauterized if still exposed, despite the absence of symptoms. There have been no published data concerning follow-up endoscopy of visible vessels, but anecdotal recounts from fellow endoscopists by and large are similar.

COMPLICATIONS

Perforation

As shown experimentally, coagulation sufficient for hemostasis may cause through-thickness necrosis in a small percentage of cases. The Nd:YAG laser has a delayed component due to the scatter effect; the full extent of damage is only reached after 48 hours or longer. Clinical perforation may not result in every instance in histologic perforation; the size as well as the location of the lesion must play a role. Healing with fibrosis, sealing, or adhesion to omentum or adjacent viscera may prevent any overt manifestation. However, when acute pain, abdominal guarding, rigidity, fever, or leukocytosis develop following electrocoagulation, perforation must be suspected. Radiologic demonstration of pneumoperitoneum confirms the diagnosis, and emergency surgical repair must be undertaken.

Failure of Hemostasis

Failure to reach the site of bleeding may be because of location, such as in the fornix of the duodenal bulb just beyond the pylorus, where only a tangential view can be obtained or in a deformed duodenum with stenosis beyond which the endoscope cannot be passed (Fig. 2-12). It may fail because of (1) inadequate visualization from torrential bleeding, (2) poor cleansing, or (3) in some cases, failure to find

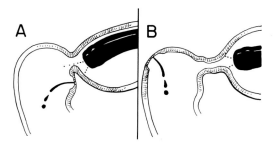

Fig. 2-12 Examples of inaccessible locations. (A) A bleeding ulcer in the fornix of the bulb visible only tangentially. (B) A bleeding ulcer in the bulb behind a stenosis.

any active sites. Most difficulties with the location are solved by using an oblique-viewing endoscope but not the lateral-viewing duodenoscope, since few probes other than the simplest electrocoagulation electrodes can clear the cannula elevator. The importance of adequate lavage, either before or during endoscopy, cannot be overemphasized. Most of the time spent on these procedures is in attaining the necessary exposure. It demands persistence and resourcefulness. One should not hesitate to remove the endoscope and reintroduce it with an overtube in order to remove the massive clots.

Truly torrential hemorrhage, with blood accumulating faster than can be removed, precludes any of the modalities of therapeutic endoscopy. Such cases should be treated with emergency surgery without further delay. For the worst possible surgical candidates, an expeditious angiographic embolization is an alternative to be considered.

When conditions appear ideal for laser treatment and yet, despite adequate energy delivered, unsatisfactory results are obtained, one should be suspicious of a large underlying vessel acting as a heat sink, preventing the adequate heat buildup necessary for coagulation. It is also reasonable to expect that a heavily calcified and atherosclerotic open artery will be more difficult to bring under control.

All renewed bleeding within 24 hours, despite apparent arrest of bleeding at endoscopy, is counted as a failure. A failure rate of 5 to 20 percent has been reported in most large series.[35,45,61,71] A clinical decision must be made at the initial assessment as to whether the bleeding is too massive to be handled with the equipment at hand and which modality is likely to be adequate if one has a choice.

Massive Exacerbation of Bleeding

This eventuality must be prepared for in all cases, although the best treatment is prevention. Too hot an electrode, resulting in sticking of an electrode to the eschar, and burning a hole in the vessel without sealing it (e.g., Nd:YAG laser) are errors in technique that can be avoided. Esophageal varices should not be treated with any of the measures described in this chapter, because they are too large (>3 to 4 mm), have thin walls, and are under pressure. The management and indication for surgery is the same as described under treatment failures.

Ulcerations: Aggravation of Existing Ulcers

An ulcer is observed immediately following laser treatment. After the Nd:YAG irradiation, the full extent of ulceration may not be reached until 48 hours after arrest of bleeding. When the ulcer is very deep, delayed perforation may occur. After electrocoagulation, extension of the ulcer may not be appreciated immediately because of the change in color, but this also becomes obvious when examined days later. Posttreatment observation for possible perforation is therefore important.

Aspiration

Aspiration is a serious threat in major bleeding, and consideration must be given to endotracheal intubation prior to undertaking endoscopy or lavage with a large tube. Other complications of endoscopy such as perforation and drug reaction must be guarded against as well.

RESULTS

There are considerable uncontrolled data in the literature, attesting to the efficacy of various endoscopic modalities for treating upper GI bleeding. However, considering the natural history that 70 to 80 percent of them stop spontaneously, an observed 95 percent efficacy in a substantial series may not reach statistical significance. The reason for the preponderance of uncontrolled data is that a properly designed randomized trial for upper GI bleeding is notoriously difficult to conduct: The wide varieties of lesions, the different magnitude of bleeding, the different local pathologic anatomy, the concomitant diseases, the difficulty in defining the end points, and the different levels of skill of the operators are all-important and may profoundly alter the outcome. Very few patients can be entered in the study if these factors are to be reasonably standardized. By the same token, the published results of randomized trials must be interpreted carefully, as not all factors can be standardized.

Papp[53] showed in a randomized trial in patients admitted with bleeding peptic ulcers bearing the visible vessel sign that monopolar electrocoagulation eliminated rebleeding and significantly reduced blood transfusions, hospitalization, and cost as compared with patients receiving only standard medical treatment. All patients with central visible vessels rebled if no treatment was given. The series is small, with eight patients in each arm, and the conclusion requires confirmation from larger series.

Vallon et al.,[76] at the Middlesex Hospital, randomized 136 patients with upper GI bleeding into argon laser photocoagulation and sham treatment, the randomization being unknown to the managing teams. Initial arrest of active spurting bleeding was effective, as evidenced by 10 of 15 successes, versus a 4 of 13 spontaneous cessation. However, there was no difference in either rebleeding, need for operative treatment, or mortality in the final analysis. If the two cases in which the deformity of the duodenum prevented the endoscopist from getting at the bleeding vessel were excluded, the treated group fared significantly better in both rebleeding and survival. Furthermore, the study was designed so that only one laser treatment session was used. If repeated laser sessions were used to treat recurrent bleeders, a different conclusion may be reached since, of the eight patients who died, six were poor operative risks. Another British group, Bown et al.,[7] ran a controlled trial utilizing the argon laser photocoagulation on patients with bleeding peptic ulcers; preliminary findings showed that although active bleeding was successfully controlled initially in all 19 patients, the rebleeding rate was 9 out of 19, compared with 9 of 20 for the control group. However, as the data accumulated, rather different results were seen. Thus, Swain et al.[71] reported significant efficacy of the argon laser treatment from the same trial (conducted in two teaching hospitals), in which patients bleeding from peptic ulcers accessible to endoscopic treatment were randomized into treatment and sham treatment groups, stratified as those with visible vessels and spurting, with visible vessel but not bleeding, and with adherent clots. These workers found a significant reduction of rebleeding in those with visible vessel treated by argon laser as compared with controls (8 of 24 vs. 17 of 28), although the reduction was not significant when only those spurting visible vessels were considered. All deaths occurred in the patients with visible vessels (28 patients), of whom 25 rebled. There was no mortality in the treated group, but 7 of 28 in the control group died. This is the first study to demonstrate significant reduction in mortality in patients with bleeding peptic ulcer treated by any endoscopic modality, compared with conventional treatment that included surgery.

A controlled trial of Nd:YAG laser photocoagulation for bleeding from the upper digestive tract was published by Rutgeerts et al.[61] Of the 46 patients in the treated group, all 70 actively bleeding (but not spurting arterial bleeding) lesions were stopped by laser photocoagulation, and significantly more lesions in the control group (40 patients) continued to bleed ($P < 0.001$). More recurrent bleeding and more operations were required in the controls, although the difference did not reach the significance level ($P < 0.1$). In 17 patients with stigmata of recent bleeding, three developed bleeding induced by the laser treatment, although only one could not be controlled. Compared with the control group of 26 patients with visible vessels (4 patients) or sentinel clots (22 patients), the treated group had less rebleeding and required fewer emergency operations, but the difference did not reach statistical significance. All actively spurting arterial bleeding lesions (23 patients) were treated by laser photocoagulation, 87 percent of which were initially controlled. Recurrence was high, however, and 61 percent required emergency surgery. The data therefore indicate that Nd:YAG laser was effective in arresting acute, nonspurting bleeding, although the recurrent bleeding and the incidence of emergency operation were not reduced. Rutgeerts et al. pointed out the relative ineffectiveness of endoscopic treatment for the spurting arterial bleeder and that such patients should be selected for early elective surgery before recurrence of hemorrhage.

The results of another controlled trial using the Nd:YAG laser have recently appeared in abstract form. Swain et al.[72] randomized 123 consecutive patients with bleeding peptic ulcers and bearing stigmata of recent bleeding into treatment and control groups. The stratification is identical to their argon laser trial and, as in that trial, only patients with accessible ulcers were included. In this series, only 5 of 62 patients rebled in the treated group, compared with 24 of 61 patients in the controls ($P < 0.005$); 4 of 34 patients with visible vessels rebled in the treated group, compared with 21 of 38 in the controls ($P < 0.005$). Even those with a spurting visible vessel fared better with treatment, as only 2 of 10 rebled compared with 7 of 9 in the controls ($P < 0.02$). Also, 5 patients in the treated group required emergency surgery, while 19 of the control group did. A significantly reduced mortality (1 of 62) was recorded for the treated group, compared with that of the controls (8 of 61) ($P < 0.05$).

Of the numerous uncontrolled studies, the results of the largest personal series probably denote the best results attainable. Papp[52] used monopolar electrocoagulation in 81 consecutive actively bleeding patients, being successful in controlling bleeding at the first attempt in 73 patients (90 percent). The failures occurred because of inaccessible ulcers and torrential hemorrhage. The rebleeding rate was 13.6%; recoagulation was successful in 40 percent of these patients. Mortality in the entire series was 2.5 percent. Gaisford's experience was almost identical in 71 patients.[24] Primary hemostasis was achieved in all patients although six patients rebled (8 percent). Only two of these patients

required surgery, since recoagulation was successful in four. No mortalities and no complications occurred.

Brunetaud et al.[8] treated 54 consecutive peptic ulcers (32 gastric and 22 duodenal ulcers) with the argon laser. Primary hemostasis was attained in 85 percent of patients, and the rebleeding rate was 11 percent. Failure of the argon laser to stop the bleeding occurred when the ulcer was inaccessible, such as hidden in the scarred duodenal bulb, when the bleeding vessel was not adequately exposed and the overlying blood absorbed most of the energy, as well as when a large artery was bleeding rapidly. There were no complications in their series.

Kiefhaber et al.[41] were successful in obtaining primary hemostasis in 94 percent of 767 acute bleeding episodes in 600 consecutive patients using the Nd:YAG laser. The 719 instances of successful control included 142 bleeding varices, 81 Mallory-Weiss tears, 415 bleeding ulcers, 74 multiple erosions, and 7 instances of bleeding in the colon. Rebleeding in varices was 30 percent, and a similar figure was quoted for ulcers, although it is unclear how many of these showed visible vessels. Eight perforations were induced by the laser therapy. Overall mortality in the bleeding ulcer patients was 33 percent, including deaths from concomitant diseases.

There are no similar studies with the bipolar electrocoagulator, the heater probe, the contact laser probe, or alcohol injection. Nor are there controlled trials comparing the efficacy of one modality with another. The data reviewed in the following section are not from prospective controlled trials but are important as they constitute the sole basis for judging which modality to invest in.

Johnston et al.[38] compared the lasers, bipolar and monopolar probes, and heater probe first experimentally; retrospectively in their own clinical experience they compared the performance of the Nd:YAG laser and heater probe and came down solidly in favor of the heater probe. What they have found so advantageous makes good surgical sense: The heater probe can be applied directly to the bleeding vessel, and the accuracy of the aim is verified if bleeding stops or is slowed markedly. By such accurate and direct heat transfer, the bleeder is sealed (coaptive sealing), causing minimal tissue damage. The surgeon is reminded of the common surgical technique with monopolar electrocautery: The bleeding vessel is first picked up with a pair of forceps, and electrocautery is then applied to the instrument by touching with the electrode; the ensuing coaptive sealing not only facilitates coagulation of the vessel but the extent of the coagulation is sharply limited to the vessel. The major disadvantage appears to be the relative slowness of the energy transfer: 10 to 15 seconds are required to seal a vessel; for anyone used to the rapidity of the electrocautery and laser photocoagulation, it definitely takes some getting used to. The monopolar coagulation forceps developed by Sugawa are based on the same principle: however, only infrequently may a bleeder be picked up by the use of forceps in endoscopic procedures. Monopolar electrocoagulation is subject to the nuisance of sticking. By contrast, the noncontact method is much more indirect; it involves a good deal of guessing where the underlying vessel runs and a certain amount of ringing with multiple shots and thus larger areas of necrosis. One must avoid cavitation and evaporation of the vessel wall with aggravation of bleeding on the one hand and inadequate coagulation with dissipation of energy by an artery with rapid flow acting as a heat sink on the other.

Sugawa et al. published their uncontrolled series of alcohol injection in the Exhibit of the American College of Surgeons Clinical Congress of 1985. Of 58 patients in their series of mostly peptic ulcers (35 of 58), only 4 failures occurred, all in the form of rebleeding; 37 of the 58 patients had visible vessels, with almost half of them actively bleeding. No deaths or major complications were attributable to therapeutic endoscopy.

Of the bewildering development of modalities for endoscopic hemostasis, which has the most potential for widespread use? The definitive consumer's guide has not been written. The enthusiastic endoscopist would do well to consider the cost, ease of use, efficacy, and safety before making the investment in both time and money. Both the argon and the Nd:YAG lasers score poor in the first two and only fair in the last two categories. These are expensive, nonportable tools with a high-maintenance requirement. Monopolar probes, especially the variant exemplified by Fruhmorgen's EHT probe, or the Swain liquid monopolar electrode, will remain in the average therapeutic endoscopist tool kit for a long time to come because it scores high in the first three categories, although fair in the fourth. By the same token, if efficacy and safety have been confirmed by wider clinical experience, 98 percent alcohol injection may well be the modality of choice in the near future. The appeal of this low-tech approach lies in its utter simplicity and universal availability, and it costs next to nothing. The heater probe is not particularly easy or difficult to use, although the equipment is much simpler, less expensive, and safer than the Nd:YAG laser. One probe, at a cost of $300, is good for only a few applications, as the nonstick coating tends to wear away. Like the laser that preceded it, the heater probe is now experiencing a surge in popularity that may well prove to be evanescent, to be superseded by simpler and less costly modalities that would surely be developed in the future. The new contact laser probes appeal to the surgeon who uses electrocautery every day; if a truly portable laser source can be manufactured (an entirely feasible technical feat since only low power is needed), it may well be the tool of choice. It appears that the current momentum in research and development of endoscopic therapeutic modalities is sustained by a firm conviction that the mortality of GI bleeding can be reduced by therapeutic endoscopy, if a safe and simple device can be found.

RESULTS OF RADIOLOGIC CONTROL OF BLEEDING

The techniques of radiologic control of bleeding are discussed in Chapter 4. Arterial embolization is especially promising in upper GI hemorrhage: 72 percent success in control has been reported.[10,43] Conditions particularly amenable to embolization appear to be hemobilia[11] and Mallory-Weiss syndrome.[10] Rebleeding within 6 months is uncommon (< 5 percent).[43] This technique is about as efficacious as therapeutic endoscopy and has similar utility in the patient unfit for surgery. It has the advantage of good exposure, since the procedure is not interfered with by blood clots in the lumen. Infarction of the stomach or duodenum, rich as they are in collaterals, have been reported, but usually after previous surgery.[43] Other complications are detailed in Chapter 4.

RESULTS OF SURGERY FOR NONVARICEAL UPPER GASTROINTESTINAL BLEEDING

The mortality of operations for the bleeding duodenal ulcer is generally lower than that for bleeding gastric ulcer,[6,20,29,34,36,39,64] typically 6 to 10 percent for duodenal and 10 to 15 percent for gastric; there is not much difference between vagotomy and drainage compared with antrectomy with vagotomy when the large series are pooled. If operative treatment had to be used for erosive gastritis, the mortality is much higher, typically between 35 and 55 percent, somewhat lower with vagotomy and drainage, and higher with gastrectomy.[6,9,12,30,31,60] For peptic ulcer disease more than 60 percent of deaths were due to cardiopulmonary complications rather than to bleeding or an inadequate operation. Complications include wound infection (8 to 33 percent),[49] leakage of anastomosis (2 to 5 percent), pulmonary (15 percent) and cardiovascular complications (20 percent) and recurrent hemorrhage (5 to 35 percent).[18,22,42,63] The last is said to be higher with vagotomy and oversewing of the bleeder than with gastrectomy, but recent data do not support this view. In Esselstyn's review,[22] for example, the figures were 5 to 26 percent for vagotomy and 8 to 33 percent for gastrectomy for bleeding duodenal ulcer. Surgical intervention for other lesions, such as plication of Mallory-Weiss tears, sub-

mucosal resection of angiomatous malformations, and miscellaneous lesions, are also subject to the same complications, but the data are not substantial enough for a true estimation.

THE ROLES OF THERAPEUTIC ENDOSCOPY AND SURGERY IN UPPER GASTROINTESTINAL BLEEDING

The impact of therapeutic endoscopy on surgery for GI bleeding is difficult to assess, as the modality has not been used community-wide for lack of therapeutic endocopists. There is a good deal of controversy regarding the best means of reducing mortality from GI bleeding. Many surgeons believe that, if high-risk patients are operated on early, mortality can be reduced.[29,30,32] Nonsurgeons, probably less aware that surgical outcome is skill dependent, point to the fact that mortality due to complications such as leakage of anastomosis accounts for a substantial percentage of the mortality, and early surgery is not the answer.[20] The reluctance of nonsurgeons to recommend surgery may well be based on an unrealistic impression of the hazards of surgery or of what constitutes a reasonable surgical candidate. Estimation of surgical risk is an imperfect art at best, one side of the equation being the technical difficulty of the task and the ability of the surgeon; it is therefore much better done jointly by the surgeon and the gastroenterologist rather than by any physician working alone, particularly one not closely involved with surgery. It is in the patient in whom survival after surgery is in doubt (e.g. the cirrhotic patient bleeding from a nonvariceal source[80]) that therapeutic endoscopy or interventional radiology is clearly indicated. For the spurting arterial bleeder, interventional radiology appears to have the edge, since rebleeding is high with therapeutic endoscopy. Therapeutic endoscopy, however, can be used to stabilize such a patient for surgery or to be used again for rebleeding. For lesser degrees of active bleeding, therapeutic endoscopy is the method of choice.

A considerable degree of therapeutic nihilism

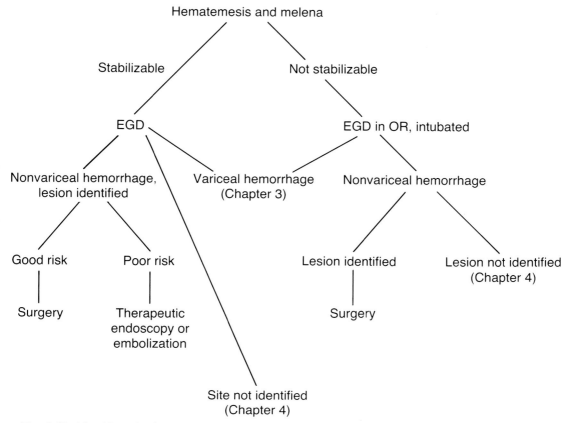

Fig. 2-13 Algorithm: An integrated approach to management of upper gastrointestinal bleeding. EGD, esophagogastroduodenoscopy.

in the management of GI bleeding is being preached by some investigators who point out that 75 percent of GI bleeding stops spontaneously and that early diagnosis, such as by deployment of endoscopy, does not improve the outcome. It is maintained that, when bleeding has stopped, knowing the diagnosis does not lead to better treatment since there is no better treatment than antacids and cimetidine.[55] What is certain is that the mortality in GI bleeding will not be changed if early diagnosis is not considered worthwhile, and therapeutic action is not based on findings. Such a policy will produce self-justifying data. Actually, a fragmented management plan of a critically ill patient is one of the more easily removed obstacles in improving the outcome of GI bleeding. For example, in the Melbourne study by Hunt et al.,[32] dramatic improvement in mortality was achieved by admitting all patients with GI bleeding into a special unit run by a team of gastroenterologists and surgeons with a defined management policy. Over a 6-year period, more than 800 patients were managed with early endoscopy, vigorous resuscitation, and defined criteria for operation. The operation rate was unchanged from before the period of study, but marked reduction of postoperative mortality (16 to 1.6 percent) contributed to a reduction in overall mortality (9 to 2.4 percent). It would be most interesting to see what effect it would have if therapeutic endoscopy is incorporated into a defined management policy in such a unit, where the full potential of therapeutic endoscopy will be realized.

While therapeutic endoscopy has had spectacular success in poor surgical candidates, the choice of this modality over surgery in low-risk patients is unclear. As the art advances, increasing numbers of competent endoscopists will extend the indications of therapeutic endoscopy to low-risk patients: After all, if it is safe for high-risk patients, why not for low-risk patients as well? This author is convinced that introduction of more effective endoscopic procedures in the future will bring about major changes in the operative armamentarium; more surgeons will become proficient in endoscopic procedures, which will replace many surgical operations.

REFERENCES

1. Allan R, Dykes PW: A comparison of routine and selective endoscopy in the management of acute gastrointestinal hemorrhage. Gastrointest Endosc 20:154, 1974
2. Allan R, Dykes PW: A study of the factors influencing mortality rates from gastrointestinal hemorrhage. Q J Med 180:533, 1976
3. Asaki S, Nishimura T, Satoh A, et al: Endoscopic hemostasis of gastrointestinal hemorrhage by local application of absolute ethanol: A clinical study. Tohoku J Exp Med 141:373, 1983
4. Avery-Jones, F: Hematemesis and melena with special reference to causation and to factors influencing the mortality from bleeding peptic ulcers. Gastroenterology 30:166, 1956
5. Blackwood WD, Silvis SE: Standardization of electrosurgical lesions. Gastrointest Endosc 21:22, 1974
6. Boulos PB, Harris J, Wyllie JH, et al: Conservative surgery in 100 patients with bleeding peptic ulcer. Br J Surg 58:817, 1978
7. Bown SG, Storey DW, Swain CP, et al: Controlled trial of argon laser photocoagulation for hemorrhage from peptic ulcers. Gut 22:A414, 1981
8. Brunetaud JM, Enger A, Flament JB, et al: Utilisation d'un laser à argon ionisé en endoscopie digestive: Photocoagulation des lesions hemorrhagiques. Rev Phys Appl 14:385, 1979
9. Byrne JJ, Guardione VA: Surgical treatment of stress ulcers. Am J Surg 125:464, 1973
10. Carsen GM, Casarella WJ, Spiegel RM: Transcatheter embolization for treatment of Mallory-Weiss tears of the gastroesophageal junction. Radiology 128:309, 1978
11. Clark RA, Frey RT, Colley DP, et al: Transcatheter embolization of hepatic arteriovenous fistulas for control of hemobilia. Gastrointest Radiol 6:353, 1981
12. Cody HS, Wichern WA: Choice of operation for acute gastric mucosal hemorrhage. Am J Surg 134:322, 1977
13. Conn HO: To scope or not to scope. N Engl J Med 304:967, 1981
14. Cotton PB, Rosenberg MT, Waldram RPL, et al: Early endoscopy of esophagus, stomach and duodenal bulb in patients with hematemesis and melena. Br Med J 2:505, 1973
15. Daikuzono N, Joffe SN: Artificial sapphire probe for contact photocoagulation and tissue vaporization with Nd:YAG laser. Med Instrum 19:173, 1984
16. Dennis MB, Peoples J, Hulett R, et al: Evaluation of electrofulguration in control of bleeding of experimental gastric ulcers. Dig Dis Sci 24:845, 1979
17. Dixon JA, Berenson MM, McClosky DW: Neodynmium YAG laser treatment of experimental canine gastric bleeding: Acute and chronic studies of photocoagulation, penetration and perforation. Gastroenterology 77:647, 1979
18. Donaldson RM, Handy J, Papper S: Five-year follow-up study of patients with bleeding duodenal ulcers with and without surgery. N Engl J Med 259:201, 1958
19. Dronfield MW, Ferguson R, McIllmurray MB, et al: A prospective randomized study of endoscopy and radiology in acute upper gastrointestinal tract bleeding. Lancet 1:1167, 1977
20. Dronfield MW, Atkinson M, Langman MJS: Effect of different operation policies on mortality from bleeding ulcers. Lancet 1:1126, 1979
21. Dronfield MW, Langman MJS, Atkinson M, et al: Outcome of endoscopy and barium radiography for acute upper gastrointestinal bleeding: Controlled trial in 1037 patients. Br Med J 284:545, 1982
22. Esselstyn CB: Surgical management of actively bleeding duodenal ulcer. Surg Clin North Am 56:1387, 1976
23. Foster DN, Miloszewski KJA, Losowsky MS: Stigmata of recent hemorrhage in diagnosis and prognosis of upper gastrointestinal bleeding. Br Med J 1:1173, 1978
24. Gaisford WD: Endoscopic electrohemostasis of

active upper gastrointestinal bleeding. Am J Surg 137:47, 1979

25. Gilbert DA, Silverstein FE, Tedesco FJ, et al: The national ASGE survey on upper gastrointestinal bleeding. III. Endoscopy in upper gastrointestinal bleeding. Gastrointest Endosc 27:94, 1981

26. Goldman ML, Land WC, Bradley EL, et al: Transcatheter therapeutic embolization in the management of upper gastrointestinal bleeding. Radiology 120:513, 1976

27. Graham DY: Limited value of early endoscopy in the management of acute upper gastrointestinal bleeding: Prospective controlled trial. Am J Surg 140:284, 1980

28. Griffiths WJ, Neumann DA, Welsh JD: The visible vessel as an indicator of uncontrolled or recurrent gastrointestinal hemorrhage. N Engl J Med 300:1411, 1979

29. Hellers G, Ihre T: Impact of change to early diagnosis and surgery in major upper gastrointestinal bleeding. Lancet 2:1250, 1975

30. Himal HS, Perrault C, Mzabi R: Upper gastrointestinal hemorrhage: Aggressive management decreases mortality. Surgery 84:448, 1978

31. Hubert JP Jr, Kieran PD, Welch JS, et al: The surgical management of bleeding stress ulcers. Ann Surg 191:672, 1980

32. Hunt PS, Korman MG, Hansky J, et al: Bleeding duodenal ulcer: Reduction of mortality with a planned approach. Br J Surg 66:633, 1979

33. Iglesias MC, Dourdourekas D, Adomavicius J: Prompt endoscopic diagnosis of upper gastrointestinal hemorrhage: Its value for specific diagnosis and management. Ann Surg 189:90, 1979

34. Inberg MV, Linna MI: Massive hemorrhage from gastroduodenal ulcer. Acta Chir Scand 141:664, 1975

35. Ihre T, Johansson C, Seligsson U, et al: Endoscopic YAG laser treatment in massive UGI bleeding. Scand J Gastroenterol 16:633, 1981

36. Jensen HE, Amdrup E, Christiansen P, et al: Bleeding gastric ulcer, surgical and non-surgical treatment of 225 patients. Scand J Gastroenterol 7:535, 1972

37. Johnston JH, Jensen DM, Mutner W, et al: Argon treatment of bleeding canine gastric ulcers: Limitations and guidelines for endoscopic use. Gastroenterology 80:708, 1981

38. Johnston JH, Sones JQ, Long BW, et al: Comparison of heater probe and YAG laser in endoscopic treatment of major bleeding from peptic ulcers. Gastrointest Endosc 31:175, 1985

39. Kaplan MS, List JW, Stemmer EA, et al: Surgical management of upper gastrointestinal bleeding in the aged patient. Am J Gastroenterol 58:109, 1972

40. Keller RT, Logan GM: Comparison of emergent endoscopy and upper gastrointestinal series radiography in acute upper gastrointestinal hemorrhage. Gut 17:180, 1976

41. Kiefhaber P, Nath G, Moritz K: Endoscopic control of massive gastrointestinal hemorrhage by irradiation with a high power neodymium YAG laser. Prog Surg 15:140, 1977

42. Langman MJS: Relationship between preoperative bleeding and perforation and bleeding after operations for duodenal ulcer. Gut 6:134, 1965

43. Lieberman DA, Keller FS, Katon RM, et al: Arterial embolization for massive upper gastrointestinal tract bleeding in poor risk surgical candidates. Gastroenterology 86:876, 1984

44. Lincheer WG, Fazio TL: Control of upper gastrointestinal hemorrhage by endoscopic spraying of clotting factors. Gastroenterology 71:642, 1979

45. MacLeod I, Mills PR, Mackenzie JF, et al: Neodymium-yttrium-aluminum-garnet laser photocoagulation for major hemorrhage from peptic ulcers and single vessels: A single blind controlled study. Br Med J 286:345, 1983

46. Matek W, Fruhmorgen P, Kaduk B, et al: The healing process of experimentally produced bleeding lesions after hemostatic electrocoagulation with simultaneous instillation of water. Endoscopy 12:231, 1980

47. Mills TN, Swain CP, Dark JM, et al: The "hot squeeze" bipolar forceps. A more effective endoscopic method for stopping bleeding from large vessels in the gastrointestinal tract. Gastrointest Endosc 29:184, 1983

48. Morgan AG, McAdam WAF, Walmisley GL, et al: Clinical findings, early endoscopy, and multivariate analysis in patients bleeding from the upper gastrointestinal tract. Br Med J 2:237, 1977

49. Nichols RL, Condon RE: Role of the endogenous gastrointestinal microflora in postoperative wound sepsis. p. 279. In Nyhus LM (ed): Surgery Annual. Appleton-Century-Crofts, New York, 1975

50. Otani T, Tatsuka T, Kanamaru K, et al: Intramural injection of ethanol under direct vision

for treatment of protuberant lesions of the stomach. Gastroenterology 69:123, 1975

51. Papp JP, Fox JM, Wilks HS: Experimental electrocoagulation of dog gastric mucosa. Gastrointest Endosc 22:27, 1975

52. Papp JP: Endoscopic electrocoagulation of actively bleeding arterial upper gastrointestinal lesions. Am J Gastroenterol 71:516, 1979

53. Papp JP: Endoscopic electrocoagulation in the management of upper gastrointestinal tract bleeding. Surg Clin North Am 62:797, 1982

54. Peterson WL, Barnett CC, Smith HJ, et al: Routine early endoscopy in upper gastrointestinal tract bleeding. A randomized controlled trial. N Engl J Med 304:925, 1981

55. Peterson WL: Gastrointestinal bleeding. p. 186. In Sleisenger MH, Fordtran JS (eds): Gastrointestinal Diseases. 3rd Ed. WB Saunders, Philadelphia, 1983

56. Piercy JRA, Auth DC, Silverstein FE, et al: Electrosurgical treatment of experimental bleeding canine gastric ulcers: Development and testing of a computer control and better electrode. Gastroenterology 74:527, 1978

57. Protell RL, Rubin CE, Auth DC, et al: The heater probe: A new endoscopic method for stopping massive gastrointestinal bleeding. Gastroenterology 74:257, 1978

58. Protell RL, Gilbert DA, Opie EA, et al: Computer-assisted electrocoagulations: Bipolar vs monopolar in the treatment of experimental gastric ulcer bleeding. Gastroenterology 80:451, 1981

59. Read RC, Huebel HC, Thal AP: Randomized study of massive bleeding from peptic ulceration. Ann Surg 162:561, 1965

60. Richardson JD, Aust JB: Gastric devascularization: A useful salvae procedure for massive hemorrhagic gastritis. Ann Surg 65:551, 1978

61. Rutgeerts P, Vantrappen G, Broecbaert L, et al: Controlled trial of YAG laser treatment of upper digestive hemorrhage. Gastroenterology 83:410, 1982

62. Sandlow LJ, Becker GH, Spellberg MA, et al: A prospective randomized study of the management of upper gastrointestinal hemorrhage. Am J Gastroenterol 61:282, 1974

63. Serebro HA, Mendeloff AI: Late results of medical and surgical treatment of bleeding peptic ulcer. Lancet 2:1462, 1966

64. Schiller KFR, Truelove SC, Williams DG: Hematemesis and melena, with special reference to factors influencing the outcome. Br Med J 2:7, 1970

65. Silverstein FE, Gilbert DA, Tedesco FJ, et al: The national ASGE survey on upper gastrointestinal bleeding. I. Study design and baseline data. Gastrointest Endosc 27:73, 1981

66. Silverstein FE, Gilbert DA, Tedesco FJ, et al: The national ASGE survey on upper gastrointestinal bleeding. II. Clinical prognostic factors. Gastrointest Endosc 27:80, 1981

67. Storey DW, Bown SG, Swain CP, et al: Endoscopic prediction of recurrent bleeding in peptic ulcers. N Engl J Med 305:915, 1981

68. Sugawa C, Shier M, Lucas CE, et al: Electrocoagulation of bleeding in the upper part of the gastrointestinal tract. Arch Surg 110:975, 1979

69. Sugawa C, Ikeda T, Fujita Y, et al: Endoscopic hemostasis of gastrointestinal hemorrhage by local injection of 98% ethanol: An experimental study. Gastrointest Endosc 30:155, 1984

70. Sugawa C: Endoscopic control of upper gastrointestinal tract bleeding, p. 35. In Dent TL, Strodel WE, Turcotte JG (eds): Surgical Endoscopy. Year Book Medical Publishers, Chicago, 1985

71. Swain CP, Bown SG, Storey DW, et al: Controlled trial of argon laser photocoagulation in bleeding ulcers. Lancet 2:1313, 1981

72. Swain CP, Bown SG, Salmon PR, et al: Controlled trial of Nd:YAG laser photocoagulation in bleeding peptic ulcers. Gastroenterology 84:1327, 1983

73. Swain CP, Mills TN, Dark JM, et al: Comparative study of the safety and efficacy of liquid and dry monopolar electrocoagulation in experimental canine bleeding ulcers using computerized energy monitoring. Gastroenterology 86:93, 1984

74. Swain CP, Mills TN: An endoscopic sewing machine. Gastrointest Endosc 31:160, 1985

75. Swain CP, Storey DW, Bown S, et al: Nature of the bleeding vessel in recurrently bleeding gastric ulcers. Gastroenterology 90:595, 1986

76. Vallon AG, Cotton PB, Laurence BM, et al: Randomized trial of endoscopic laser photocoagulation in bleeding peptic ulcer. Gut 22:228, 1981

77. Volpicelli NA, McCarthy JD, Bartlett JD, et al: Endoscopic electrocoagulation: An alternative to operative therapy in bleeding peptic ulcer disease. Arch Surg 113:483, 1978

78. Wara P, Hojsgaard A, Amdrup E: Endoscopic electrocoagulation—An alternative to operative

hemostasis in active gastroduodenal bleeding? Endoscopy 12:237, 1980

79. Wara P: Endoscopic prediction of major rebleeding—A prospective study of stigmata of hemorrhage in bleeding ulcer. Gastroenterology 88:1209, 1985

80. Wirthlin LS, Urk HV, Matt RB, et al: Predictors of surgical mortality in patients with cirrhosis and non-variceal bleeding. Surg Gynecol Obstet 139:65, 1974

3

The Role of Sclerotherapy in Management of Esophageal Variceal Bleeding

The treatment of esophageal variceal hemorrhage has gone through more changes in fashion than most major entities in clinical medicine, a reflection of the lack of uniformly satisfactory results obtainable from any single modality advanced so far. The early history of therapeutic effort has recently been reviewed by Donovan.[21] Table 3-1 lists the contributions that significantly affected therapeutic practice for bleeding varices in chronologic order, covering the past eight decades. Early development focused mainly on treatment of the local lesion, such as tamponade of the bleeding vessel or injection sclerosis, but the original concept of portal diversion for decompression was almost as old.[20] During the mid-1940s, the rationale of reduction of the portal hypertension as the basis for lasting cure of recurrent hemorrhage from varices received most attention, culminating in the introduction of portacaval shunting by Whipple.[79] The seemingly impeccable logic was supported as much by uncontrolled data as enthusiasm and, because of its clinical efficacy in prevention of variceal hemorrhage, the procedure was widely used. Twenty to 30 years later, however, when portacaval shunt was examined by prospective randomized controlled trials it became clear that

shunting was not a uniformly satisfactory treatment, as it offered no advantage in survival.[34,58] While patients with patent shunts may be free of bleeding, they often develop hepatic encephalopathy; the incidence and the severity depended on the manner in which it was reported. It was demonstrated that diversion of portal flow from the impaired liver brought about the deterioration,[4,77] a fact recognized as early as the 1890s by Pavlov, who coined the term *meat intoxication*.

To avoid total diversion of portal flow upon which the diseased liver is critically dependent, selective shunting of the gastroesophageal varices was proposed. The distal splenorenal shunt (Warren) is such an operation, designed to separate the venous drainage of the gastroesophageal area artificially from the rest of the portal system and shunting it into the systemic venous circulation via the left renal vein.[78] It is not known how permanent such selectivity can be maintained since, if collaterals develop between the portal and systemic circulation in response to a pressure gradient, the same would be expected to occur between the artificially separated portions of the portal system. Indeed, radiologic studies show that the selectivity of the shunt

39

Table 3-1. Treatment of Esophageal Varices: Major Historical Developments

Technique	First Use
Omentopexy	Talma (1889)
Splenectomy	Banti (1894)
Balloon tamponade	Wesphal (1930)
Sclerotherapy	Crafoord and Frenckner (1939)
Portacaval shunt	Whipple (1945)
Esophagogastrectomy	Phemeister (1947)
Transesophageal ligation	Borema (1949)
Sengstaken-Blakemore tube	Sengstaken-Blakemore (1950)
Portoazygous disconnection	Tanner (1950)
IV Pituitrin	Kehne (1956)
Distal splenorenal shunt	Warren (1966)
Devascularization	Sugiura (1973)

in many instances did not last.[5,29,48] Collaterals do develop from the hypertensive portion into the shunted portion, increasing the flow at the splenorenal shunt. The pancreatic blood flow has been shown by Warren's group to play a major role and act as a siphon,[29] although the collaterals in the gastric wall may act likewise. Alcoholic cirrhotics, in particular, are likely to lose such selectivity.[29] The incidence of encephalopathy in selective shunts is variable, but truly low incidence are reported in a few centers.[17,30,60] Today selective shunting is generally recognized among surgeons as the preferred elective treatment for long-term control of variceal bleeding, particularly in nonalcoholic cirrhosis, with an efficacy comparable to portacaval shunts in prevention of recurrent hemorrhage, and yet has a lower encephalopathy rate.[30] These results are considered generally attainable given certain standards in surgical skills.

The opinion is still divided regarding emergency shunting as a treatment of acute hemorrhage. The only agreement appears to be that high surgical mortality can be expected. In a patient who is actively bleeding with an ailing liver, more and more surgeons have come to realize the futility of treating a complication of liver disease by incurring further insults to the liver—and at a staggering cost.[13,49] For this

situation, there has been a trend to return to nonshunt surgical techniques, an example is the elaborate devascularization procedure such as the Sugiura procedure,[70–72] consisting of splenectomy, meticulous devascularization of the greater and lesser curvatures of the stomach with preservation of the coronary vein, transection and reanastomosis of the esophagus, and selective vagotomy and pyloroplasty, all done through a thoracoabdominal incision. If such procedures can be accomplished expeditiously with reasonable loss of blood, judged to be within the limits of tolerance by the impaired liver, there may indeed be a role for them in the therapeutic armamentarium for variceal hemorrhage, but such surgeons exist mostly in other institutions. It is procedures like this that make the less invasive modalities appear superior by comparison, irrespective of proven efficacy. Among these are the simplified portoazygous disconnection such as ligation of the coronary vein and transection of the esophagus or stomach with the stapler,[14,19,64] sclerotherapy with modern endoscopes,[26,43,80] percutaneous transhepatic embolization of the variceal channels,[2,67] and the use of β-blockers to reduce the portal flow and pressure.[42] Many of these are still unproven, and some have already been shown to be ineffective. Of these, sclerotherapy is the only modality that has been tested with randomized controlled trials and is currently by far the most widely used nonsurgical treatment for esophageal varices. It would appear that the therapeutic possibility has gone full circle in half a century; it was in 1939 that sclerotherapy was first introduced.[18] On the basis of the premise that sclerotherapy does not further injure the liver, is relatively simple to perform, and does not preclude future shunt surgery, it has a decided role in management of bleeding esophageal varices, especially in the acutely bleeding patient.

INDICATIONS

Randomized controlled trials have demonstrated that sclerotherapy is useful in several situations:

1. *To stop active bleeding:* In experienced centers, sclerotherapy is more than 90 percent successful in arresting active bleeding and is superior to the use of Sengstaken-Blakemore balloon tamponade in efficacy, morbidity, mortality, and patient acceptance. No other nonoperative measures can live up to this claim.

2. *To eradicate varices or prevent future bleeding episodes when undertaken as a chronic regimen with maintenance injections:* Controlled trials so far indicate that sclerotherapy is moderately successful in attaining this objective. Although there is no trial comparing chronic sclerotherapy with shunting, it is likely that sclerotherapy is less effective than portacaval shunt in preventing rebleeding but has far less morbidity. Survival has been shown to be increased in two series and no difference in four others (see Results). It seems reasonable to offer this as the definitive treatment for high-risk patients who are likely to succumb to an operation and to those whose liver disease is likely to progress. Sclerotherapy is the preferred treatment when the patient cannot be easily shunted anatomically, as after failure of a previous portasystemic shunt.[11] In the case of occlusion of a selective distal splenorenal shunt, the varices can be very large, and sclerotherapy is the treatment offering the least complicated solution.

3. *To be used prophylactically in patients with large varices that have never bled before.* As yet there are only limited data to support this indication. Recent data have correlated the likelihood of future bleeding with the size and length of varices. Prophylactic injection may be justified in patients with high portal pressure and large varices and also in those with poor liver function in whom the first attack of bleeding carries a high mortality. An example is the patient who has large varices and intractable ascites for which peritoneal venous shunt is contemplated. The resulting volume expansion is likely to bring on variceal rupture which carries a high mortality in such a patient. Prophylactic sclerotherapy seems justified for this situation.

Other factors may tip the scale in deciding whether the patient should be treated by shunt surgery or chronic sclerotherapy, such as the availability of a skilled sclerotherapist or surgeon and the follow-up care and the patient's own desire. A special consideration of the patient's occupation is relevant here: A professional highly dependent on critical intellect is likely to be severely handicapped by minor degrees of encephalopathy that may be passed as insignificant for a worker of manual skill.

CONTRAINDICATIONS

Sclerotherapy, like any other therapeutic endoscopic procedure for gastrointestinal (GI) hemorrhage, should be done only in a hemodynamically stable patient. When the patient is in shock, the first priority is resuscitation. Diverting the manpower to get ready for endoscopy is not in the patient's best interest.

Infrequently truly massive hemorrhage from esophageal varices may make it difficult to see clearly. Such patients are generally hemodynamically unstable and sclerotherapy is contraindicated on that basis. Vasopressin infusion and/or Sengstaken-Blakemore balloon tamponade may be used to decrease the rate of bleeding, while resuscitation catches up in order to optimize the chances for a successful injection.

Gastric variceal hemorrhage, when shown coming clearly from an area well away from the gastroesophageal junction, contraindicates sclerotherapy to the esophageal varices. Injecting the esophageal varices will not only not stop the bleeding but will actually aggravate it by blocking the outflow of the varix. There is no satisfactory endoscopic means of treating gastric varices at present. The gastric mucosa is quite different from the esophageal mucosa in that the veins move with the folds, making it difficult to inject. Using the conventional end or oblique viewing endoscope, the veins just distal to the gastroesophageal junction can only be examined by reverse gastroscopy; injection in this position is hazardous as the needle is almost perpendicular to the veins, making it easy to penetrate the stomach (Fig. 3-1A). Although this difficulty can be solved by the use

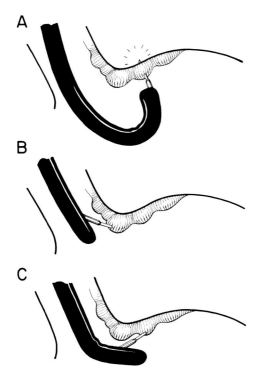

Fig. 3-1 Injection of gastric varices is difficult with conventional equipment. (A) By retroflexion of the end-viewing endoscope, the injector is at right angles to the varices, risking penetration of the gastric wall. (B, C) The duodenoscope is a possible solution as shown on these diagrams, but the conventional injectors often cannot clear the cannula elevator at the opening of the instrument channel.

of a lateral viewing endoscope (Fig. 3-1B,C), the available injectors do not perform well in this position. The short rigid needle-housing mechanism of the injector cannot be passed over the cannula elevator of the duodenoscope. Smaller gastric varix may be coagulated carefully with the Nd:YAG laser with reverse gastroscopy, but the endoscope is easily damaged if the beam hits it inadvertently; besides, most laser experts would hesitate to treat varices with the laser.

Sclerotherapy should not be used to treat bleeding from deep ulcers resulting from inaccurate injection. Often such bleeding comes from the collaterals in the musculature (see Complications), and injection into the depth of the ulcer

in an attempt to get at the offending vessel only worsens the necrosis. Perforation may result.

Serious coagulopathy is a relative contraindication to sclerotherapy. Elective injections should not be undertaken until the abnormality is at least partially corrected, but one can seldom afford this luxury in emergency settings. A 20 to 30 percent prolongation of the prothrombin time is acceptable.

Sclerotherapy is not the therapy of choice for variceal hemorrhage secondary to thrombosis of the splenic vein, following trauma or pancreatitis. Since splenectomy is curative for this condition, the role of sclerotherapy is confined to stopping acute bleeding.

MECHANISMS OF ACTION

Both experimental studies[69] and postmortem histopathologic studies of injected varices[22,32] have clearly demonstrated extensive thrombosis of submucosal esophageal varices proximal and distal to injection sites. Even though this was seen in patients who died 48 hours after injection and clinically thrombosis can be demonstrated endoscopically in patients receiving chronic injections, it is not known whether thrombosis is also the mechanism of action accounting for the instantaneous action of sclerotherapy. Animal studies suggest that the detergent nature of the sclerosants is capable of irreversibly damaging the endothelium and producing instantaneous thrombosis[57] but, considering that sclerosants are washed rapidly via the collateral flow into the systemic circulation, the considerable dilution factor may have prevented instantaneous thrombosis. Also, paravariceal injection has been reported to be effective in stopping bleeding acutely, indicating that other mechanisms may be operative as well. Intravariceal manometry during sclerotherapy revealed some interesting observations.[12] In patients undergoing sclerotherapy, the intravariceal pressure was measured by attaching a manometer to the injector through a three-way stopcock. Injection of each variceal column at two levels was undertaken successively (Fig. 3-2, P1, P2, followed

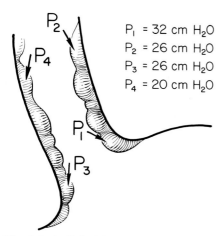

$P_1 = 32$ cm H_2O
$P_2 = 26$ cm H_2O
$P_3 = 26$ cm H_2O
$P_4 = 20$ cm H_2O

Fig. 3-2 A clinical investigation of changes of variceal pressure due to sclerotherapy. Each column of varices was injected at two levels (P1, P2) before moving on to the next column (P3, P4). When the needle entered the varix, the pressure reading was first obtained, followed by injection of the sclerosant. For example, at P1, pressure was 32 cm H_2O. At P2, pressure was 26 cm H_2O, after sclerosant had been injected at P1. In a separate column, the pressure at P3 was 26 cm H_2O before injection, same as P2. Therefore, the uninjected column had the same pressure as the injected column. P4 was 20 cm, after injecting at P3. (Data from Chung RS, Lewis JW: Injection slerotherapy for recurrent variceal hemorrhage following failure of operative treatment. Gastroenterology 80:1125, 1981 (abs.).)

by P3, P4), immediately preceded by measurement of intravariceal pressure at these points. A fall in the variceal pressure, for example, at P2, (P2 minus P1) was always recorded in the column that had just been injected distally (at P1). However, on inserting the needle at P3, it was found that the pressure in an uninjected column also decreased, and to the same extent as the injected column (P3=P2). Anatomic studies[7,68] have shown that the coronary inflow (situated on the serosal aspect of the stomach) traverses the muscular layers of the esophagus at the gastroesophageal junction (Fig. 3-3) in reaching the submucosal position to form columns of gastroesophageal varices. If sustained esophageal spasm occurs as a result of the irritating action of the sclerosants injected, the inflow

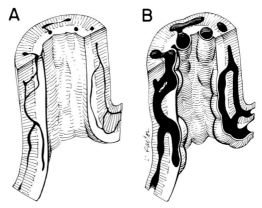

Fig. 3-3 Relationship of the variceal channels to the esophageal musculature at the gastroesophageal junction. (After Stelzner F, Lierse W: Der angiomuskulare dehnverschlub der terminalen speiserohre. Langenbecks Arch Klin Chir 321:35, 1968.) (A) Normal. (B) Portal hypertension.

may be significantly reduced by compression of the veins in their intramuscular course (Fig. 3-4). This explanation is compatible with the observed changes in intravariceal manometry. Clinically transient but intense esophageal contraction is routinely observed at sclerotherapy. Thus muscular contraction of the lower esophagus may at least in part account for the effect of instantaneous cessation of bleeding.

Camara et al.[9] studied the systemic cardiovascular action of larger clinical doses of sclerosants such as sodium morrhuate, and also tetradecyl sulfate (unpublished data) in the dog. A profound but transient decrease in cardiac output,

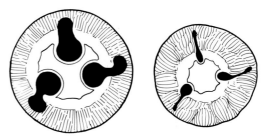

Fig. 3-4 Hypothesis of the acute effect of sclerotherapy. Esophageal muscular contraction (e.g., spasm induced by sclerotherapy) temporarily compresses the inflow to the varices at the gastroesophageal junction, reducing the pressure and flow to the varices.

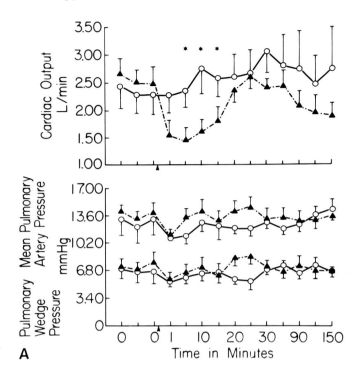

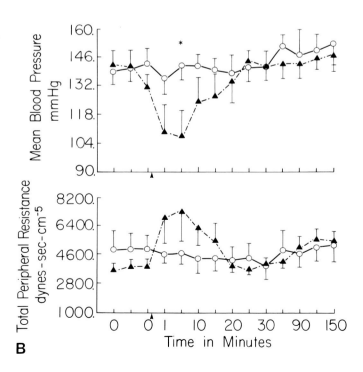

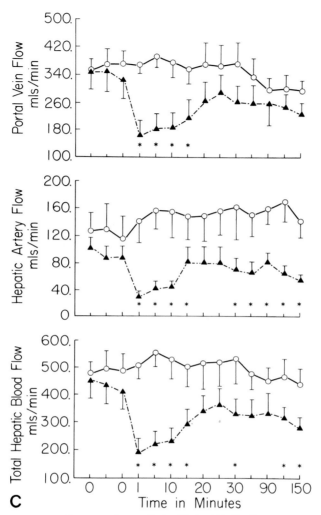

Fig. 3-5 Effects of intravenous sodium morrhuate (0.4 ml/kg). (A) Cardiac output, mean pulmonary artery pressure, and pulmonary wedge pressure. Note decreased cardiac output without significant change in pulmonary wedge and artery pressure. (B) Arterial pressure and peripheral resistance. Note sharp fall in blood pressure and increase in peripheral resistance. (C) Portal vein flow, hepatic arterial flow, and total hepatic blood flow. Note marked transient decrease in all flow measurements after injection. (*Figure continues.*)

systemic pressure, and portal venous and total flow was induced (Fig. 3-5). An identical but even more transient effect is seen with tetradecyl sulfate (unpublished data). Since increase and decrease in flow produce large changes in pressure in the cirrhotic liver, it is conceivable that a decrease in cardiac output induced by Na morrhuate may result in decrease in portal pressure, just as propranolol reduced portal pressure by reducing cardiac output.[41,42] Such hemodynamic changes may conceivably have contributed to the clinical success in the arrest of acute variceal hemorrhage.

A completely different rationale underlies the practice of paravariceal injection, where the sclerosant is specifically deposited outside of the veins, the *esophageal wall sclerosis* described by Wodak.[82,83] As practiced currently

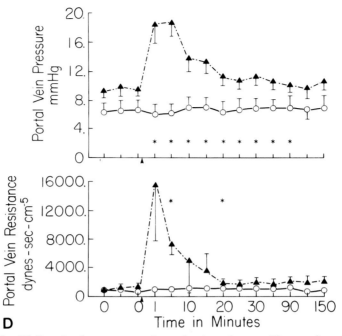

Fig. 3-5 (*Continued*). (D) Portal vein pressure and portal vein resistance. The transient sharp rise of portal pressure and resistance is most likely the result of greater outflow than of inflow reduction, but the total flow is greatly diminished. (Figs. A-D from Camara DS, et al: Hemodynamic effect of the sclerosant Na morrhuate in dogs. Surg Gynec Obst 161:327, 1985.)

in some European centers, the sclerosant is given in more dilute concentrations and smaller volumes but by more numerous injections (30 to 40) into the submucosa alongside the varices, in order to provoke tissue reaction, fibrosis and thickening of the mucosa over the varices to prevent rupture while preserving them as collateral channels. Paquet and Oberhammer[52] published impressive results with this technique, while others reported much less success.[37] Smith and Rose[66] compared the two methods and demonstrated that while the sclerosant remained in the submucosa for as long as 90 minutes when given paravariceally, it was not very thrombogenic. A greater risk of ulceration and full-thickness necrosis of esophageal wall is associated with this technique.

Some endoscopists hold a middle view. They reason that because it is difficult to achieve accurate intravenous injection, and even accurate injection may be followed by some extravasation when the needle is withdrawn, it really does not matter whether injection has been intra- or extravariceal. The argument is quite foreign to surgical thinking. It is like saying to the surgeon that if wound infection commonly occurs following certain operations, good surgical techniques matter little.

TECHNIQUE

Equipment

As in any procedure for GI hemorrhage, a strong light source is essential, not only because one may have to look through a film of blood, but also because of the need to provide a view for the assistant to coordinate the maneuvers through a teaching attachment. The endoscope must have a large channel so that suction is not diminished after an injector has been inserted in it. A built-in forceps elevator is useful in aiming the injector in some circumstances but not essential. A built-in water jet, on the other hand, saves so much time in clearing the view that it is almost mandatory.

The injector is made of a catheter sheath, 120 to 140 cm long, with a retractable needle, 4 mm long, and No. 23 or 25 gauge at the tip. The original Olympus reusable injector still has certain advantages, not the least of which is that it is sturdy and well machined, with good balance and the correct amount of flexibility. The needle is lockable in the extended position with a positive click. However, it does not stand up to many cycles of sterilization, the piano wire sheath is difficult to clean, and the needle becomes dull. All the many disposable injectors on the market handle like any disposable instruments, and some are so flexible that it is almost impossible to direct or aim. The retraction mechanism may not be dependable, but the advantage is convenience.

Many sclerosants have been used, and the selection and concoction are often based on conjecture rather than experimental data. Thus antibiotics have been added on the basis that it would combat bacteremia, 50 percent dextrose because it is thrombogenic (to slow-flowing peripheral veins), and thrombin because of its clot-promoting property. When tested systematically in in vivo experiments, only ethanol, sodium morrhuate, sodium tetradecyl sulfate, and ethanolamine are effective sclerosants. In general, efficacy (thrombogenicity) and ulcerogenicity go hand in hand: The more destructive it is to the endothelium, the more necrotizing it is when it is extravasated. Absolute alcohol appears to be the most sclerotic, but it is so necrotizing that it is difficult to use safely for this purpose; however, it shows promise when used in very small amounts for bleeding gastric ulcers (see Chapter 2). Ethanolamine is the least thrombogenic of the four sclerosants. Both sodium morrhuate (5 percent) and sodium tetradecyl (1 percent, 3 percent) are formulary items and have about equal efficacy. Tetradecyl is colorless and resembles water in consistency, while the morrhuate is yellowish, smells like cod liver oil, and is slightly more viscous. Both agents can cause anaphylaxis and allergic reactions. Both

are extensively used in the United States, but ethanolamine is also commonly used in the United Kingdom.

Patient Preparation

EMERGENCY MANAGEMENT FOR ACTIVE BLEEDING

Sclerotherapy is clearly effective in arrest of active bleeding and, as such, is a valuable first-line treatment. It is more effective than Sangstaken-Blakemore balloon tamponade.[1,54,40] However, when performed under such circumstances, the procedure is quite demanding of skill and experience, and not many centers are staffed to offer this service 24 hours a day. As a practical necessity, active bleeding may first be slowed or controlled with ancillary measures such as vasopressin infusion, 0.4 units/min in 5 percent dextrose via a central line following a bolus dose of 20 units in 100 ml of dextrose over 20 minutes, or balloon tamponade with the Senstaken-Blakemore tube, or both. A new analogue, triglycyl lysine vasopressin (terlipressin), has been shown to be more effective in a randomized trial.[25] It has a more sustained action on the smooth muscles and does not affect the myocardium. A placebo-controlled double-blind trial[76] showed that, when used in conjunction with sclerotherapy and balloon tamponade in a standardized regimen, it is superior to placebo in reducing blood requirement, duration of balloon tamponade, treatment failures, and mortality. Simultaneous administration of nitroglycerin (0.4 mg sublingually, q 30 min) has been shown to enhance the action of vasopressin by further reduction of the wedged hepatic venous pressure while preserving cardiac output.[28] When the balloon is used, sclerotherapy should be performed within 12 hours to limit the trauma to the esophageal mucosa. The Minnesota tube, the modification whereby a fourth lumen provides for continuous suction of the saliva, is preferred. A new tube should always be used and even then should always be tested under water for air tightness of the balloons. The lubricated tube is first passed in the deflated state via the mouth with proper pharyngeal anesthesia or via the nose if the patient is already intubated with an oral endotracheal tube. Stiffening the Sengstaken-Blakemore tube with a guidewire sometimes helps pass the high-resistance area of the endotracheal cuff. The tube is inserted almost all the way, and the gastric area is auscultated for bubbling sound when air is instilled into the aspirating lumen. The gastric balloon is then slowly inflated with 250 to 300 ml of air. During inflation, if the patient shows signs of discomfort, inflation must stop, as the gastric balloon may be in the esophagus. When fully inflated, the tube is pulled back until it catches, indicating that it is abutting the cardia. This is confirmed by radiography, followed by application of 1 to 1.5 lb of traction by some means of anchoring, such as to a football helmet, worn by the patient. The esophageal balloon is only inflated when hemorrhage still continues as determined by aspiration of the gastric lumen. Inflation to 35 mmHg is recommended, but this must not be maintained for more than 24 hours without deflation, even if sclerotherapy is not intended. If balloon tamponade is routinely and skillfully used as part of the management of acute variceal bleeding, the patient can be endoscoped when optimal manpower and expertise is available. The view is usually clear for accurate injection when the tube is removed.

When temporizing measures are not used, and sclerotherapy is used to treat active bleeding, the first essential preparation is lavage, provided the patient is stable hemodynamically. Consideration should be given to endotracheal intubation if bleeding is truly massive. The patient's torso should be elevated to 45 degrees so that blood is easily cleared from the esophagus by flowing into the stomach.

In many instances a cooperative patient anxious to have bleeding controlled may not require sedation, but in most patients diazepam should be given intravenously. Pharyngeal anesthetization should be thorough, as the endoscope or lavage tube may have to be inserted more than once. Meperidine is given during injection to reduce pain.

In an uncooperative or intoxicated patient, consideration should be given to performing the procedure under general endotracheal anesthesia. The airway is protected and movements minimized, facilitating accurate injections.

Endoscopic Techniques

THE FREE-HAND TECHNIQUE

After checking the functions of the endoscope, the injector is inserted into the instrument channel before passing the endoscope (Fig. 3-6). This is to eliminate the period of delay between discovery of an active bleeder and the insertion of the injector, since exposure time is precious. The needle remains retracted until shortly before injection.

After passing the cricopharyngeus, the entire esophagus is surveyed for the number, size, and vertical span of the varices. A shooting jet of blood or vigorous oozing is immediately dealt with by injecting 2 ml of 1.5 percent tetradecyl or 2 ml of 5 percent sodium morruhate into the varix, preferably distal to the bleeding point, but it is often expedient to enter proximally, as the jet of blood prevents easy access to the distal varix. Figure 3-7 shows how the sclerosant may be injected without loss from the bleeding point, even though the needle entered proximally. More than 90 percent of the time, this single injection suffices; bleeding slows down to a trickle, and then stops within a minute. A second injection or even a third may be given distally, if needed, to attain complete hemostasis, but it is important to allow plenty of time to make sure it is clearly needed. This author disagrees with the often-advocated practice of injecting by the side of the bleeding point outside the varix to attempt compression with the edema induced: It is not only unnecessary but may actually be harmful.

In the absence of active bleeding, the stigmata of recent bleeding are searched for. An adherent clot on one varix, "cherry spots" (actually sealed rupture points), raised white spots (most probably platelet–fibrin plugs), are as significant as the visible vessel sign in bleeding ulcers.

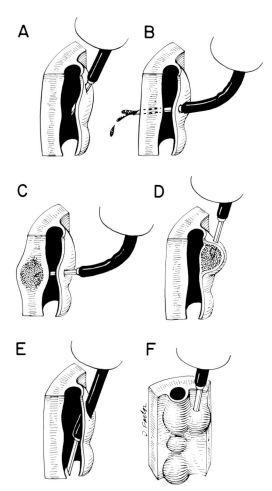

Fig. 3-6 Free-hand injection: techniques and errors. (A) Accurate intravariceal injection. (B) Full-thickness penetration. (C) Intramuscular injection—too deep. A vertical entry of the needle in (B) and (C) had been brought about by extending too much of the injector outside of the channel, combined with forward movement of either the endoscope or the injector. (D) Too superficial, swelling on top of varix. (E) Cannulation—the sheath of the injector has entered the varix. (F) Paravariceal injection—a "miss."

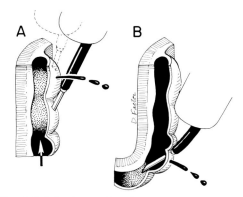

Fig. 3-7 Injecting a bleeding varix. (A) Injection should be distal to the bleeding point. (B) However, it is at times expedient to enter proximally, but the sclerosant should be deposited into the vein distal to the point of rupture.

These must be accurately injected in the same way as the active bleeder. Other signs, such as the blue signs, or the varices upon varices, are indicative of the severity of the varices and are more correctly called signs of impending hemorrhage.[3] These varices must also be similarly treated.

Sometimes no apparent site of bleeding can be found in the esophagus, yet there are fresh clots in the stomach. Before concluding that bleeding comes from a site in the stomach, it is well to examine the gastroesophageal junction just beyond the esophagus. Oozing, cherry-red signs and small clots can be hidden by the edge of the esophagus as it opens into the cardia. It can be seen better on reverse gastroscopy or with a lateral-viewing endoscope. If such a site is found, it can be effectively sclerosed by injecting the variceal column just at the gastroesophageal junction. However, if the site is found to be more than 2 to 3 cm away into the cardia, such injection may not work. This constitutes true gastric variceal bleeding, an unusual event for which eosphageal variceal sclerosis gives poor results.

Often the bleeding varix is in a hiatus hernia, and the bleeding location is at the hiatus. This is readily accessible to the endoscope and should be injected in the same manner as for esophageal varices. Considerable skill is required, however, if much sliding movement occurs with respiration. It should also be noted that the Sengstaken-Blakemore balloon may not be effective in this location.

Examination of the rest of the upper GI tract is mandatory for the patient presenting for the first time. Gastric erosions, ulcers, Mallory-Weiss tears, and other sources account for at least 30 percent of all upper GI bleeding complicating portal hypertension. The strategy in getting the entire territory covered is no different from that used for diagnosis of other acute GI bleeding (see Chapter 2).

When, after exhaustive search, no other pathology is found except for clots in the stomach and clean-looking esophageal varices, the varices can be assumed to be the source with considerable certainty, especially when these are long and tortuous or prominent. In such cases, and in all cases in which the actively bleeding varix has been successfully dealt with, the endoscope is positioned at just above the gastroesophageal junction, where all variceal columns are systematically injected, using 2 ml of the sclerosant for each column. This done, the endoscope is withdrawn for 5 cm and the column injected for a second round. Failure to inject all varices may account for the high incidence of rebleeding within a few days, since the flow may be channeled to the uninjected varix or varices.

In repeat sessions it is necessary to differentiate patent varices from thrombosed ones. Patent varices change in size with phases of respiration; they appear to have thin walls and indent readily with the tip of the injector. A thrombosed varix has a thick whitish wall and does not indent when probed gently with the injector (needle retracted) but moves away like a cord. Moreover it is difficult to penetrate with the needle and, when finally penetrated, it offers great resistance to injection. After withdrawal of the needle, only a dimple marks the site, sometimes followed by some oozing of the sclerosant but little blood.

Much has been written about the ulcerogenicity of the sclerosants, but most studies are faulted because the accuracy of the injections has not been documented. Accurate intranvenous injection is critical if the objective is to cause intimal damage and avoid ulcerations. To achieve this, aiming passes may be made with the needle retracted, to get a feel for the direction of the injector. A helpful trick for the novice is to put a hairline behind the eyepiece at the focal plane marking the exact position where the injector would emerge from the instrument channel, to be used as a gunsight. The endoscope is simply jockeyed into position, and the target varix lined up with the gunsight. The injector is then moved out of the channel and the needle extended. With a short jab, the varix is entered either right on top or from its side. A little momentum is necessary for penetration and, since the target moves with respiration and transmitted cardiac pulsation, it takes considerable skill to be consistently accurate. However, if the needle is judged to be paravariceal despite the best effort, a trial injection of 0.2 ml is warranted; an immediate swelling confirms the suspicion. The needle may then be withdrawn without causing hemorrhage and another injection attempted. When the needle is truly intravenous, it should be evident in the endoscopic view: The varix is slightly dimpled at the site of entry, no swelling occurs with injection, the resistance to the plunger is not excessive, and needle withdrawal is followed by a small stream of blood. The novice is likely to be concerned on first encountering such bleeding. If the sclerosant has been injected intravenously, such needle puncture bleeding always stops within 30 seconds, and neither tamponade nor reinjection is necessary. The situation is quite different if the varix has been punctured or lacerated without injecting any sclerosant. Brisk bleeding may result but, since the endoscope is already in position, prompt injection of sclerosant distal to the puncture readily corrects the blunder. It is critical to remain calm and to refrain from repeatedly injecting the same area when bleeding appears to be ongoing. It usually takes a little time, perhaps 30 seconds or more (although it may feel like minutes), for the bleeding to stop. Injection should be discontinued if swelling appears, indicating extravasation. Since the varix can always be entered elsewhere, risking ulceration is uncalled for. The needle may be left extended in going from one varix to another, since it assists in aiming and eliminates another set of commands to the assistant, who should only operate the plunger.

There are several methods to jockey the injector to get at a varix on the opposite wall. The most convenient is to use the directional controls to maneuver the tip to line up with the target.

This approach diminishes the acuteness of the angle of entry, a minor disadvantage compared with the convenience. A second method is to rotate the endoscope for 90 to 180 degrees in order to substantially change the position of the instrument channel with respect to the varix. The disadvantage is that the controls are now operated by an unfamiliar hand, unless the endoscopist goes over to the other side of the table. A third way is to insert the injector into the other instrument channel, if a twin-channel instrument is used. With some practice, complete injection of all varices at two levels in a nonbleeding patient takes no more than 10 minutes, and the total blood loss rarely exceeds 50 ml.

If the endoscopist is disciplined to systematically follow a clockwise or counterclockwise pattern, all varices will be injected in sequence. A useful adjunct, however, is addition of dilute methylene blue to the sclerosant, but then it is not so much as to mark the site of injection as to ensure intravariceal injection, since a considerable portion of the variceal column becomes blue when intravariceal injection has been successful.

THE SHEATH TECHNIQUE

The sheath technique is an English method originating with Williams and Dawson,[80] who developed a semiflexible sheath with a side slot near the tip for the target varix to protrude into. The principle is that if a varix is thus fixed in the slot, it is a veritable sitting duck and is therefore hard to miss. The sheath is made of polyurethane measuring 50 cm long with an internal diameter of 2 cm and an external diameter of 2.5 cm. The slot is 3 cm × 0.5 cm and is located 2 cm from the tip. A foreoblique endoscope, the Olympus GIF-K, is recommended, but any end-viewing endoscope will do as well. General anesthesia is advised for the novice, as the large tube can be difficult to slide down the esophagus, but in expert hands local anesthesia and sedation will suffice in many cases. The sheath is mounted over the endo-

scope, which is passed in the usual manner. Endoscopy of the upper GI tract should first be performed before sliding the sheath into position. Slow rotation of the sheath enables a varix to protrude into the window or slot. The target is centered on the endoscopic view and the endoscope anchored within the sheath by flexing the tip and locking the controls. The varix is now injected with 5 percent ethanolamine oleate until it fairly oozes, taking usually 5 ml or so. The sheath is then rotated to compress on the one just treated, until the next varix protrudes into the window and injection is repeated. The first level of injection is done at the gastroesophageal junction but, because of swelling, usually only four injections can be made. If the swelling is severe, rotating the slot may risk lacerating a varix; it can then be advanced into the stomach, rotated, and brought back into place to snare another varix. A second round of injections is next performed 5 cm or so proximally. The sheath is left in place for several minutes at the end of the procedure for more compression.

THE RIGID ENDOSCOPE TECHNIQUE

The technique of rigid endoscopy is discussed in Chapter 1. This is the original technique used by Crafoord and Frenckner[18] in 1939. General anesthetic is required. Terblanche modified a Negus esophagoscope with a slot 0.5 × 4 cm cut near the tip, opposite the beak. The advantages claimed include good suction and a proximal lighting immune to obsuration by blood clots. The injector is the Macbeth needle, a long, thin, hollow steel tube offset at the hub so that the syringe does not get in the endoscopist's way. It is used just like the sheath technique: The endoscope is rotated to allow a varix to protrude, fixing it for injection. Indeed this is a much simpler technique than the sheath method. Many surgeons have used the Jackson esophagoscope without any modification and find such injection uncomplicated. This author prefers a Hopkins rod–lens telescopic attachment if the rigid endoscope is used. Without the telescope, the error of parallax with such a narrow-viewing angle is so great as to render accuracy unattainable, especially when the view is further partially blocked by the injector. A set of accessories including the telescopic attachment, a flexible injector and its grooved guide, or a rigid injector and its carrier is available from Storz, popular in some European centers. The flexible injector is mounted with a 1-cm-long 19-gauge needle. This author finds it useful only for research projects where the variceal pressure has to be measured by manometry. The optics of the Hopkins rod–lens system are excellent, although the angle of view is still not as wide as desirable. The major difficulty with the use of the rigid esophagoscope, in the opinion of this author, is working at the gastro-esophageal junction. The esophagus gradually passes to the left and anteriorly as it approaches the stomach (see Chapter 1). The endoscopist (or rather the headholder) may rotate the patient's head to the right and extend the neck, which helps the endoscope deviate to the left and anteriorly, but determining the exact junction is not as straightforward as with flexible endoscopy. A few patients were referred to this author after previous sclerotherapy by rigid endoscopy. In some patients the injection had been performed much higher than ideal, often at 32 to 34 cm from the incisor. Recurrent bleeding occurred at 40 cm, almost as though no treatment had been given.

CRITIQUE OF TECHNIQUES

It is impossible to be objective in evaluating techniques since, if one is well satisfied with the technique, one does not switch to another just for the sake of making a fair evaluation. Experts at any method produce equally superior results. The disadvantages of rigid endoscopy have been mentioned (see Chapter 1); one objection is that it is more difficult to learn and that perforation is significantly higher even in expert hands. The use of anesthesia is not so bad in

acute hemorrhage, and endotracheal intubation may be required in massive hemorrhage anyway. However, if maintenance injection is also to be done under anesthetic, a number of general anesthetics in short succession may not be so innocuous. With the sheath method, the sheath itself is difficult to put down in the anesthetized patient, let alone when the patient is awake. The most serious drawback, in this author's opinion, is the absolute lack of view: The sheath is an unbelievable handicap to those not used to working with it. It effectively hides puncture site bleeding and does not provide very convincing compression, which is not achievable even with balloons. The sclerotherapist with an average degree of hand–eye coordination finds it easy to inject intravenously when allowed a clear view. The sclerotherapist also finds quickly that puncture site bleeding stops spontaneously without any need for compression. As is well known to surgeons, the simplest technique is always the most elegant, if not the best.

Postinjection Management

Continued hemostasis is monitored by vital signs, serial hematocrits, and bowel movements, but an indwelling nasogastric tube is best avoided. Tachycardia is almost always present when the patient is experiencing postinjection chest pain, which should improve within a few hours. The patient is kept NPO as long as dysphagia remains. In most cases liquids can be started within 6 to 12 hours and soft diet the next day. Analgesics are given for postinjection pain as required. Other measures, such as prevention of encephalopathy, treatment of tense ascites, correction of coagulopathy, and treatment of insipient renal failure are important adjuncts. Fever without demonstrable source is treated symptomatically (see Complications). The use of antibiotics is not predicated on objective data but is based on the arguments that (1) sclerotherapy is not a sterile procedure, (2) transient bacteremia are demonstrable, (3) the patient is often susceptible to infection because of hypovolemia, malnutrition, and chronic liver disease, and (4) it would be disastrous to allow the chemical thrombophlebitis of the varices to become septic. Correction of hypovolemia may be accomplished with transfusion of fresh frozen plasma to simultaneously correct the clotting deficiencies. In a euvolemic patient, however, one must refrain from overzealous correction of clotting deficiencies by this means, as volume expansion may lead to high portal pressure and blowout of the varix.

Timing of Subsequent Sessions: Frequency of Injections

Confusion and empiricism are the order of the day in this area. In centers that experience a high rate of recurrent bleeding after the initial session, frequent injection is instituted in an attempt to improve results. Others are satisfied with fewer injections and claim that complications are thereby kept low. Thus in Cello's study[10] involving Child's C patients with alcoholic cirrhosis, injections were given 1, 4, 7, and 14 days after the first injection. On the other extreme, Reilly et al.[56] reinject every 6 weeks until varices disappear. The Copenhagen Sclerotherapy Group inject every 3 days for three sessions, then every 6 weeks.[36] In the Mayo Clinic it is once every 4 to 6 weeks after the first injection.[31] Common sense may prove a better guide. The goal is to prevent rebleeding on the one hand and to avoid subjecting the esophagus to repeated chemical inflamation before it has a chance to recover from the previous one. We have found that since recurrent bleeding is most common after the first 4 days and that symptoms take at least that many days to clear after the first injection, the second session is scheduled between 4 and 7 days. The third through fifth sessions are done at monthly intervals. Thereafter it is either 3 or 6 months, depending on the size of residual varices. The recurrent bleeding rate after 6 months in our

experience is very low, a finding in good agreement with most series.[26,31,36,56]

Complications

PAIN

Pain is more a symptom than a complication of the therapy. It begins immediately and lasts a few hours. It is a dull, aching, crushing, precordial type of visceral pain, radiating to the back between the scapulae, sometimes to the root of the neck. It is even relieved by nitroglycerin. Marked extravasation is associated with more pain and sustained spasm, but increasing pain and dysphagia and odynophagia are worrisome, as perforation must be suspected (see Perforation).

HEMORRHAGE FROM NEEDLE PUNCTURE

Backbleeding following successful intravariceal injection never causes problems if the sclerotherapist has learned to refrain from taking repeated panic shots at the same site. However, laceration of a varix without actually injecting the sclerosant can be frightening. Fortunately this is readily stopped by injection distal to the laceration. Cannulation of the varix, that is, ramming the sheath of the injector into the vein, is a serious technical error that may result in much bleeding when the injector is withdrawn. Some claim that a square-ended injector prevents this. However, if it is realized that cannulation has occurred, excessive bleeding can usually be avoided if an adequate (but not excessive) amount of sclerosant has been deposited, and the injector is not removed until 20 to 30 seconds have elapsed.

PYREXIA

Low-grade fever develops in 20 percent of our patients, lasting a day or two. Transient bacteremia has been reported following sclerotherapy,[8] although it is not regarded as serious. There is no evidence that pyrexia is related to bacteremia, and neither requires treatment. However, a case can be made to give prophylactic antibiotics to patients with valvular disease undergoing sclerotherapy.

PULMONARY CHANGES

Pleural effusion and basal atelectasis are the most common pulmonary changes, found in 20 percent of patients undergoing emergency sclerotherapy, resolving in a few days. The etiology of pleural effusion is unknown. Possible causes include sympathetic effusion from phlebitis of paraesophageal veins or even pulmonary embolization of droplets of the sclerosant. Pulmonary embolism has only recently been reported in an abstract, but the details are obscure. Considering the large number of injections done in the past 5 years, this must be rare. Symptoms suggestive of adult respiratory distress syndrome (ARDS) have been reported when a large amount of sclerosant has been injected in critically ill patients.

The syndrome of tachycardia, chest pain, dysphagia, pyrexia, and pleural effusion is suggestive of esophageal perforation and mediastinitis. Esophagram is invariably normal but does not negate minor perforation. Indeed, the only sure differentiation is to observe spontaneous improvement within 6 hours. The surgeon familiar with the syndrome of phlebitis often wonders whether this may be the syndrome of phlebitis in the mediastinal veins.

ULCERATIONS

The incidence of this complication varies between 10 and 20 percent in large series. In smaller series, the incidence is much higher, up to 50 percent or more. Even within the large series, the incidence falls as the number of treated patients, and presumably expertise, accumulates. Both accuracy and the amount of sclerosant employed are involved; just looking at the amount used may not reveal the relationships.[60] As accuracy improves, the amount of sclerosant used tends to decrease and further decreases the risk of ulcerations.

It is clinically useful to distinguish two kinds of ulcerations: superficial and deep. Superficial ulcers from necrosis of the submucosa heal readily and have little clinical significance. Epithelialized depression and epithelial tags may remain for months. Deep ulceration, on the other hand, results from necrosis down to the muscle coats and is associated with much more sinister consequences. Recalcitrant bleeding in the form of oozing has been reported from deep ulcers, probably from collaterals in the muscular layers. This should not be treated with further injections, which cause more necrosis as the offending vessel is deep inside the muscle, quite out of reach (Fig. 3-8). The heater probe is a possible solution, although no one has any substantial experience to report as yet. The surer way to prevent exsanguination, when the ulcer has been bleeding continuously, is to ligate the bleeder by open operation. This complication is preventable. Repeated injections at the same spot, a

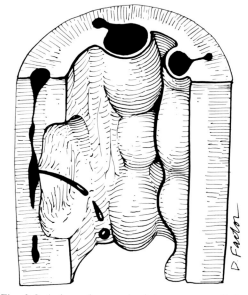

Fig. 3-8 A deep ulcer erodes into a venous collateral in the muscular coat, giving rise to recalcitrant bleeding.

panic move in treating a bleeding site (including bleeding from the needle puncture), must be avoided as this is the usual scenario leading to the development of deep ulcers.

DYSPHAGIA

About 25 percent of patients complain of dysphagia sometime in the course of sclerotherapy. The symptom usually appears 2 to 3 months after the initiation of therapy. The usual complaint is occasional and unpredictable regurgitation of swallowed food, often red meat, or a sensation of food sticking behind the sternum. A small percentage of these patients (about 1 in 5) have actual strictures, a few others may have a persistent ulcer, while most have no apparent cause demonstrable with radiologic or endoscopic evaluation. Symptoms disappear after a few months without any treatment, although this author has empirically treated some patients by passing a 50 Fr. Hurst dilator with remarkable success.

The changes in esophageal motility have been studied by manometry following acute[12] and chronic injections.[39,50,63] Acute changes diagnostic of esophageal spasm occur in 30 percent of patients when tested immediately after injection, although most experienced sclerotherapists recognize sustained contraction after each session. Chronic changes are more variable. One study claimed that the function of the lower esophageal sphincter (LES) is adversely affected and may predispose to reflux,[50] while others reported little long-term change.[39,63] The motility changes may well be the basis of dysphagia in the group with no endoscopic or radiologic signs.

STRICTURES

The incidence is variable, ranging from 4 to 27 percent.[70] The etiology is most likely transmural fibrosis induced by sclerotherapy. While individual response to the sclerosant may vary, it is likely that excessive amount and inaccurate injections may have contributed to a large degree as well. The stricture always occurs at the level corresponding to the recorded site of injection and is associated with pronounced fibrosis of the mucosa with complete disappearance of varices. One may regard this as a sign of overtreatment, but it is undeniably a sign of success. Such strictures are readily dilatable; once dilated to 46 to 50 Fr., there is no recurring need for dilation, unlike peptic strictures (see Chapter 9). There is no risk of causing variceal bleeding in the dilation of such strictures, since there are no varices.

PERFORATION

Most perforations related to sclerotherapy have a delayed onset except for instrumental injuries, which occur more frequently with the use of rigid endoscopes. The difference between deep ulceration, stricture formation, and delayed perforation is one of degree. Full-thickness necrosis gives rise to perforation, while full-thickness inflammation results in fibrosis and stricture. Deep ulceration results from the same process of necrosis as involved in perforation, except that it is more limited in extent.

The full-blown manifestations of mediastinitis take 2 to 3 days to develop. The first clue is that the postinjection chest pain is unusually severe and fails to abate within a few hours, as it usually would. Odynophagia and dysphagia may actually increase, and increased salivation is a worrisome sign. Tachycardia, fever, hiccoughs, and mediastinal air shown on chest radiographs should make the diagnosis obvious. Contrast esophagram may reveal a diverticulum-like localized leak. Conservative treatment with broad-spectrum antibiotics, NPO, and a policy of watchful preparedness for intervention is usually successful (see Chapter 9). Surgical drainage is required for radiologically demonstrated nonlocalized perforation or unchecked mediastinitis. Thoracotomy via the right or left chest (depending on the side of perforation) with T-tube diversion (see Chapter 9) and intercostal drainage and feeding enterostomy is indicated.

Unlike instrumental perforation, primary repair is never feasible however early the intervention.

RECURRENCE OF UPPER GASTROINTESTINAL HEMORRHAGE

The incidence of recurrence of bleeding may be as high as 40 percent within 7 days in some early series, prompting the practice of routine injection a second time within this period. In our early experience, this was shown to come from varices bearing no injection marks, indicating that this is a technical error of omission. It is surmised that increased flow was diverted to the single patent varix when all others were thrombosed. It is also possible that a small varix, thought to be inconsequential and not injected at the first session, may become prominent as a result of the altered flow and eventually bleed. Since we have instituted the routine of injecting a second session within a week, early recurrent bleeding has been greatly reduced. In a survey of the American Society for Gastrointestinal Endoscopy (ASGE) in 1981, this complication ranked second to ulcerations as reported by sclerotherapists around the country.

Bleeding can arise from ulcers secondary to sloughing. Superficial ulcers rarely bleed but when they do, it is from erosion into the nearby varix for which the injection was originally intended. Most troublesome hemorrhage comes from deep ulcers: Here intramuscular collaterals are of high pressure and inaccessible by the needle (see under Ulceration) (Fig. 3-8).

GASTRIC VARICEAL HEMORRHAGE

Most series report that the incidence is not as high as expected on pure theoretical conjecture.[45] However, this early optimism may not bear out, since long-term follow-up data are still scarce. In our experience, oozing from an area of mucosa immediately distal to the gastroesophageal junction, tangential to the view of the conventional endoscope, is the commonest cause of minor bleeding in patients maintained on sclerotherapy within the first 6 months. Often the endoscopist may not find any actively bleeding areas, although there can be no question that the patient has been actively bleeding, unless reverse gastroscopy is routinely performed. Many of these episodes do not require transfusion, as spontaneous cessation is the rule. Many times the patient may report classic malena for a day or two with no other manifestation, with perhaps a hematocrit in the low 30s. Whether or not this is true, gastric variceal hemorrhage or congestion in the mucosa with erosion bleeding is a matter of conjecture.

FAILURE OF SCLEROTHERAPY TO CONTROL BLEEDING

In the rare case in which massive bleeding continues despite sclerotherapy, the endoscopist must be suspicious of gastric variceal hemorrhage (see Contraindications) or of hemorrhage from deep esophageal ulcers and, even more rarely, of multiple points of rupture of esophageal varices with bleeding so rapid that a clear view was not obtainable, sheath or rigid endoscopic method notwithstanding. All these conditions may be temporized with Sengstaken-Blakemore tamponade, but emergency surgical plication of the bleeding points, with some form of expeditious portoazygous disconnection, should be considered. Such operation may be combined with operative sclerotherapy using an ordinary syringe and 25-gauge needle injecting the gastric and esophageal varices at the gastroesophageal junction, exposed via an incision in the anterior gastric wall.[14]

RESULTS

The results of sclerotherapy, now 7 to 8 years after the revival of this technique, may be discussed under the headings of (1) arrest of acute hemorrhage, (2) prevention of recurrent hemorrhage, and (3) prophylactic use to prevent the first episode of variceal rupture.

Treatment of Acute Hemorrhage

Since all upper GI hemorrhages have a propensity to stop spontaneously, the true effect of sclerotherapy is only assessible with randomized trials. Many investigators are convinced of the unethical nature of such trials, and few truly controlled data are available despite the abundance of uncontrolled data. Barsoum et al.[1] compared rigid esophagoscopy intravariceal injections against Sengstaken-Blakemore balloon tamponade in variceal bleeding mainly secondary to schistosomiasis. Sclerotherapy was successful in stopping bleeding in 74 percent of patients compared with a 42 percent success with tamponade, a significant difference. Using the fiberoptic technique, Korula, Larson, and colleagues compared acute injection against standard medical treatment consisting of either balloon tamponade or vasopressin infusion and found injection to be significantly more effective than medical treatment in stopping bleeding.[37,40] Although there was no difference in survival in the short-term life-table analysis,[37] acute sclerotherapy conclusively decreased the number of bleeding episodes, the rebleeding incidence, and the blood transfusion requirement. The latter was true even for Child's C patients and for those actively bleeding at the time of randomization, primarily due to the singular drop in transfusion after sclerotherapy.[40] This is as conclusive objective evidence as can be obtained to support what the early sclerotherapists have known all along: Bleeding simply stops as soon as the bleeder is injected. Paravariceal injection is less effective for acute control. In fact, no significant effect was demonstrated by even the most ardent proponents. Thus, Paquet and Feussner,[54] who use paravariceal injection, found that 95 percent of active bleeding was controlled by injection compared with only 73 percent controlled by tamponade; however, the difference was not statistically significant. Using paravariceal injection also, the Copenhagen Esophageal Varices Sclerotherapy Group found that sclerotherapy was not more effective than medical treatment in stopping acute bleeding, as the transfusion requirement and the duration of hemorrhage were the same, while the complications due to sclerotherapy were considerable.[36] To this author, the studies simply reinforce the surgical concept of control of bleeding in general, a concept not so apparent to nonsurgeons. The most effective termination of bleeding is to control the bleeding vessel itself, not the tissue around it. The fact that paravariceal injection is not effective for acute control but intravariceal simply emphasizes that accuracy of injection makes all the difference.

A large amount of uncontrolled data show that 90 to 95 percent of success can be attained with sclerotherapy, superior to any form of treatment.[35,44,52,56] Surveying both controlled and uncontrolled results, the use of sclerotherapy as the first line of treatment of variceal bleeding is well supported. It confers the same advantages as photo- or thermocoagulation for bleeding ulcer. From the surgeon's point of view, this is the most important use of this modality.

Chronic Sclerotherapy

Most series addressing this aspect start with sclerotherapy for acute bleeding, followed by various regimens of reinjection to aim at long-term control. Again only randomized controlled trials comparing chronic sclerotherapy with conventional medical or surgical treatment give meaningful data. In particular, comparing results from geographically widely separated areas is full of pitfalls, as the underlying liver disease, as well as the severity of disease, can be very different.

The first report of a randomized controlled trial on the efficacy of chronic sclerotherapy was from Terblanche's group at Cape Town.[74] Sclerotherapy, performed with the rigid endoscope under general anesthesia in 37 patients, was compared with a control group of 38 patients that also received sclerotherapy but only for the acute episode, while the treatment group received scheduled sclerotherapy as long as varices were still visible. The design was influenced by the feeling that it would be unethical to give medical treatment to patients acutely bleeding from varices, regarded by some surgeons as no treatment. Despite the bias for the control group, the treatment group had a significantly lower rebleeding rate. Ninety-five percent of the patients in the treated group had eradication of varices, which remained free of varices for a mean of 22 months. Most recurrent bleeding was seen in those patients before the varices were obliterated. In 1983 Terblanche updated the 5-year results, analyzing cumulative recurrent bleeding and survival.[75] Although there were fewer rebleeding episodes and less blood was transfused in the treated group, the difference failed to reach significance level. The two groups had identical survival curves, so no advantage was enjoyed by the treated group in longevity.

The King's College Hospital group published their 5-year results of a randomized trial comparing chronic sclerotherapy against medical treatment.[45] This group used the sheath method, injecting ethanolamine. Of the 56 patients in the sclerotherapy group, 55 percent rebled, compared with 82 percent rebled in the control group (60 patients), a highly significant difference; 74 percent of the recurrent bleeding in the treated group occurred before eradication of varices. A median of four sessions was required for eradication. Very few patients bled after eradication of the varices. Analysis of cumulative survival by the life-table method showed significantly improved 5-year survival compared with control: 18 deaths in the treated group against 32 in the control.

The Copenhagen Esophageal Varices Sclerotherapy Group[36] also looked at the long-term survival of their patients who underwent paravariceal injections. In contrast to the early result, when sclerotherapy was not better than in the conventional medically treated group in stopping acute bleeding, and the mortality at 2 months was 50 percent for both, survival at 40 months was significantly better in the sclerotherapy group (35 percent vs. 22 percent). This improvement was noted after the first 3 months. It was also noted that the group randomized to sclerotherapy had more severe encephalopathy and tense ascites.

The latest prospective randomized controlled study came from the University of Southern California,[37] in which 120 patients were randomized, following the initial variceal bleeding, into sclerotherapy (63 patients) and control (57 patients). Mean follow-up was 12.5 months and 14.9 months for sclerotherapy and control groups, respectively; 21 percent of each group was lost to follow-up. For recurrent bleeding, shunt surgery was offered to both groups. The treated group required significantly fewer transfusions and had longer bleeding free intervals, especially in those with variceal obliteration. Cumulative life-table analysis of survival revealed no difference in survival in the two groups. However, if the patients who underwent shunt operations in both groups were removed from the analysis (6 percent for sclerotherapy and 28 percent for control groups), the injection treatment provided significantly prolonged survival ($P < 0.05$).

From Cairo a randomized trial was reported comparing fiberoptic sclerotherapy using ethanolamine as the sclerosant, against either conventional medical treatment or splenectomy and devascularization procedure (when the patient was considered a good surgical risk) in a population with mostly schistosomiasis liver disease.[84] The groups were comparable in hepatic reserves rating. In the 1-year result analysis, 13 percent of the treated group rebled, compared with 29 percent of those treated with conventional measures, including devascularization. The mortalities were 9 percent and 24 percent, respectively, for the sclerotherapy and non-sclerotherapy groups. The difference in both the rebleeding rate and the mortality was significant, in favor of sclerotherapy.

Surveying the randomized studies published to date, chronic sclerotherapy has been shown to be capable of eradicating varices and preventing rebleeding in those in whom varices had been obliterated.[37,45] Recurrent bleeding, however, is not completely eliminated, and it is not certain whether injected patients live longer. Considering that no greater claim can be made by portacaval shunts, sclerotherapy is clearly an important contribution, at a much reduced cost and without inducing hepatic encephalopathy.

Prophylactic Sclerotherapy

Understandably, the efficacy of this use of sclerotherapy is difficult to prove. The predictors of impending hemorrhage are not absolutely predictive, even though size and vertical length of varices have been said to give some degree of correlation, in addition to certain signs mentioned previously.

Paquet and Oberhammer[52] reported the results of a controlled study of prophylactic paravariceal sclerotherapy. Based on the endoscopic finding of stigmata of impending hemorrhages, 32 patients were randomized to paravariceal injection, while 33 served as controls. During the 3 years of the study, 87 percent of the controls bled, 64 percent of whom died. In the treated group, 9 percent bled and 18 percent died. The difference was highly significant, and the study had to be terminated at 3 years.

Witzel from West Berlin recently published the results of a larger controlled trial of prophylactic intravariceal sclerotherapy that ran for 25 months.[81] Patients were stratified into three categories in each group according to the size of the varices and the Child's classification in hepatic reserve. In the control group, over 25 months, hemorrhage occurred in 35 percent of patients with small varices, 53 percent in those with larger varices, and 83 percent in those with the largest varices. This is compared with only a total of 9 percent of patients who bled in the entire group treated prophylactically. Overall mortality was 23 percent for the treated group and 55 percent for the controls, also a significant difference.

If these preliminary findings suggesting that prophylactic injection successfully prevents variceal hemorrhage are confirmed, this may become the most important role of sclerotherapy, or for that matter, the most promising treatment for esophageal varices. A 12-center Veterans Administration cooperative study examining the efficacy of sclerotherapy, with one of the arms addressing prophylactic use, is currently under way, and this important question may be answered in the next several years.

RESULTS OF β-ADRENERGIC BLOCKADE TREATMENT: PROPRANOLOL

Based on the hemodynamic action of reduction of cardiac output with decreased splanchnic flow, thereby lowering the portal pressure, propranolol has been shown to have a significant effect in prevention of rebleeding in good risk patients. Lebrec[40,41] used a dose (40 to 360 mg/day) that produced a 25 percent reduction of pulse rate in a single-blind trial and obtained convincing data demonstrating reduction in rebleeding incidence (1 in 38 in the propranolol-treated group vs. 16 in 36 in the placebo group) by 1 year and in mortality as well by the second year (11 vs. 56 percent by the Kaplan-Meier method). However, the results were not confirmed by another well-documented single-blind controlled trial from the Royal Free Hospital.[6] In this study, 12 of 26 patients on propranolol rebled, while 11 of 22 in the controls did. Four patients in the propranolol-treated group died (all from hemorrhage) compared with two in the placebo group. The side effects of propranolol are not inconsequential: In addition to lethargy, impotence, and Raynaud's phenomenon, among other problems, hemorrhaging patients may fail to increase their heart rate in response to hypovolemia. Propranolol-induced hepatic encephalopathy has also been reported due to decrease in flow to the critically impaired liver. Abrupt withdrawal may cause dysrhythmia and sudden death or rupture of varices. The efficacy of this treatment is still not proven and must await further data.

RESULTS OF SURGICAL TREATMENT

The significance of these results of sclerotherapy must be examined against the results of surgical treatment. Portacaval (end-to-side)

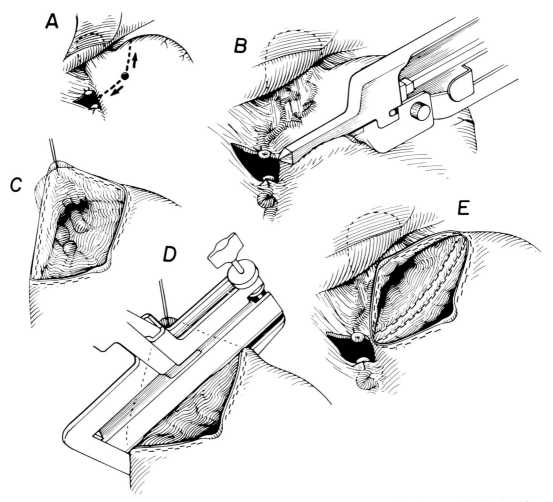

Fig. 3-9 Simplified portoazygous disconnection combined with operative sclerotherapy. (A–C) Anterior gastrostomy to be accomplished by GIA stapler. Gastroesophageal varices well exposed for operative sclerotherapy. (D–E) Posterior gastric wall stapled with two applications of TA 90 stapler. Care was taken to close the staples tightly to reduce their height. Coronary veins divided. Operation to be completed by closing the anterior gastrostomy. (Chung RS, Camara DS: Simplified portoazygous disconnection (Tanner's operation) combined with operative sclerotherapy for bleeding varices. Am J Surg 148:389, 1984.)

shunting performed electively is still the most effective treatment in the prevention of recurrent variceal bleeding.[59] Orloff [51] reviewed the results of the major series, which had an operative mortality of 2 to 23 percent (mostly 12 percent) and a rebleeding rate of 0.5 to 19 percent, with an average of about 3 percent. The encephalopathy reported in Orloff's own series is 21 percent in a 5-year follow-up overall,[51] although many maintain that it is present in all patients to some degree, the severity being determined by many variables. The only prospective study of encephalopathy following portacaval shunt[47] recorded an incidence of 53 percent, compared with 38 percent in controls receiving medical treatment.

The results of the distal splenorenal shunt were recently updated.[30] Reported experience in more than 25 centers showed an overall operative mortality of 9 percent, with shunt patency and bleeding control rates in excess of 90 percent, encephalopathy 0 to 18 percent, and a 5-year survival of 50 to 60 percent. Five prospective randomized trials comparing the selective shunt with various total shunts confirmed the claim of advantage of the selective shunt in survival and incidence of encephalopathy, while operative mortality, recurrent hemorrhage, and shunt occlusion (when recorded) are about the same.[17,24,38,55,60] Nonalcoholic cirrhosis appeared to have a higher 5-year survival with this operation (70 to 80 percent), as compared with alcoholic liver disease (45 percent).[85] Esophageal varices diminish in size in most and disappear in some, but in 20 percent of patients they may remain unchanged.[33] The leukopenia and thrombocytopenia of hypersplenism are ameliorated.[23]

The results of devascularization procedures are more difficult to interpret, if it were only for the numerous variations and permutations. The lack of standardization combined with small numbers makes comparison of published data almost meaningless. Since one purported use is as an emergency measure for poor-risk patients, the method must be expedient. Tanner's portoazygous disconnection, in its various modifications, is one of these. Recurrence of bleeding is about 50 percent.[73] This author has combined coronary vein ligation and stapling of the gastric walls with operative sclerotherapy of the gastric varices for poor-risk patients who failed sclerotherapy[14] (Fig. 3-9A–E). Early recurrent bleeding was encountered at the staple lines on two occasions, and was thought to be due to inappropriate closure height of the staples, which are designed for two thicknesses rather than one. Attention to this detail seems to have corrected the problem. Esophageal transection with the EEA stapler is associated with a mortality of at least 23 percent[65] and much higher (e.g., 83 percent[10]) in Child's C patients who most often require it, and with a rebleeding rate of 1 percent, reflecting selection by high operative mortality. Serious complications (26 percent) of leakage, stenosis, wound infection,

and ascitic leak belie the apparent simplicity of the operation. Elaborate and time-consuming devascularization procedures are more appropriate for treating the variceal bleeder electively and for prevention of encephalopathy. In 1984 Sugiura and Futagawa[72] updated the results of their series of 671 patients undergoing his procedure of esophagogastric devascularization, esophageal transection, splenectomy, selective vagotomy, and pyloroplasty. Operative mortality was 13.3 percent when used as an emergency measure, 3 percent when used electively and 4.9 percent overall. Rebleeding was 1.5 percent. In the United States, the experience of this operation is scattered and not substantial. The results of a recent series[27] from New York University reported an operative mortality of 9.5 percent for elective operations and 53 percent for emergency operation, when an actually lesser procedure (the thoracic Sugiura procedure) was performed. The average operating time is 9.5 hours for the elective complete Sugiura procedure from this series. A variceal bleeding rate of at least 37 percent was recorded in the complete Sugiura procedure and 67 percent in those who had only the thoracic portion.

SCLEROTHERAPY IN AN INTEGRATED APPROACH TO VARICEAL HEMORRHAGE

Reviewing the sea of data of surgical treatment of variceal bleeding, the most unsatisfactory results are for those cases with continued bleeding despite transfusion, vasopressin, and balloon tamponade. The main contribution of sclerotherapy is for this situation, being the most effective and the least risky to the patient of any methods advanced so far. In the author's own practice, emergency sclerotherapy has been employed routinely for treatment of acute variceal bleeding since 1978 by design of the protocol in the early stages of development of the technique. This practice has conserved the resources of the surgical service, favorably affecting the deployment of manpower, operating room time, blood banking, and occupation of

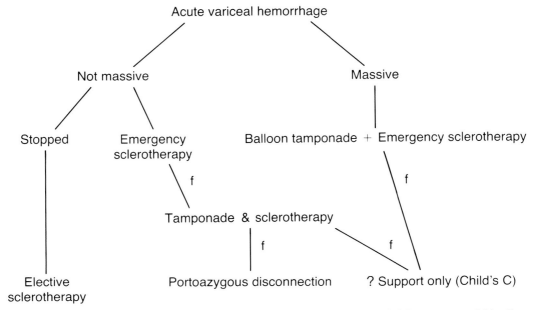

Fig. 3-10 Algorithm for management of acute bleeding esophageal varices. f–failure to control bleeding.

intensive care beds. Chronic sclerotherapy is used as the definitive treatment for patients referred for failure of shunts and other forms of surgical treatment. Particularly after occlusion of a distal splenorenal shunt, the varices are extremely engorged, for which skilled and intensive sclerotherapy is probably the least complicated solution. It is also used in patients with poor hepatic reserve referred from elsewhere as resistant to sclerotherapy or having difficult anatomy. In low-risk patients, the choice of selective shunt or chronic sclerotherapy is less clear; the patient's preference is given some consideration, as it is a choice made largely from subjective reasons. To date this author has not practiced prophylactic sclerotherapy, al-

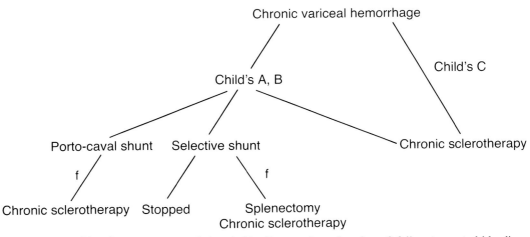

Fig. 3-11 Algorithm for management of chronic bleeding esophageal varices. f–failure to control bleeding.

though this indication is growing stronger with accumulation of data. The algorithm shown in Figure 3-10 highlights the role of sclerotherapy in an integrated program of management of bleeding esophageal varices.

It would appear that sclerotherapy, an old idea that was not adequately tested due to the limitations of technology, has finally established its place in therapeutics through improved instrumentation. It is simple in concept but is actually a demanding technique, requiring much practice to perfect. As in all skill-dependent procedures, early results are really not a fair indication of the potential of the procedure. In interpreting the literature, inordinately bad early results indicate more the desire to publish early rather than the lack of merit of the procedure. As skill accumulates, the results improve. In the 6 to 7 years since reintroduction of this procedure, a great difference is already obvious in the apparent efficacy and incidence of complications. The complication rates published in 1981 and 1982 are no longer representative of today's experience. The most valuable contribution of sclerotherapy may well be in the prevention of variceal hemorrhage when used prophylactically. This, however, has yet to be established by experience.

REFERENCES

1. Barsoum MS, Bolous FI, El-Roody AA, et al: Tamponade and injection sclerotherapy in the management of bleeding esophageal varices. Br J Surg 69:76, 1982
2. Bengmark S, Borjesson B, Hoevels J, et al: Obliteration of esophageal varices by PTP: A follow-up of 43 patients. Ann Surg 190:549, 1979
3. Beppu K, Inokuchi K, Koyanagi N, et al: Prediction of variceal hemorrhage by esophageal endoscopy. Gastrointest Endosc 27:213, 1981
4. Britton RC, Voorhees AB, Price JB: Perfusion of the liver following side-to-side porta-caval shunt surgery. Surgery 62:181, 1967
5. Burchell AR: Hemodynamic evaluation of shunting techniques. p. 83. In Orloff MJ, Stipa S, Zipara V (Eds): Medical and Surgical Problems in Portal Hypertension. Academic Press, New York, 1980
6. Burroughs AK, Jenkins WJ, Sherlock S, et al: Controlled trial of propranolol for the prevention of recurrent variceal hemorrhage in patients with cirrhosis. N Engl J Med 309:1539, 1983
7. Butler H: The veins of the esophagus. Thorax 6:276, 1951
8. Camara DS, Gruber M, Barda CJ, et al: Transient bacteremia following endoscopic injection sclerosis of esophageal varices. Arch Intern Med 143:1350, 1983
9. Camara DS, Caruana JA, Chung RS, et al: Hemodynamic effects of the sclerosant sodium morrhuate in dogs. Surg Gynecol Obstet 161:327, 1985
10. Cello JP, Crass R, Trunkey DD, et al: Endoscopic sclerotherapy versus esophageal transection in Child's class C patients with variceal hemorrhage. Comparision with results of portacaval shunt. Preliminary report. Surgery 91:333, 1982
11. Chung RS, Lewis JW: Injection sclerotherapy for recurrent variceal hemorrhage following failure of operative treatment. Gastroenterology 80:1125, 1981 (abs.)
12. Chung RS, Pohl H: Sclerotherapy: How does it work? Clin Res 30:686A, 1982 (abs.)
13. Chung RS, Lewis JW: Cost of treatment of bleeding esophageal varices. Arch Surg 118:482, 1983
14. Chung RS, Camara DS: Simplified portoazygous disconnection (Tanner's operation) combined with operative sclerotherapy for bleeding varices. Am J Surg 148:389, 1984
15. Clark AW, Westaby D, Silk DBA, et al: Prospective controlled trial of injection sclerotherapy in patients with cirrhosis and recurrent variceal hemorrhage. Lancet 2:552, 1980
16. Cohen LB, Korsten MA, Scherl EJ, et al: Bacteremia after endoscopic injection sclerosis. Gastrointest Endosc 29:198, 1983
17. Conn HO, Resnick RH, Grace ND: Distal splenorenal shunt versus portal-systemic shunt: Current status of a controlled trial. Hepatology 1:151, 1981
18. Crafoord C, Frenckner P: New surgical treatment of varicose veins of the oesophagus. Acta Otolaryngol 27:422, 1939
19. Delaney JP: A method for esophagogastric devascularization. Surg Gynecol Obstet 150:899, 1950
20. Donovan AJ, Covey PC: Early history of the

portacaval shunt in humans. Surg Gynecol Obstet 147:423, 1978

21. Donovan AJ: Surgical treatment of portal hypertension: A historical perspective. World J Surg 8:626, 1984

22. Evans DMD, Jones DB, Cleary BK, et al: Esophageal varices treated by sclerotherapy: A histopathological study. Gut 23:615, 1982

23. Ferrara J, Ellison EC, Martin EW Jr, et al: Correction of hypersplenism following distal splenorenal shunt. Surgery 86:570, 1979

24. Fischer JE, Bower RH, Atamian S, et al: Comparison of distal and proximal splenorenal shunts—A randomized prospective trial. Ann Surg 194:531, 1981

25. Freeman JG, Cobden I, Lishman AH, et al: Controlled trial of terlipressin (glypressin) versus vasopressin in the early treatment of esophageal varices. Lancet 2:66, 1982

26. Goodale RL, Silvis SE, O'Leary JF, et al: Early survival after sclerotherapy for bleeding esophageal varices. Surg Gynecol Obstet 155:523, 1982

27. Gouge TH, Ranson JHC: Esophageal transection and devascularization for bleeding esophageal varices. Am J Surg 151:47, 1986

28. Groszman RJ, Kravetz D, Busch J, et al: Nitroglycerin improves the hemodynamic response to vasopressin in portal hypertension. Hepatology 2:757, 1982

29. Henderson JM, Millikan WJ, Wright-Bacon L, et al: Hemodynamic differences between alcoholic and non-alcoholic cirrhosis following splenorenal shunt—Effect on survival? Ann Surg 198:325, 1983

30. Henderson JM, Millikan WJ, Warren WD: The distal splenorenal shunt: An update. World J Surg 8:722, 1984

31. Hughes RW Jr, Larson DE, Viggiano TR, et al: Endoscopic variceal sclerosis: A one year experience. Gastrointest Endosc 28:62, 1982

32. Hunt BL, Mitros FA, Lewis JW: Histologic changes in esophagus after injection sclerotherapy. Gastrointest Endosc 28:137, 1982 (abs.)

33. Hutson DG, Pereiras R, Zeppa R, et al: The fate of esophageal varices following selective distal splenorenal shunt. Ann Surg 183:496, 1976

34. Jackson FC, Perrin EB, Felix WR: A clinical investigation of the portacaval shunt. V. Survival analysis of the therapeutic operation. Ann Surg 174:672, 1971

35. Johnston GW, Rodgers HW: A review of 15 years experience in the use of sclerotherapy in the control of acute hemorrhage for esophageal varices. Br J Surg 60:797, 1973

36. Kjaergaard J, Fischer A, Miskowiak J, et al: Sclerotherapy of bleeding esophageal varices. Long-term results. Scand J Gastrointest 17:363, 1982

37. Korula J, Balart LA, Radvan G, et al: A prospective randomized controlled trial of chronic esophageal variceal sclerotherapy. Hepatology 5:584, 1985

38. Langer B, Rotstein LE, Stone RM, et al: A prospective randomized trial of the selective distal splenorenal shunt. Surg Gynecol Obstet 150:45, 1980

39. Larson GM, Vandertoll D, Netscher DT, et al: Esophageal motility: Effects of injection sclerotherapy. Surgery 96:703, 1984

40. Larson AW, Cohen H, Zweiban B, et al: Acute esophageal variceal sclerotherapy: Results of a prospective randomized controlled trial. JAMA 255:497, 1986

41. Lebrec D, Poynard T, Hillon P, et al: Propranolol for prevention of recurrent gastrointestinal bleeding in patients with cirrhosis. N Engl J Med 305:1371, 1981

42. Lebrec D, Poynard T, Bernuau J, et al: A randomized controlled study of propranolol for prevention of recurrent gastrointestinal bleeding in patients with cirrhosis: A final report. Hepatology 4:355, 1984

43. Lewis JW, Chung RS, Allison JG: Sclerotherapy of esophageal varices. Arch Surg 115:476, 1980

44. Lewis JW, Chung RS, Allison JG: Injection sclerotherapy for control of acute variceal hemorrhage. Am J Surg 142:592, 1981

45. Macdougall BRD, Westaby D, Theodossi A, et al: Increased long term survival in variceal hemorrhage using injection sclerotherapy. Lancet 1:124, 1983

46. McIndoe AH: Vascular lesions of portal cirrhosis. Arch Pathol Lab Med 5:23, 1928

47. Mutchnick MG, Lerner E, Conn HO: Portalsystemic encephalopathy and portacaval anastomosis: A prospective, controlled investigation. Gastroenterology 66:1005, 1974

48. Nabseth DC, Widrich WC, O'Hara ET, et al: Flow and pressure characteristics of the portal system before and after splenorenal shunts. Surgery 78:739, 1975

49. O'Donnell TF, Gambarowicz RM, Callon AD, et al: The economic impact of acute variceal bleeding: Cost-effectiveness implications for

medical and surgical therapy. Surgery 88:693, 1980

50. Ogle SJ, Kirk CJC, Bailey RJ: Esophageal function in cirrhotic patients undergoing injection sclerotherapy for esophageal varices. Digestion 18:178, 1978

51. Orloff MJ: Elective therapeutic porta-caval shunt. p. 127. In Orloff MJ, Stipa S, Zipara V (eds): Medical and Surgical Problems of Portal Hypertension. Academic Press, New York, 1980

52. Paquet KJ, Oberhammer E: Sclerotherapy of bleeding esophageal varices by means of endoscopy. Endoscopy 10:7, 1978

53. Paquet KJ: Prophylactic endoscopic sclerosing treatment of the esophageal wall in varices—A prospective controlled randomized trial. Endoscopy 13:4, 1982

54. Paquet KJ, Feussner H: Endoscopic sclerosis and esophageal balloon tamponade in acute hemorrhage for esophagogastric varices: A prospective controlled randomized trial. Hepatology 5:580, 1985

55. Reichle FA, Fahmy WF, Golsorkhi M: Prospective comparative clinical trial with distal splenorenal and mesocaval shunts. Am J Surg 137:13, 1979

56. Reilly JJ Jr, Schade RR, Roh MS, et al: Esophageal variceal sclerosis. Surg Gynecol Obstet 155:497, 1982

57. Reiner L: The activity of anionic surface active compounds in producing vascular obliteration. Proc Soc Exp Biol Med 62:49, 1946

58. Resnick RH, Iber FL, Ishihara AM, et al: A controlled study of the therapeutic portacaval shunt. Gastroenterology 67:841, 1974

59. Reynolds TB, Donovan AJ, Mikkelsen WP, et al: Results of a 12 year randomized trial of portacaval shunt in patients with alcoholic liver disease and bleeding varices. Gastroenterology 80:1005, 1981

60. Rikkers LF, Rudman D, Galambos JT, et al: A randomized controlled trial of the distal splenorenal shunt. Ann Surg 188:271, 1978

61. Rikkers LF, Miller FT, Christian P: Effect of portasystemic shunt operations on hepatic portal perfusion. Am J Surg 141:169, 1981

62. Rose JDR, Crane MD, Smith PM: Factors affecting successful endoscopic sclerotherapy for esophageal varices. Gut 24:946, 1983

63. Sauerbruch T, Wirsching R, Leisne B: Esophageal function after sclerotherapy for bleeding varices. Scand J Gastrointest 17:745, 1982

64. Skinner DB: Transthoracic, transgastric interruption of bleeding esophageal varices. Arch Surg 99:447, 1969

65. Smith G: Portal hypertension. p. 513. In Shackelford RT, Zuidema G (eds): Surgery of the Alimentary Tract. Vol. 3. WB Saunders, Philadelphia, 1981

66. Smith PM, Rose JDR: Endoscopy in portal hypertension. p. 63. In Salmon PR (ed): Gastrointestinal Endoscopy. Advances in Diagnosis and Treatment. Williams & Wilkins, Baltimore, 1984

67. Smith-Liang G, Scott J, Long RG, et al: Role of percutaneous transhepatic obliteration of varices in the management of hemorrhage from gastroesophageal varices. Gastroenterology 80: 1031, 1981

68. Stelzner F, Lierse W: Der angiomuskulare dehnverschlub der terminalen speiserohre. Langenbecks Arch Klin Chir 321:35, 1968

69. Sugawa C, Okumura Y, Lucas CE et al: Endoscopic sclerosis of experimental esophageal varices in dogs. Gastrointest Endosc 24:114, 1978

70. Sugiura M, Futagawa S: A new technique for treatment of esophageal varices. J Thorac Cardiovasc Surg 66:677, 1973

71. Sugiura M, Futagawa S: Further evaluation of the Sugiura procedure in the treatment of esophageal varices. Arch Surg 112:1317, 1977

72. Sugiura M, Futagawa S: Esophageal transection with paraesophagogastric devascularization (the Sugiura procedure) in the treatment of esophageal varices. World J Surg 8:673, 1984

73. Tanner NC: The late results of porto-azygos disconnection in the treatment of bleeding from esophageal varices. Ann R Coll Surg Eng 28:153, 1961

74. Terblanche J, Northover JMA, Bornman D, et al: A prospective evaluation of injection sclerotherapy in treatment of acute bleeding from esophageal varices. Surgery 85:239, 1979

75. Terblanche J, Bornman PC, Kahn D, et al: Failure of repeated injection sclerotherapy to improve long term survival after esophageal variceal bleeding: A five year prospective controlled trial. Lancet 2:1328, 1983

76. Walker S, Stiehl A, Raedsch R, et al: Terlipressin in bleeding esophageal varices: A placebo-controlled, double-blind study. Hepatology 6:112, 1986

77. Warren WD, Muller WH: A clarification of some

hemodynamic changes in cirrhosis and their surgical significance. Ann Surg 150:413, 1959

78. Warren WD, Zeppa R, Foman JJ: Selective transplenic decompression of gastroesophageal varices by distal splenorenal shunt. Ann Surg 166:437, 1967

79. Whipple AO: The problem of portal hypertension in relation to hepatosplenopathies. Ann Surg 122:449, 1945

80. Williams KGD, Dawson JL: Fiberoptic injection of esophageal varices. Br Med J 2:766, 1979

81. Witzel L. Wolbergs E, Merki H: Prophylactic endoscopic sclerotherapy of esophageal varices: A prospective controlled study. Lancet 1:773, 1985

82. Wodak E: Osophagusvarizenblutung bei portaler hypertension: Ihre therapie und prophylaxe. Wien Med Wochenschr 110:581, 1960

83. Wodak E: Akute gastrointestinale blutung. Resultate der endoskopischen sklerosierung von osophagusvarizen. Schweiz Med Wochenschr 109:591, 1979

84. Yassin YM, Sherif SM: Randomized controlled trial of injection sclerotherapy for bleeding esophageal varices—an interim report. Br J Surg 70:22, 1983

85. Zeppa R, Hutson DG, Levi JV, et al: Factors influencing survival after distal splenorenal shunt. World J Surg 8:733, 1984

4

Bleeding from Small and Large Intestines: The Role of Diagnostic and Therapeutic Endoscopy

THE ROLE OF ENDOSCOPY: DIAGNOSTIC MORE THAN THERAPEUTIC

Management of the patient who has continued to bleed from a source in the gastrointestinal (GI) tract below the ligament of Treitz is an exercise in logical thinking, since establishing the precise diagnosis often requires sequential and timely deployment of endoscopy, radiology, scintiscanning, or operation in any combination. Resection of a solitary lesion of the intestine harboring a group of bleeding lesions is relatively simple; it is the localization that is difficult. No logical and effective operation can be performed if the bleeding source has not been localized. The role of therapeutic endoscopy is overshadowed by its role in diagnosis, since surgical treatment is often straightforward by comparison.

There are other reasons, mostly anatomic, as to why therapeutic endoscopy does not play as important a role in the colon as it does for the upper GI tract. The colon requires preparation for clear visualization (possibly except for continuous massive bleeding, see below). Lesions are more often multiple and, when discovered in the quiescent period, it is difficult to know which was the source of bleeding. For that matter, the actual source may well be somewhere in the small intestine, mostly out of reach of the conventional endoscope. Technically, too, therapeutic endoscopy via the colonoscope is more difficult: The colon is thin and more easy to perforate, exposure during active bleeding is more problematic, and application of modalities developed for upper GI hemorrhage has only just begun. Consider, for instance, bleeding from diverticulum due to erosion of an arteriole situated at the neck, 1 or 2 mm from the serosa. The potential for perforation is great when treated by any of the current available endoscopic techniques.

MANAGEMENT SCHEME

Even more important than in the case of upper GI bleeding, the history provides vital clues to start the clinician on the right track of investi-

67

gation. No matter how much blood it contains, the presence of brown stools in the movement indicates a site in or distal to the left colon. This observation is based on the fact that bleeding from the right colon and above tends to be mixed with the intestinal contents, which is semiliquid in the right colon, whereas bleeding from the left colon merely coats the solid contents unevenly, so that blood and stool are obviously separated and readily recognized by most patients. Passage of red blood in a patient with hemodynamic instability and active bowel sounds is suggestive of an origin higher than the colon, and sources in the upper GI tract must be considered. Recurrent small amounts of red blood staining the toilet bowl is likely to originate from the anal canal; spurting or dripping after a normal evacuation is characteristic of hemorrhoids, while fissures tend to be accompanied by pain as well. Bleeding from carcinoma in the same area certainly can mimic these common conditions. Orderly investigation follows different routes depending on whether the patient (1) is actively and massively bleeding at the time of presentation; (2) has just bled massively but now has stopped; or (3) has been chronically, slowly, or intermittently bleeding in the past several months. The pace of management is dictated by the severity of bleeding. For chronic blood loss in the stool, colonoscopy can be performed electively, and as much time as necessary can be devoted to preparation. Patients who have just bled massively but who are not actively bleeding and those who are still actively bleeding are two special categories discussed separately in this chapter as they require distinctly different approaches, differing not only in preparation but also in timing and technique.

The Actively Bleeding Patient

Common to the management of all massive GI bleeding, the first priority is to attain cardiovascular stability. If the patient is bleeding so massively per rectum that, despite all efforts to resuscitate, the vital signs cannot be stablized for any duration, emergency angiography should be done with laparotomy to follow should the lesion revealed by angiography be unsuitable for interventional radiology (e.g., aortoduodenal fistula). The role of the endoscopist then is to stand by for operative endoscopy as required by operative findings (see Operative Endoscopy).

If a nasogastric tube had been passed when the patient was actively bleeding and no blood was recovered, only the esophagus and stomach are exonerated but the duodenum is not. Since an expeditious upper GI endoscopy takes just about as long, this is preferred to inserting the tube. In skilled hands the duodenum up to the third portion can be exonerated by direct inspection, especially if the history is compatible with aortoduodenal fistula. The ampulla of Vater can be inspected for fresh blood. Uncommonly gastroesophageal varices can bleed massively and stop as suddenly, manifesting solely as blood passed per rectum. In such case only the stigmata of recent bleeding on one varix gives away the clue, as the fundus and the rest of the upper GI tract may be cleared of blood, accounting for a negative nasogastric aspirate. Therefore, in all such patients the author prefers esophagogastroduodenoscopy as a first step of investigation.

The next quick step that should be taken is rigid sigmoidoscopy. This achieves three objectives. First, it rules out a major bleeding source in the anorectal region, which is quite common with fresh blood per rectum. Second, it permits suction removal of clots in the rectal ampulla, paving the way for the next investigation. Last, but not least important, it shows whether blood is continuously coming from above. If active bleeding is confirmed by this finding, either emergency colonoscopy or angiography should be performed. If no blood appears after waiting for a period of time, while other signs indicate cessation of bleeding, the patient should be given a good bowel preparation (such as whole gut lavage) for a total colonoscopy.

When active bleeding has been confirmed at sigmoidoscopy, the angiography team should be informed, but while the patient is still in the endoscopy suite, a colonoscope should be inserted, aiming to get as much contributory information as circumstances allow. In most centers it will require, depending on the time of day, at least one hour for mobilization of the angiographic team. When the patient is actively passing blood emergency colonoscopy without preparation is surprisingly feasible, a situation to be clearly distinguished from the patient who has just recently bled and has stopped for several hours. Emergency colonoscopy should only be undertaken by the experienced endoscopist. In such hands, not only is visualization possible, but the diagnostic yield has been shown to be quite high in this clinical setting.[19,27] The colon is stimulated to move by large quantities of blood in the lumen similar to the action of whole gut lavage (volumogenic diarrhea), and the lumen is readily negotiable. Once the bleeding has slowed and the bowels have stopped, however, the clots are stagnant and water absorption renders the content viscid, sticky, and very difficult to irrigate. Furthermore, the entire colon and even the terminal ileum can be filled with altered blood by the segmentation movement of the colon even when the actual source of bleeding is in the sigmoid, making the deduction as to the location of bleeding impossible.

In the absence of adequate endoscopic facility, ^{99m}Tc-sulfur colloid scintiscanning is rapid and helpful. Intravenous injection is followed by detection of the extravasated radioactivity in the gut within minutes when there is active bleeding. When the scans are taken sequentially, the localization value is enhanced. For example, radioactivity appearing at the right upper abdomen may be either the duodenum or hepatic flexure. But if the transverse and descending colon is subsequently outlined and appears to be continuous with the initial spot, the bleeding site is identified as the hepatic flexure. Some radiologists insist that a technetium scan be positive before embarking on angiography, which carries a significant risk of inducing renal failure due to toxicity of the contrast medium in a hypovolemic patient. For further discussion the reader is referred to the section on the diagnostic role of arteriography and scintiscanning in this chapter.

Recent Massive Bleeding, but Quiescent at the Moment

The choice of diagnostic modality is much less of a controversy: Upper GI endoscopy and colonoscopy are clearly the procedures of choice. Upper GI series and double-contrast enemas, the traditional investigations, have a much lower yield and interfere with angiography as well as scintiscanning, should the patient bleed massively again.

While an upper endoscopy can be performed at any time, these patients need a good colon preparation before colonoscopy can be carried out. Time and effort should be expanded to do this thoroughly before an examination is feasible. There is always the urgent desire to know what one is dealing with and to do so before the next episode of active bleeding. The best method is to use whole gut lavage as it is gentle, rapid, and well tolerated unless it is contraindicated by renal failure, congestive heart failure, or high-grade obstruction. The sulfate-containing electrolyte solutions (Colyte; Golytely) are administered by nasogastric tube at 2 L/hr for 3 hours or until the effluent is clear. The examination is performed about 1 hour after the last movement. Previous barium studies are helpful as a road map just as in other diagnostic colonoscopy. The goal of colonoscopy is to examine the entire colon, and the technique of colonoscopy does not differ from any other elective situation.

Although there is a much better chance of identifying abnormalities in a well prepared colon, it is not uncommon to find multiple lesions. Furthermore, because the small bowel is not within reach of the examination, one should be cautious in assigning a lesion found as being the probable source of a recent massive bleeding. For example, the presence of a patch of angiodysplasia in the right colon and numerous diverticula in the left make it difficult to know which one had been bleeding, unless some stigmata, such as an adherent clot, are observed. Even so, the findings are all significant as they must be all be considered in planning treatment. Results from large series show that 40 percent will have specific lesions identified on colonoscopy. The most common of these lesions are polyp (15 percent), carcinoma (10 percent), unsuspected inflammatory bowel disease (7 percent), and angiodysplasia (5 percent).[19,27]

Chronic Bleeding

An entirely negative upper gastrointestinal endoscopy is the first prerequisite to proceed further. Rectal examination, followed by protosigmoidoscopy will elucidate all lesions in the anal canal and rectum. No preparation is necessary for sigmoidoscopy; indeed, it is preferable to examine the mucosa in the undisturbed state so that subtle findings are not confused with artifacts. For example, mild degrees of inflammation, presence of pus, or mucus are important clues and some of the material may be available for culture or microscopy.

Colonoscopy is the next logical step. Radiological contrast study is not a good substitute: A positive study may not identify the bleeding lesion while a negative or equivocal study must still be followed by total colonoscopy after adequate preparation. In bleeding unexplained by proctosigmoidoscopy and barium enema, 40 percent of positive yield of a causative lesion from colonoscopy is expected, and one quarter of these are carcinomas.[27] For elective therapeutic endoscopy for lesions so discovered, see elsewhere in this chapter.

Technique of Colonoscopy During Active Bleeding[19,41]

For the actively bleeding patient, no preparation other than clearance of clots from the rectal ampulla is needed, which has been done through the sigmoidoscope. The instrument of choice is a double-channel colonoscope with a built-in water channel, although some prefer a smaller-caliber, more flexible endoscope with a wide channel. This author believes in the use of a colonoscope rather than the 60-cm sigmoidoscope; too often the endoscopist wished he had a colonoscope in his hands when he ran out of length but found the way ahead wide open and stained with fresh blood. If a colonoscope had been used and the going turned out to be difficult above the sigmoid colon, the examination could have been terminated and nothing lost. The procedure is best performed under fluoroscopy. Unlike ordinary diagnostic colonoscopy, fluoroscopy is invaluable for localizing an area discovered to be actively bleeding since the usual landmarks may all be obliterated. This author does not use diazepam for this procedure; but if blood pressure permits, small doses of meperidine are given intravenously as needed.

The endoscopist and assistant must be appropriately capped and gowned since this is an emergency procedure that is far from tidy. Most of the initial difficulty can be readily overcome if it is realized that the rectal ampulla, which collects the blood coming continuously from above, must be cleared first before insertion. Repeated insertion of the rigid sigmoidoscope may be necessary for this purpose, and may actually prove to be time saving. Utilizing the technique of travelling above the blood level, with the lumen insufflated only when needed, the endoscope is advanced without allowing the tip to get tangled with the clots, which are to be dispersed with the water jet when they get in the way, rather than aspirated. Mucosal slide by is avoided if possible, and straightening of the sigmoid loop with repeated withdrawals will facilitate subsequent insertion. At times a solid wall of clot lies ahead, with no clue whatever as to where the lumen lies. The WaterPik irrigation attachment may then be used to ''blast'' away some clots in order to see the mucosa, and to deduce where the center of the lumen is. The initial goal is to insert as far as possible as long as fresh blood is seen. Once a blood-free area is entered, and no bleeding comes down ahead, the endoscope need not be inserted any further as the goal is to localize the area first, the pathology second. Total colonoscopy is not attempted in this setting. If the cecum is reached with blood still coming from above before the angiography suite is ready, the angiography team is advised to concentrate on selective superior mesenteric arteriogram. If insurmountable difficulty is encountered from blood continuously blocking the view despite clearance, for example, in the sigmoid flexure, that by itself is an important piece of information.

Although the findings are noted as insertion is in progress, the real examination begins on withdrawal. To make the most out of the information, the findings are best categorized as follows:[19]

1. Active bleeding site identified
2. Adherent clot in one spot
3. Fresh blood in one segment, nonbloody contents proximally
4. Fresh blood in one segment, unable to get above it; or entire colon has fresh blood in it
5. Failure to localize bleeding

The reliability of the first three categories of findings has been shown to be very high.[19] The chances of obtaining useful information, localizing the bleeding area to a confined segment of the colon is more than 75 percent. Depending on the nature of the lesions identified, therapeutic endoscopy can be performed for categories 1 and 2 (see p. 72). Even the information in category 4 is helpful to the surgeon: A blind subtotal colectomy, for example, will not solve the problem if bleeding is actually coming from the small bowel.

The most common cause of unsatisfactory examination is the presence of stool or altered blood, indicating that the patient is not actively bleeding, or that the bleeding is so slow that the cathartic effect is not observed. The information is still of some value, as now time can be taken to prepare the patient who is to be treated as a recent massive bleeder but quiescent at the moment.

THERAPEUTIC COLONOSCOPY

Indications

If, in the course of emergency colonoscopy for bleeding, a discrete source is identified, it would be rare indeed for the endoscopist not to wish to be able to do something to stop the bleeding. The broad indications are similar to therapeutic endoscopy for upper GI bleeding. The first indication is when an open operation is to be avoided if at all possible, and other nonoperative methods (e.g., interventional radiology) are not available or cannot be applied. The second is that the lesions should be accessible to the endoscope and are amenable to being treated by the available modalities, such as photocoagulation. The third requirement is that the lesions must have been shown to be the source of bleeding, or at least clinically appear to be the presumptive source, or that recurrent bleeding has been demonstrated or is highly likely in the future. The major consideration governing safety is the thickness of the gut wall in the area to be treated. Since the colonic wall is thin, the therapeutic margin is small. Even so, clinical perforation is not necessarily as high as suggested by acute experimental studies, since the processes of sealing and healing may modify the pathologic response. The lesions amenable to therapeutic endoscopy include angiodysplasia and related lesions, polyps, bleeding from the stalk after a polypectomy, idiopathic ulcers, and sometimes discrete bleeding from a necrotic tumor. Lesions not suitable for therapeutic endoscopy include diverticulosis and most multiple acute bleeding ulcers in ulcerative colitis or Crohn's disease. When the lesions are concentrated over a segment of the intestine, operation is indicated rather than endoscopic methods. While bleeding may be helped temporarily by therapeutic endoscopy in ischemic colitis, inflammatory bowel disease and radiation colitis, there are no data in the literature to support its use, and in theory at least, endoscopic therapy may be meddlesome if surgery is unavoidable.

Technique of Endoscopic Control of Colonic Bleeding

All the therapeutic modalities described for upper GI bleeding may be applied for colonic and small intestinal bleeding. Because of the difference in anatomy and difficulty of exposure, there is considerably less experience in the use of these modalities in treating colonic bleeding. For detailed descriptions of the individual techniques the reader is referred to Chapter 2. Some lesions are more suited to one technique than others. The following are the more common entities.

BLEEDING STALK FROM A RECENT POLYPECTOMY

The history is quite typical and the diagnosis is usually without doubt. The patient is often bleeding actively at presentation and is suitable for emergency colonoscopy by the technique described above. The endoscope is passed to the location of the polypectomy and the diagnosis confirmed. A spurting central arteriole can be seen at the transected stalk, and is best strangulated by the polypectomy snare. Coagulation current is applied to the stump until it turns white. There is some risk of injury to the colonic wall if overdone. An acceptable alternative is to allow strangulation for 15 minutes without coagulation, followed by touching the center of the stump with the monopolar probe after the snare has been removed. When the stump is too short and snaring is unsuccessful, other modalities must be used. A monopolar electrocoagulation probe is probably more risky of perforation than other means, but can be used successfully with skill. An insulated coagulating forceps (serrated grasping forceps modified for electrocautery) will sometimes work well, if the arteriole is grasped while the current is passed, but the stalk is usually too thick for the forceps to encompass, and the arteriole is usually retracted rather than protruded. Argon laser photocoagulation is probably ideal for a stubby stump.

BLEEDING POLYPS

These are also removed by snares (see Chapter 8). Blood accumulation may make exposure of the polyp difficult, but if the endoscope is advanced to just beyond the bleeding point and the loop opened under direct vision in a clear area, the snare can be dragged over the clot and polyp by withdrawing the endoscope slowly. The snare is closed with the tip of the catheter at the base of the stalk. Bleeding stops instantly with strangulation of the polyp and the view can be further improved with air insufflation. Polypecotmy is then performed in the usual manner.

SMALL ANGIOMATOUS LESIONS (ANGIODYSPLASIA, ARTERIOVENOUS MALFORMATIONS)

These lesions can be coagulated with the insulated coagulating biopsy forceps using the technique of hot biopsy. Even large patches can be dealt with by patiently taking small bites, that is, performing as many as 15 to 30 hot biopsies over a wide area. Many endoscopists dispense with biopsy, fearing provocation of hemorrhage, and rely on the characteristic gross appearance. The tissue taken with the hot biopsy technique is quite readable by the usual histologic examination. The angiodysplasia lesions are flat, bright red, with characteristic foot processes of extension. Sometimes fingerlike projections may be seen radiating from a central spot. It may appear as a single lesion, but often multiple lesions are encountered over a distance of 10 cm or more. The surface is glistening like normal mucosa. Whitish flecks near the center of the lesion, not removable with irrigation, represent erosions. Angiodysplasias are friable and bleed easily and vigorously upon contact, clearly distinguishing them from suction artifacts. The most frequent location is in the cecum opposite the ileocecal valve, but they are also commonly found in the right colon and less commonly in the terminal ileum. They vary from 2 to 3 mm to 2 to 3 cm in diameter.

Using the coagulating forceps, however, hot biopsy can be obtained with the first bite, followed by systematic destruction of the angiodysplasic lesion with a low setting of coagulating current. A medium sized bite is first obtained at the periphery of the largest lesion. With a tenting action (Fig. 4-1) to elevate it slightly above the level of the rest of the mucosa, current is applied with 1- to 2- second bursts until bubbling and whitening is seen at the tip of the forceps. The forceps is withdrawn and the tissue held inside the cups is removed for pathologic examination. Thereafter the process is repeated. Bleeding areas resulting from these bites may be further coagulated with the forceps, or a ball-tipped monopolar probe with water irrigation via a central lumen as described in Chapter 2.

Simple monopolar electrocoagulation with or without liquid instillation via the central lumen of the probe may be applicable to small lesions

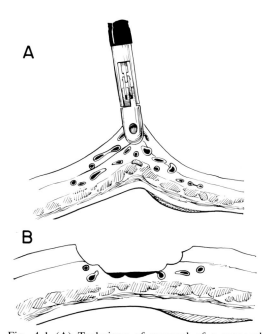

Fig. 4-1 (A) Technique of removal of a mucosal angiodysplastic lesion by piecemeal hot biopsies. (B) If the lesion extends into the muscularis and beyond, complete removal cannot be achieved by endoscopic means. This is the postulated mechanism of recurrent hemorrhage.

(less than 1 cm^2). The heater probe appears to have a good margin of safety in this situation provided distention is avoided. For a large lesion, one may coagulate from the periphery towards the center or vice versa. There is no published experience to indicate which is more preferable. The technique of using the heater probe is described in Chapter 2.

Argon laser photocoagulation is another useful modality for ablation of angiodysplasia lesions. The penetration is relatively defined and controllable (1 mm), the energy is specifically absorbed by the blood-carrying vessels, and it is a noncontact method quite easy to use. Many reports have substantiated its efficacy and safety,[6,22,26] provided care is exercised to avoid distention. The cecal wall is 1 to 2 mm thick in the normal condition, except in the tenias, where it may be 3 mm. This thickness will be further decreased with the coaxial CO_2 flow from the laser waveguide unless a very low flow rate is used and with adequate venting. With a power setting of 6 to 8 watts, a treatment distance of 2 cm (spot size 3 mm), using 1- to 5- second pulses, the periphery of the lesion is hit directly until it turns white. The laser is next moved to an adjacent peripheral spot and so on to cover the outer circumference of the lesion. After this the beam is moved more centrally until the entire lesion has been photocoagulated. Endoscopy should be repeated in 2 to 3 days to evaluate the completeness of the treatment, but also to treat missed lesions. Deep extensions are common and may be photocoagulated if small vessels are seen at the base of the previously treated areas. Extreme care must be exercised if repeat coagulation is undertaken as the risk of perforation is increased.

The Nd:YAG laser has also been used in Europe for bleeding lesions in the colon, such as angiodysplasias. There is inadequate experience to guide its routine use for colonic angiodysplasias. In view of its depth of penetration and in view of the need to use the effect of the scatter to coagulate the vessels, this modality is not easy to use for large lesions.

Sugawa has obtained good results by injection of 0.2 ml of 98 percent alcohol directly into the lesions (Chapter 2). Blanching marks the injected portion of the angiodysplasic lesion. A total of 0.8 ml may be used over the largest lesion. No perforations have occurred.

Failure of therapeutic endoscopy to eradicate the lesions is an indication for surgical resection, provided there is a reasonable clinical certainty that the lesions are responsible for the ongoing chronic blood loss.

BLEEDING ULCERS

A solitary ulcer of the cecum or the sigmoid colon may be the source of bleeding. Unlike peptic ulcer disease, in which major bleeding often comes from a discrete vessel exposed in the base of the ulcer, bleeding from solitary ulcers in the colon tends to come from the edge of the mucosa. In this author's experience, touching the ulcer edge with electrocautery is effective. The ulcer may have been enlarged thereby, but presumably healing is rapid if the predisposing conditions are treated. This includes uremia, sepsis, shock, congestive failure, and immunosuppression. Diffuse bleeding from pseudomembranous colitis is treated specifically with vancomycin and supportive treatment rather than any meddlesome topical modalities, which only worsen the lesions.

VARICES (INTESTINAL AND STOMAL) AND HEMORRHOIDS

Varices are demostrable at colonoscopy, usually in the sigmoid, in the cirrhotic but rarely are they large or the source of persistent bleeding. Duodenal varices are reported too, and have shown to be a rare cause of bleeding.[42]

Stomal varices are not uncommon, and are usually found around a colostomy after abdominal perineal resection for rectal cancer performed at least 1 to 2 years previously. This is often a source of troublesome recurrent bleeding, subjecting the patient to considerable risks of exsanguination. Similar varices are found around an ileostomy.[1] The first sign is blood filling the colostomy bag, without any other symptoms. Endoscopy through the stoma should

be considered if blood is evenly mixed in the contents of the bag, which suggests that the bleeding source is higher than the stoma. Colostomy revision is followed by recurrent formation of varices. Sclerotherapy however, is very feasible and should be considered as the alternative treatment, particularly if operation is hazardous. New varices may form, but these can be treated the same way.

Figure 4-2 shows the appearance of varices around a colostomy stoma. They resemble the roots of a tree coming close to the soil surface. The author has had good success by injecting them on the mucosal aspect with a 25-gauge needle mounted on a 2-ml syringe, injecting 0.5 to 1 ml of 1 percent sodium tetradecyl sulfate solution (Sotradecol) per varix. After verifying that the needle is intravenous by aspirating blood freely, the solution is injected into the varix followed by application of pressure for several minutes on the varix itself. There should be no swelling if there has been no extravasation. The same result can be attained by injecting from the cutaneous aspect, but this is painful and may result in small ulcerations.

Prominent hemorrhoids, even when they have bled repeatedly, should not be treated by sclerotherapy. This author has been referred cases in which the hemorrhoids have been mistakenly injected by endoscopists who have treated them as esophageal varices. All developed necrosis,

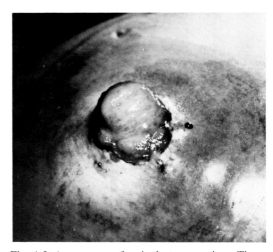

Fig. 4-2 Appearance of pericolostomy varices. Three rootlike varices are visible; small bleeding points mark the cutaneous punctures site of sclerotherapy.

infection, edema, pain, and recurrent bleeding. The proper injection treatment of hemorrhoids depends on the stimulation of perivenous fibrosis to prevent prolapse by injection into the submucosa above the dentate line, and not on thrombosis of the hemorrhoids. For patients with portal hypertension and troublesome bleeding hemorrhoids, this author recommends hemorrhoidectomy as it is still the best treatment, when performed skillfully, for the severe and complicated lesion.

LEIOMYOMA

A leiomyoma within the reach of the endoscope can be coagulated by any of the modalities available: The bleeding point is in a thick portion of the tumor, usually at the bottom of a crater and perforation is thus less likely. Elective surgery should be undertaken when the patient has recovered from the bleeding episode as it is difficult to differentiate a benign from a malignant lesion.

SUTURELINE BLEEDING

Even though this may theoretically occur following colonic anastomoses, it is much rarer than following gastric anastomoses; and then it is usually foreshadowed by other complications such as abscess, leakage and peritonitis. Therapeutic endoscopy has no recognized role in the treatment of this complication, which should be dealt with by reoperation.

Complications

In addition to complications due to diagnostic colonoscopy, the therapeutic procedures carry certain specific risks.

PERFORATION

Excessive air distention with marked thinning of the bowel wall predisposes to full-thickness injury with any modality of therapeutic endos-

copy. Overinsufflation usually results from attempts to obtain exposure. It is important to check the function of the gas vent when the laser is used prior to shooting, and suction to reduce the colonic lumen should always be used before using the heater probe or electrocoagulation.

Other mechanisms of perforations are due to colonoscopy itself. Serosal splitting that extends to a full-thickness tear can result from the stretching force imparted to the colon by the bend of the endoscope. Perforation of a diverticulum by the tip of the endoscope is a well-recognized hazard.

The typical symptom is sudden onset of sharp abdominal pain, well localized to the site of suspected perforation during or shortly after the procedure. Shoulder pain follows shortly, accompanied by signs of peritonitis. Pneumoperitoneum is demonstrable on the chest radiograph. Urgent operation is mandatory to reduce the severity of fecal peritonitis. Primary repair is feasible if there is minimal fecal loading in the colon and if the bowel has been well prepared. Exteriorization of the area of injury in the form of diversion colostomy is the safest procedure if the peritonitis is marked, if there has been delay in diagnosis, or if the colon is loaded with feces.

EXPLOSION ASSOCIATED WITH ELECTROCAUTERY

This has been shown to be totally preventable if the bowel is well prepared, and if mannitol-containing fluid is avoided in the preparation (see Chapter 8). Prior to using electrocautery, the colonoscopist should insufflate with CO_2 if the lesion is in a poorly prepared colon.

RECURRENT BLEEDING

Following treatment of angiodysplasia lesions, a percentage of patients may develop recurrent bleeding at the site of coagulation. The postulated mechanism is shown in Figure 4-1. If the vascular abnormality extends deep into the muscularis, it may not be possible to remove or coagulate all feeding vessels of the lesion. Hemorrhage results from lysis of the clots in the vessels. Repeat coagulation may be successful, but is hazardous of perforation. This complication should be regarded as a failure of therapeutic endoscopy and surgical treatment is indicated.

PROVOCATION OF MASSIVE BLEEDING

This is likely to follow efforts at piecemeal removal of a hemangioma that consists of a mass of vessels extending deep into the submucosa, or even through to the serosa. Protruding vascular malformation should not be treated with therapeutic endoscopy. Less suspicious lesions must be approached with extreme care: The Argon laser or the heater probe is preferred to piecemeal removal with multiple hot biopsies.

SPLENIC INJURY

When the colonoscope puts the splenic flexure on a stretch the attachment to the splenic capsule may be torn, resulting in intraabdominal hemorrhage. The first symptom is sharp pain, at first at the left upper quadrant, but quickly spreads to the entire abdomen. Left shoulder pain, shortness of breath, and collapse may follow. Abdominal tap confirms hemoperitoneum. Immediate laparotomy is indicated.

INTRAABDOMINAL HEMORRHAGE

By a mechanism similar to the causing splenic injury, internal hemorrhage may arise as a result of minor lacerations of the liver capsule, mesenteric tears, or tears of adhesions. Persistent abdominal pain, ileus, tenderness of the abdomen, and a falling hematocrit constitute the characteristic syndrome. Operative treatment is usually not necessary if hemodynamic stability is maintained, as the symptoms usually improve with watchful conservative treatment.

ILEUS

Overdistention may be followed by prolonged ileus of several days' duration. Some surgeons have observed serosal tears as a result of excessive distention in these patients when operated on for other reasons.

Results

There are no randomized trials specifically addressing the efficacy of therapeutic colonoscopy for actively bleeding lesions. It is not known, for example, how often the endoscopist fails to visualize the lesion and therefore is unable to do anything about it. Jensen and Bown[27] reported 70 percent success in identifying bleeding lesions in 40 patients who had successful emergency colonoscopy; 35 percent of these were telangiectasia or angiodysplasia and all responded to argon treatment, without subsequent rebleeding or complications.

A few studies specifically dealt with elective treatment of angiodysplasia and related lesions in the colon, using the transfusion requirement before and after treatment as a measure of efficacy. Howard, Buchanan and Hunt[23] reported 20 good results out of an experience of 23. Jensen and Bown[27] reported reduction in the frequency of bleeding, emergency admissions, total transfusions, and improvement in the hematocrit after treatment with argon laser. Others[7,45,46] have made similar quantification of the efficacy of the argon laser.

THE ROLE OF ARTERIOGRAPHY AND SCINTISCANNING

Arteriography

Since the first application of angiography for the diagnosis in 1963,[36] this diagnostic tool has become so important that most centers provide continuous coverage for this service. Extravasation of the contrast agent into gut lumen is demonstrable with arterial bleeding at a rate exceeding 0.5 ml/min. Similar extravasation is observable with venous bleeding at and above this rate. An exception is esophageal variceal bleeding, which is rarely visualized as extravasation, possibly due to rapid transport into the stomach. Selective arteriography will demonstrate major bleeding, such as bleeding duodenal or gastric ulcers, but superselective injection is needed to demonstrate diffuse capillary sources and even slower rates of bleeding. Even if the bleeding point is too small to be seen, the collected contrast in the lumen of the gut seen in serial films will also help localize the bleeding site. When a small stream of contrast has collected between the mucosal folds, it may take on the appearance of an anomalous vessel, sometimes called a pseudovein.[39]

In those patients not actively bleeding, abnormal vessels provide indirect evidence of the bleeding source. Angiodysplasias (arteriovenous malformations, vascular ectasias, telangiectasias) are demonstrated as a slight distal dilation of the feeding artery, a vascular tuft or blush, and rapid emptying into an early draining vein, visualized during the late arterial phase. The discovery of these lesions does not provide incontestable evidence that they were responsible for the episodes of bleeding; nevertheless, the information has proved extremely useful in the management of chronic bleeding.

Angiography was the only means of localizing the source of acute GI bleeding before the widespread use of endoscopy, but now the diagnostic role of angiography has been largely superseded by endoscopy except for three areas where angiography remains the preferred method. These are hemobilia, bleeding into the pancreatic duct, and bleeding in the small intestine. The capability to treat many specific bleeding sites by selective embolization has widened the indications for angiography for acute GI hemorrhage. The role and timing of angiography are discussed in the management scheme in the section, The Actively Bleeding Patient.

The angiographic catheter is inserted into a major limb artery (usually the femorals) by the Seldinger technique and advanced into the visceral arteries: the celiac, superior, or inferior mesenteric. Selective study is by injection of any one of these major arteries, the usual initial study for bleeding. Superselective injections, by cannulation of the secondary or even tertiary branches in the celiac and superior mesenteric, are performed as required, especially when embolization is contemplated. Rarely is it necessary to perform superselective angiography on the inferior mesenteric. Further yield may be possible with supplemental techniques such as magnification or subtraction angiography when indicated. The contrast injection is performed by a mechanized injector at a rate adjusted for the size of the vessel, and rapid sequential films are typically taken at two per second for the first 3 seconds, followed by one every 2 seconds for 24 seconds.

The exact anatomical localization of the segment of small bowel bearing the bleeding lesion, for example, a patch of angiodysplasia, may be difficult. If surgery is to be performed, the angiographer may superselectively catheterize the feeding artery and inject 1 ml of methylene blue to stain the bowel prior to laparotomy.

Scintiscanning

Scintiscanning by injection of ^{99m}Tc-sulfur colloid is a noninvasive yet rapid method for localization of the bleeding source in the presence of brisk bleeding. The radiopharmaceutical is rapidly cleared from the circulation by the reticuloendothelial system, with a circulatory half-life of 2 minutes. After an IV dose of 5 to 10 mCi, sequential anterior images are obtained with the scintillation camera at 5-minute intervals for 30 mintues. When blood is lost into the gastrointestinal tract, radioactivity collects in the lumen and is recognizable as an increased area of radioactivity distinct from the liver, spleen, and bone marrow. Serial films following the progress of the collection helps to identify the region of the gut where bleeding originated. The method is rapid; extravasation may be recognizable 15 minutes after IV injection and is free of the hazards of angiography.

If ^{99m}Tc-labeled heat-treated red cells are

used instead of the sulfur colloid, the activity remains in the circulation for a longer period of time: Intermittent bleeding may then be identifiable by repeat scanning within a 24-hour period whenever renewed bleeding is clinically evident. A dose of 15 to 30 mCi is given, and scanning is repeated at various intervals. Vascular structure will be seen in the earlier images, including major blood vessels, kidneys, liver, and spleen. Later, most of the activity is sequestered in the spleen due to heat pretreatment of the red cells. Any activity that is distinct from these structures represents hemorrhage. Slow or intermittent bleeding, at a rate as low as 10 to 20 ml/hr, may be detectable by this means. If scanning has been infrequent, however, intermittent blood loss may be localized more distally than the true origin. The sigmoid colon, for example, may show activity when the actual source may be much higher up in the gut. When the patient is actively bleeding, the ^{99m}Tc-sulfur colloid should be used instead, as the tagged red cells light up the vascular structures which tend to interfere with the discrete imaging of the bleeder.

OTHER NONOPERATIVE TREATMENT

Supportive Treatment

Correction of hypovolemia, coagulation abnormalities, central and peripheral circulatory failure, and renal failure must be attended to as the investigation of bleeding proceeds. Patients with a history of aspirin use and demonstrating prolongation of bleeding time must be treated with platelet transfusion. In this author's experience, emergent surgery has been averted more than once by this expediency.

Vasopressin

Vasopressin infusion, originally used for esophageal variceal hemorrhage given by the IV route, is effective in constriction of visceral arteries when delivered selectively to the bleeding artery. In patients with hypovolemia, hypoperfusion, and generalized vasoconstriction, the agent is unlikely to be of use. It is definitely contraindicated in the presence of coronary arterial disease, previous myocardial infarction, and unstable cardiac dysrhythmias. An analogue of vasopressin, triglycyl lysine vasopressin (terlipressin), has more sustained action on contraction of the smooth muscle without affecting the heart, and has been successfully used for variceal bleeding.[17] It is likely to be useful for other gastrointestinal bleeding where the volume status has been adequately maintained but as yet there is no data in the literature to support this use.

Interventional Radiology

One radiologic aid is selective intraarterial infusion of vasopression (vasoconstrictive technique). The splenic artery is said to be most responsive, but the gastroduodenal, superior, and inferior mesenteric also respond well. When diagnosis of a bleeding artery is confirmed by selective angiography, the intraarterial catheter is utilized for intraarterial vasopressin infusion, which is given at the rate of 0.2 units/min for 20 minutes, followed by repeat angiogram. For colonic bleeding in the territory of the inferior mesenteric artery, it is not necessary to further selectively catheterize the branch. If cessation of bleeding is confirmed, the treatment can be continued for 24 hours and then weaned off. If this dose is unsuccessful in stopping bleeding, the infusion can be increased to 0.4 units/min and the result checked by another angiogram after 20 minutes. For continued catheter care the patient must be nursed in an intensive care unit with a staff that is knowledgeable and experienced in the care of indwelling arterial catheters. Failure to control bleeding at 0.4 units/min indicates failure of this method of treatment, and an alternative must be sought.

Superficial mucosal lesions such as erosive gastritis respond well to superselective infusion of vasopressin into the left gastric artery, a success rate of 80 to 90 percent is expected. Bleeding from larger vessels, such as from peptic ulcer disease, responds less well to this therapy. Similarly, in lower GI bleeding such as diverticulosis and angiodysplasias, selective infusion of vasopressin into the inferior mesenteric artery will control 90 percent of left colonic bleeding, and superselective infusion into the ileocolic, right, or middle colic will control right colonic bleeding in the vast majority of cases.[3]

Selective embolization (a vaso-occlusive technique) is an alternative method, and is preferred by many angiographers in many situations. Its success depends on accurate localization of the bleeding branch and direct superselective catheterization of this branch. In the upper GI tract, infarction is unlikely to result from successful embolization because of the rich collaterals; by the same token, embolization of one feeding artery, such as one end of the gastroduodenal artery in bleeding duodenal ulcer, may not be sufficient to arrest bleeding; occlusion of the bleeding branch itself, a tertiary or even smaller branch, is required—quite a technical challenge. Unlike the vasoconstrictive technique, the therapy cannot be halted or reversed if signs and symptoms of ischemia develop; inadvertent occlusion of other major vessels is a definite risk if there is reflux or alteration of flow pattern due to catheterization.

Autologous blood clots, gelfoam, polyvinyl alcohol, steel coils, and isobutyl cyanoacrylate (a glue) are the commonly used agents for embolization. Clot lysis is rapid and so is not often used today, but gelfoam is the favorite of many radiologists as it is easy to use and lasts sufficiently long to be clinically useful. Recanalization after gelfoam embolization occurs in 7 to 20 days, but permanent occlusion results from the use of polyvinyl alcohol or isobutyl cyanoacrylate and steel coils. A recent development is the catheter with detachable balloons, a technique that allows very controllable embolization of smaller vessels, as a misplaced balloon can be retrieved and repositioned.

In lower GI hemorrhage, embolization is not indicated except as a last resort, as the risks of bowel infarction are great.[5]

Complications of angiography are not incon-

sequential. In skilled hands thrombotic complications at the site of arterial puncture may be expected to occur 1 in 1,000.[22] Other complications include hematoma, vascular spasm, pseudoaneurysm, and arteriovenous fistula, for a total incidence of less than 1 percent, and should be avoidable with adequate attention to technical details and post procedure care. Subintimal injection of visceral arteries are usually recognized early and rarely lead to significant clinical symptoms.

In hypovolemic patients, diabetics, and those with decreased renal function, there is a significant incidence of renal toxicity due to the use of excess amount of contrast media, manifesting as transient but marked increase of creatinine and BUN.[38] This complication has received less attention in the radiologic literature, partly because the patient is cared for after the procedure in another service. Even with modern contrast agents and vigorous intravenous hydration, 11.3 percent of a series of 400 consecutive patients undergoing aortography developed acute renal dysfunction, with a 1.5 percent incidence of renal dialysis.[37] In those patients with preexisting abnormal renal function, 42 percent developed such dysfunction, with 8.3 percent of them requiring dialysis. This factor should be taken into consideration prior to angiography, and volume restoration should be optimal in all patients before this procedure is undertaken.

OPERATIVE MANAGEMENT OF BLEEDING FROM OBSCURE SITES

Despite the most rigorous and logical sequential deployment of endoscopy, scintiscanning, and angiography, an occasional patient may still come to emergency surgery because of continued bleeding and without a definite diagnosis of the site of bleeding.

The surgical management of such a situation actually begins with a careful review of the diagnostic data accumulated so far with emphasis on the known negatives. Has the upper GI tract been exonerated completely? Has the esophagus, especially esophageal varices, been absolutely ruled out? Are the patient's clotting parameters in order? The surgeon must only undertake exploration of the abdomen when he is absolutely sure that the bleeding source is not in the extraabdominal portion of the alimentary tract.

Operative Strategy

The operation is begun with a midline incision centered at the umbilicus, ready to be extended in either direction as indicated. A large-bore nasogastric tube should be in place. The stomach, duodenum, pancreas, and liver should be thoroughly examined, particularly for evidence of less commonly encountered causes of bleeding, including aortoduodenal fistula, pseudocysts, and abnormalities of the liver. If blood is aspirated from the nasogastric tube, but no external evidence of gastroduodenal disease exists, an anterior gastrostomy is made at the antrum. The clots are evacuated, the pylorus packed, and the interior of the stomach inspected and palpated. A bleeding artery is frequently palpable as a small "lead shot" that stands out from the normal soft mucosa. If blood appears to come from the cardia, the incision is extended in order to inspect the fundus and the lower esophagus. If no active bleeding is found in the stomach, the likely source is the duodenum; the pylorus pack is removed and the first, and sometimes the second, portion of the duodenum can be palpated. If negative, operative duodenoscopy can be performed without risking a duodenostomy. Inspection is quite feasible with the choledochoscope (either rigid or flexible, preferably the flexible), in the author's experience. The endoscope is inserted through a pack in the pylorus, and a bowel clamp is placed at the jejunum just after the ligament of Treitz. The entire duodenum is filled with saline from the infusion port of the choledochoscope. The first and second portions of the duodenum are clearly and easily inspected, including the ampulla. Blood streaming into the saline-filled lumen is much easier to recognize than oozing into the empty lumen. The more distal duode-num cannot be inspected with the rigid choledochoscope, but complete duodenoscopy can be accomplished with the fiberoptic choledochoscope.

If no blood is aspirated from the nasogastric tube, bleeding is distal to the pylorus. Inspection of the small intestine loops should reveal dark fluid in the lumen. Blue color suggests blood, but it is difficult to differentiate from bile without aspiration. After identifying the highest level of the dark fluid by following the intestine proximally, the luminal content is aspirated with a 19-gauge needle. The significance of this finding is that blood is coming from a site at or higher than this level. If there is no dark fluid in the small intestine, no conclusion can be drawn.

The entire intestine is palpated bidigitally to appreciate soft or hard luminal structures such as polyps and other tumors. Leiomyomata are usually evident on the serosal aspect as well, as are carcinoids and the rarer metastatic lesions such as melanoma. If a Meckel's diverticulum is found, it is carefully palpated to appreciate if any induration exists, especially at the base. An entirely soft diverticulum without thickening is likely to be innocent. The colon is similarly examined although it is more difficult to palpate thoroughly, as it is wider and partially retroperitoneal. Next, the mesenteric attachment is examined for evidence of a leash of prominent vessels, especially near the right colon, as sometimes, although not invariably, larger arteriovenous malformation in the adjacent bowel is suggested by such vessels.

A number of maneuvers are available to further identify the bleeding site if active bleeding is still ongoing, as evidenced by distention of the intestine and hemodynamic instability. Five to six atraumatic intestinal clamps can be applied on the small intestine dividing it into six to seven segments of approximate equal length. Continued bleeding will manifest as one segment getting more distended than others, and the bleeding site is localized to that segment. Patience is essential, since if bleeding is slow, it may take some time for the distention to become obvious. This move is frustrated, of course, if bleeding is no longer active by the time this maneuver is performed. Under this circumstance, intraoperative endoscopy is warranted. If bleeding in the colon is suspected, as by clot distention in the presence of a clean small bowel, compartmentalization with multiple clamps may aid localization, but this is not as important as in the small bowel, since subtotal colectomy is usually the most expedient procedure.

When a segment is identified as containing the bleeding lesion, it should be opened after insertion of a pursestring suture. Blood is evacuated and the lumen irrigated. The lesion should be easily identifiable by endoscopic examination with a choledochoscope after distending the lumen with saline as described for the duodenum.

If there are no clues at laparotomy as to the site of bleeding after careful search of the serosal aspect of the intestines and thorough palpation of the entire gut, and yet bleeding is not active enough to render the method of segmental occlusion effective, operative endoscopy is indicated. Only a few lesions remain to be excluded, such as angiodysplasias of the small bowel or the telengiectasias of the Osler-Weber-Rendu variety, intestinal varices, and other esoteric entities. The surgeon should have anticipated such a possibility and made appropriate arrangements with an endoscopist beforehand.

Rationale and Indication of Intraoperative Enteroscopy

The small intestine is inaccessible to the conventional endoscope and enteroscopy at present is only clinically practical when performed in conjunction with laparotomy. When a source of chronic blood loss is suspected to be present in the small intestine, after exhaustive negative investigations such as upper and lower GI endoscopy, angiography, and small bowel contrast study, elective operative enteroscopy, done in conjunction with exploratory laparotomy, may be utilized to locate mucosal lesions that may account for the chronic blood loss. In the emergency setting, operative enteroscopy is used to locate actively bleeding lesions in the small in-

testine, an integral step in the operative strategy for bleeding from obscure sites. It does not replace colonoscopy or esophagogastroduodenoscopy as operative endoscopy is a more difficult examination and yields less optimal results.

Technique of Intraoperative Enteroscopy

The equipment required is a 180-cm colonoscope, disinfected with soaking in glutaraldehyde solution.[6,18] A videocamera attachment is essential, since it is hard to communicate verbally to the surgeon all the findings, positive or negative, that would substantially affect management on a continuous basis. A teaching attachment is not a satisfactory alternative; it usually requires the surgeon to step away from the operating field. The procedure is performed in two parts: first, per oral enteroscopy, followed by per anal colonoscopy.

A bowel clamp is placed across the pylorus to prevent air distention of the intestine rendering operation difficult. The colonoscope is passed into the esophagus, facilitated by the anesthesiologist holding the patient's jaws forward. Examination of the esophagus and stomach is followed by passage to the pylorus, when the clamp must be removed. It is more expeditious for the endoscopist to intubate the pylorus without external aid. The surgeon may aid intubation of the second portion of the duodenum externally, guided by the view on the monitor. After the duodenum is intubated, passage of the colonscope tends to form a large loop in the body of the stomach. The surgeon must counter this by supporting with one hand on the body of the stomach, and one on the second portion of the duodenum, while the endoscopist should pull back to eliminate the loop already formed (Fig. 4-3).

The jejunum is next entered, aided by the surgeon presenting the loop to the endoscope, assuming the ligament of Treitz had been taken down from previous exploration. The endoscopist now steadily and slowly advances the colonoscope, while the surgeon lifts up the intestine

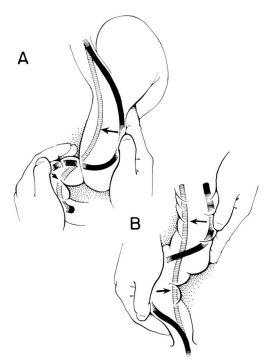

Fig. 4-3 Technique of externally supporting the endoscope to minimize loop formation during operative endoscopy. Loops will form in the stomach and sigmoid unless steps are taken to prevent them as shown. (A) Preventing loop formation in the stomach. (B) Preventing loop formation in the sigmoid.

and straightens it to present an axial view to be seen on the monitor. When the colonoscope has been fully inserted, 80 cm or so of it would have passed beyond the ligament of Trietz. The rest of the small intestine can be easily telescoped over the 80 cm or so of the shaft for a complete enteroscopy. Suspicious areas should be marked with a stitch on the serosa.

Some experts recommend transillumination of the entire small bowel after completion of enteroscopy as the vascular pattern can be clearly seen in a darkened room. In case of doubt, artifacts may be differentiated by reverse transillumination.[6] The light source is turned off, and a bright spot light, such as the surgeon's head light, is focused on the area in question. An abnormal vascular pattern is clearly visible on the videomonitor by this technique. If the lesion is a hematoma or bruising produced by

trauma the normal vascular pattern is preserved; in fact, the hematoma would be nearly invisible with this illumination. As the endoscope is withdrawn suction is applied to collapse the bowel.

The withdrawn colonoscope is rinsed and the functions checked. It is to be inserted via the anus for examination of the colon. The operating drapes should be arranged to form a tent to prevent contamination by the endoscopist. The surgeon should mobilize the splenic flexure while the equipment is being moved for the per anal examination. A bowel clamp is placed at the terminal ileum. The technique is similar to enteroscopy except that the endoscope moves into the intestine rather than the intestine over the endoscope. The surgeon's task is to support with his hands the sigmoid and the splenic flexure to counter loop formation, and to warn of too much air distention (Fig. 4-3). The procedure is considerably more difficult than regular colonoscopy, contrary to what the surgeon generally believes, particularly when the endoscopist happens to be teamed with an impatient surgeon who insists on maniuplating the tip from outside. An advantage of the videomonitor is that the surgeon immediately sees how disastrous it is to the view to be meddlesome. The air-distended colon tends to balloon into the wound once the counterpressure of the abdominal wall is lost. Transillumination and reverse transillumination are more useful here as the clots and fecal matter tend to be more confusing than in the small bowel. If the terminal ileum was not examined during the preceding operative enterscopy, the bowel clamp is repositioned to a higher location, and the ileal intubation is aided by the surgeon. Withdrawal of the endoscope is always accompanied by suction to collapse the bowel.

Skeptical surgeons often ask, "How often is intraoperative enteroscopy of help?" Many believe that if intraoperative endoscopy is successful in localization of a lesion, such a lesion would have been localizable by means other than enteroscopy. Unfortunately there are no objective data to answer this important question; even how often operative enteroscopy has failed to localize a source of bleeding is unclear. Considering the gamut of pathologic entities, this author is convinced that small vascular lesions and nonpalpable mucosal lesions in the small intestine defy localization by any other means. However, the chief virtue of this procedure may well come from another direction. The worst operative mistakes are made when the surgeon is forced to operate with no diagnosis; and when no signs of bleeding are evident at laparotomy, the surgeon's best option is to do nothing. It may be that the most valued aspect of a negative operative enteroscopy is to assure the surgeon of the correctness of this decision. This is not likely to be appreciated by those who have not personally experienced the difficulty of the situation.

Choice of Surgical Operations and Results

The surgical operation performed depends on the findings. If the site of bleeding cannot be localized, usually when active bleeding has stopped, no resection should be done. Some advocate a loop ileostomy in mid- or terminal ileum to aid localization in case bleeding recurs, since the bowel is now accessible by enteroscopy into both limbs. The drawback is that the patient may not bleed again for many weeks, to recur only after closure of the ileostomy.

When bleeding has been localized to the stomach and duodenum, the operation performed depends on the pathology identified. For bleeding from chronic peptic ulcers, an expeditious ulcer operation should be performed in addition to careful ligation or plication of the bleeder, if it has not been excluded from the gastrointestinal tract. The principle of local operations for local pathology is a safe one for all other mucosal bleeding lesions. For gastric or esophageal varices, intraoperative sclerotherapy via the gastrotomy is feasible and injection can be accurately done as the exposure is good.[9] In addition some form of expeditious portoazygous disconnection, such as stapling of the gastric walls and division of the coronary veins for interrup-

tion of flow to the varices should be accomplished.[9]

If bleeding has been localized to the small bowel, local resection of the segment bearing the lesion solves the problem. When bleeding has been accurately localized in the colon, segmental resection is the operation of choice. When localization is imprecise but the rectum is known to be normal, the most expeditious operation appears to be a subtotal colectomy with ileorectal anastomosis, a relatively simple operation with a good functional result and most effective in preventing recurrent colonic bleeding.[2,4,12,34] After a short period of adaptation, patients with ileorectal anastomosis have no more than two to three formed bowel movements a day. Drapanas et al.[12] compared the operative mortality of 11 percent for subtotal colectomy with ileorectal anastomosis to a mortality of 30 percent for segmental colectomy, with as many as 30 percent recurrent bleeding observed in those having segmental resection. McGuire et al.[34] supported this approach and showed that the procedure can be performed with a low operative mortality even in the elderly bleeding patient. A right hemicolectomy for known angiodysplasia bleeding, as advocated by Boley,[4] is not necessarily followed by a high recurrence rate, as 80 to 90 percent of patients do not rebleed even if diverticula are found on the left colon in some of these patients.

Failure to identify a source of bleeding occurs at about 10 to 20 percent in many series of massive gastrointestinal hemorrhage[15,24,29] without the use of operative enteroscopy. It is not known whether the number can be improved with the orderly deployment of the current investigative tools as outlined in this chapter, but this author believes it would. For those patients coming to laparotomy because of continued bleeding, the failure to identify the source was usually because active bleeding had just stopped by the time the incision was made. Stigmata of recent hemorrhage is likely to be detectable with operative enteroscopy, just as it is for endoscopy of the upper GI tract, enhancing the chance of a positive diagnosis. If hemorrhage recurs following a negative laparotomy and operative enteroscopy, the entire diagnostic procedures following the algorithm must be repeated, but with even more aggression if the source is to be located. In this author's experience, gastric variceal hemorrhage (one patient) and colonic variceal hemorrhage (one patient) was ultimately found to be the cause in two such patients, both of whom had obliteration of esophageal varices from sclerotherapy.

COMPLICATIONS

Postoperative complications following procedures for GI hemorrhage are well known and have been quoted as the deterrent for recommending early surgery, but such complications are more likely to follow inadequate resuscitation, repeated transfusion, commonly seen in patients making their way eventually to the surgeon. A high wound infection rate following surgery for massive GI hemorrhage has been documented.[32,35] For gastric surgery, contamination by the anacidic gastric content has been cited as a reason although how much the contributory role of shock plays in the pathogenesis is unclear. In emergency colon surgery, contamination is definitely a factor. Leakage of anastomosis is a major contribution to mortality in many series of bleeding from either the upper or lower GI tract.[2,12,13,24,25] Emergency gastric and colonic surgery is extremely demanding of surgical skill and judgment and must not be undertaken lightly by the inexperienced.

Nonspecific complications as a result of massive blood loss include hypovolemic shock and the sequelae of inadequate resuscitation. Fatal delay in resuscitation has been quantified as continued hemorrhage when the subject has already bled down to one-half of his blood volume, even though continued hemorrhage is replaced pari passu.[8] Such a situation has been shown to be incompatible with life. Myocardial ischemia, stroke, and renal failure occur in compromised patients long before this stage is reached and carry a high mortality. Complications of blood transfusion must also be considered. Following massive blood replacement, coagulopathy may occur if clotting factors are

not appropriately replaced. Transmission of disease is the most common serious complication due to transfusion, including hepatitis and, rarely, acquired immune deficiency syndrome (AIDS). Hyperkalemia, acidosis, and hypothermia are but a few of the host of possible but preventable complications.

Pulmonary Complications

This is a particularly common complication for this clinical situation. ARDS may complicate hypovolemic shock and massive blood replacement. Aspiration pneumonitis is always a major concern. The occurrence of postoperative atelectasis and pneumonia is not different from any other major emergency surgery.

Recurrent Hemorrhage

Recurrent hemorrhage following surgical treatment for upper GI bleeding is a substantial problem,[11,31,44] and much argument has gone on for years about the efficacy of different types of procedures. However, even for the same operation of vagotomy and pyloroplasty with plication of the bleeder, recurrent bleeding has been quoted as high as 20 to 36 percent[21,29] on the one extreme, and as low as 1 to 8 percent.[16,20] The results of the more recent series are, however, much more optimistic, typically 3 percent.[15] For bleeding from the colon, recurrence is 10 to 30 percent (even higher in a few series) except where a subtotal colectomy had been performed.[4,12] In view of the usual multiplicity of lesions in bleeding from the lower gut, this is not surprising. Both diverticula and angiodysplasias are multiple lesions, and recurrent or new lesions may continue to develop, since the lesions are degenerative in nature. Boley et al.[4] showed that, in the presence of both diverticular disease and angiodysplasia, a right hemicolectomy is successful in prevention of rebleeding in 80 to 90 percent of cases. Data from another retrospective series[14] indicated that left colectomy for presumed diverticular bleeding is a particularly poor operation, with a rebleeding rate of more than 80 percent within 2 weeks of the procedure, and a reoperation rate of more than 60 percent, for either rebleeding or (less commonly) for anastomotic leak.

Mortality

Overall surgical mortality has not declined in recent years but in most series the proportion of patients with variceal hemorrhage increased, while those with ulcers decreased. The overall surgical mortality is about 25 percent,[10,15,43] but for nonvariceal hemorrhage it is about 10 percent,[10,13,15,24,25,33] somewhat higher for gastric ulcers.[26,43] For massive lower GI bleeding, the overall mortality is 10 percent.[4,12,14,34,47]

ELECTIVE THERAPEUTIC ENDOSCOPY FOR POTENTIAL BLEEDING LESIONS

There are only two main groups of lesions with natural history well known enough to warrant consideration of elective treatment when the lesions are not actively bleeding: gastroesophageal varices and mucosal angiomatous malformations, including angiodysplasias and the telangiectasias of the Osler-Weber-Rendu syndrome. Esophageal varices are discussed in Chapter 3. The treatment of nonbleeding angiomatous malformation depends on the nature and extent: For extensive lesions such those found in Osler-Weber-Rendu syndrome where the entire GI tract may be involved, the only treatment feasible is palliative therapeutic endoscopy. Many and all of the modalities discussed in Chapter 2 can be applied, but argon photocoagulation seems particularly appropriate. In fact, more than one therapeutic endoscopist obtained expertise by treating a single patient with extensive lesions over numerous sessions. New lesions develop in time and require more treatment. Most reports in the literature focused on the use of argon laser photocoagulation for these lesions. Heater probe, monopolar electrocoagulation with the hot biopsy forceps technique,[40] and Nd:YAG laser[28,30] have also been successfully used (techniques described in Chapter 2).

When the small bowel is extensively involved, these lesions may be reached through operative enteroscopy and photocoagulated with the Argon laser. When lesions are concentrated in one segment of the gut, surgical resection is the most expeditious method even though future recurrence is likely.

Isolated angiodysplasias is indicated for therapeutic endoscopy even though it may be difficult to prove directly that it had been responsible for previous bleeding episodes. Freedom from rebleeding cannot be guaranteed, since even apparent success for many years may be followed by recurrence due to development of new lesions. Nor is it possible to exclude similar lesions in the ileum beyond the reach of the conventional endoscope and yet too small to be evident on angiography. It is therefore difficult to evaluate the clinical efficacy of therapeutic endoscopy for this situation. However, if the endoscopist is confident in clearing the right colon of angiodysplasias, for example, it is a more logical choice than a right hemicolectomy, since new lesions may develop elsewhere. Since this lesion affects mostly the elderly population, with associated diseases such as aortic valve disease, previous valve replacement requiring chronic anticoagulation, chronic renal failure, chronic hemodialysis, and other medical conditions multiplying the risks for surgery, therapeutic endoscopy is particularly useful.

The clinical experience reported so far has been favorable, with minimal complications.[7,23,27,28,45,46] Table 4-1 lists the series published so far. Apparent short-term success can be claimed for 66 to 98 percent of cases treated, bearing in mind the difficulty in interpretation of the results.

THE ROLE OF ENDOSCOPY IN THE INTEGRATED APPROACH IN MANAGEMENT OF GI BLEEDING FROM OBSCURE SITES

The algorithm (Fig. 4-4) summarizes the discussion of this chapter. The contributions of radiology and endoscopy have reduced, although not completely eliminated, the diagnos-

Table 4-1. Laser Photocoagulation for Vascular Lesions

Reference	No. of Patients	Laser	Complication	Rebleeding
Waitman et al.[46]	250	Argon	0	5
Bowers and Dixon[7]	13	Argon	0	*
Howard et al.[23]	23	Argon	0	3
Jensen and Bown[27]	15	Argon	0	*
Johnston[28]	22	Nd:YAG	0	3
Sudry et al.[45]	15	Argon	0	5

* Not stated.

tic difficulty posed by the bleeder from obscure sites in the GI tract. Especially in acute crisis brought on by major bleeding, an orderly integrated approach greatly reduces management mistakes exemplified historically by "blind" gastrectomy or colectomy. Since surgery is still the main treatment currently available when bleeding fails to stop, the ultimate role of endoscopy in this clinical condition is to facilitate accurate surgical treatment.

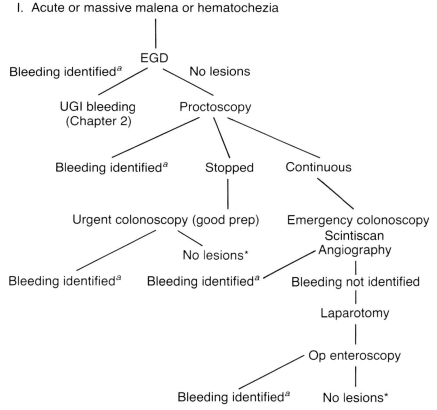

Fig. 4-4 Algorithm showing management of obscure bleeding from the gastrointestinal tract. EGD, esophagogastroduodenoscopy. (*), repeat workup all over if rebled in future. ([a]), see algorithm III. f = failed. (Figure continues.)

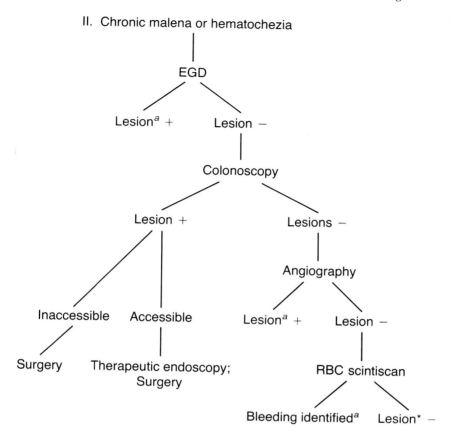

II. Chronic malena or hematochezia

EGD

Lesion[a] +   Lesion −

Colonoscopy

Lesion +   Lesions −

Inaccessible   Accessible   Angiography

Surgery   Therapeutic endoscopy;   Lesion[a] +   Lesion −
            Surgery

RBC scintiscan

Bleeding identified[a]   Lesion* −

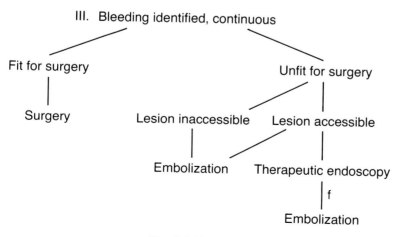

III. Bleeding identified, continuous

Fit for surgery   Unfit for surgery

Surgery   Lesion inaccessible   Lesion accessible

Embolization   Therapeutic endoscopy

f

Embolization

Fig. 4-4 (*Continued*).

REFERENCES

1. Adson MA, Fulton RR: The ileal stoma and portal hypertension. An uncommon site of variceal bleeding. Arch Surg 112:501, 1977
2. Alexander-Williams J: Surgical management of acute intestinal bleeding. p. 357. In Dykes PW, Keighley MRB (eds): Gastrointestinal Hemorrhage. Wright PSG, Bristol, 1981
3. Athanasoulis CA, Waltman AC, Novelline RA, et al: Angiography: Its contribution to the emergency management of gastrointestinal hemorrhage. Radiol Clin North Am 14:265, 1976
4. Boley SJ, DiBiase A, Brandt LJ: Lower intestinal bleeding in the elderly. Am J Surg 137:57, 1979
5. Bookstein JJ, Naderi JJ, Walter JR: Transcatheter embolization for lower gastrointestinal bleeding. Radiology 127:345, 1978
6. Bowden TA Jr: Intraoperative endoscopy of the gastrointestinal tract. p. 167. In Dent TL, Strodel WE, Turcott JG (eds): Surgical Endoscopy. Year Book Medical Publishers, Chicago, 1985
7. Bowers JH, Dixon JA: Argon laser photocoagulation of vascular malformations in the GI tract: Short term results. Gastrointest Endosc 28:126, 1982
8. Collins JA: Massive blood transfusion. Clin Hematol 5:201, 1976
9. Chung RS, Camara DS: Simplified Portoazygous disconnection (Tanner's operation) combined with operative sclerotherapy for bleeding varices. Am J Surg 148:389, 1984
10. Darle N, Haglund U, Larsson I, et al: Management of massive gastroduodenal hemorrhage. Acta Chir Scand 146:277, 1980
11. Donaldson RM Jr, Handy J, Papper S: Five-year follow-up study of patients with bleeding duodenal ulcers with and without surgery. N Engl J Med 259:201, 1958
12. Drapanas T, Pennington DG, Kappelman M, et al: Emergency subtotal colectomy: Preferred approach to management of massive diverticular disease. Ann Surg 177:519, 1973
13. Dronfield MW, Atkinson M, Langman MJS: Effect of different operation policies on mortality from bleeding peptic ulcer. Lancet 1:1126, 1979
14. Eaton AC: Emergency surgery for acute colonic hemorrhage—A retrospective study. Br J Surg 68:109, 1981
15. Elerding SC, Moore EE, Wolz JR, et al: Outcome of operations for upper gastrointestinal tract bleeding: an update. Arch Surg 115:1473, 1980
16. Farris JH, Smith GK: Vagotomy and pyloroplasty: A solution to the management of bleeding duodenal ulcer. Ann Surg 152:416, 1960
17. Freeman JG, Cobden I, Lishman AH, et al: Controlled trial of terlipressin (glypressin) versus vasopressin in the early treatment of esophageal varices. Lancet 2:66, 1982
18. Forde K: Intraoperative colonoscopy. p. 189. In Hunt RH, Waye JD (eds): Colonoscopy Techniques. Year Book Medical Publishers, Chicago, 1981
19. Forde, KA, Treat MR: Colonoscopy for lower gastrointestinal tract bleeding. p. 26. In Dent TL, Strodel WE, Turcott JG (eds): Surgical Endoscopy. Year Book Medical Publishers, Chicago, 1985
20. Forster JH, Hall AD, Dumphy JE: Surgical management of bleeding ulcers. Surg Clin North Am 46:387, 1966
21. Herrington JL Jr: Vagotomy-pyloroplasty for duodenal ulcer: A critical appraisal of early results. Surgery 61:698, 1967
22. Hessel SJ, Adams DF, Abrams HL: Complications of angiography. Radiology 138:273, 1981
23. Howard OM, Buchanan JD, Hunt RH: Antiodysplasias of the colon. Lancet 2:16, 1982
24. Hunt PS, Hansky J, Korman MG: Mortality in patients with hematemesis and melena: A prospective study. Br Med J 1:1238, 1979
25. Hunt PS, Korman MG, Hansky J, et al: Bleeding duodenal ulcer: Reduction in mortality with a planned approach. Br J Surg 66:633, 1979
26. Inberg MV, Linna MI: Massive hemorrhage from gastroduodenal ulcer. Acta Chir Scand 141:664, 1975
27. Jensen D, Bown S: Gastrointestinal angiomata. p. 151. In Fleischer D, Jensen D, Bright-Asare P (eds): Therapeutic Laser Endoscopy in Gastrointestinal Disease. Martinus Nijhoff, Boston, 1983
28. Johnston JH: Complications following endoscopic laser therapy. Gastrointest Endosc 28:135, 1982
29. Kelley HG, Grant GN, Elliott DW: Massive gastroduodenal hemorrhage. Changing concepts of management. Arch Surg 87:6, 1963
30. Kiefhaber P, Nath G, Moritz K: Endoscopic control of massive gastrointestinal hemorrhage with a high power neodymium-YAG laser. Prog Surg 177:15, 1977
31. Langman MJS: Relationship between preopera-

tive bleeding and perforation and bleeding after operations for duodenal ulcer. Gut 6:134, 1965

32. Lewis RI: Wound infection after gastric duodenal operations: A ten year review. Can J Surg 20:435, 1977

33. McGregor DB, Savage LE, McVay CB: Massive gastrointestinal hemorrhage: A twenty-five years experience wth vagotomy and drainage. Surgery 80:530, 1976

34. McGuire HH, Hayes BW: Massive bleeding from diverticulosis of the colon: Guidelines for therapy based on bleeding patients observed in fifty cases. Ann Surg 175:847, 1972

35. Nichols RL, Smith JW: Intragastric microbial colonization in common disease states of the stomach and duodenum. Ann Surg 182:557, 1975

36. Nusbaum M, Baum S: Radiographic demonstration of unknown sites of gastrointestinal bleeding. Surg Forum 13:374, 1963

37. Paredero MV, Dixon SM, Baker D, et al: Risk of renal failure after major angiography. Arch Surg 118:1417, 1983

38. Pomeranc MM: Acute renal failure in association with the administration of radiographic contrast material. JAMA 239:125, 1978

39. Ring EJ, Athanasoulis CA, Waltman AC, et al: The pseudovein. An angiographic appearance of arterial hemorrhage. Can J Radiol 24:242, 1973

40. Rogers BHG: Endoscopic electrocoagulation of vascular abnormalities of the gastrointestinal tract in 51 patients. Gastrointest Endosc 28:2, 1982

41. Rossini FP, Ferrari A: Emergency colonoscopy. p. 289. In Hunt RH, Waye JD (eds): Colonoscopy Technique. Year Book, Chicago, 1981

42. Sauerbruch T, Weinzierl M, Deitrich HP, et al: Sclerotherapy of a bleeding duodenal varix. Endoscopy 14:187, 1984

43. Schiller KFR, Truelove SC, Williams DG: Hematemesis and melena with special reference to factors influencing the outcome. Br Med J 2:7, 1970

44. Serebro HA, Mendeloff AI: Late results of medical and surgical treatment of bleeding peptic ulcer. Lancet 2:1462, 1966

45. Sudry P, Brunetaud JM, Paris JC, et al: Treatment of digestive angiomas with Argon laser. Gastroenterol Clin Biol 5:426, 1981

46. Waitman AM, Grant DZ, Chateau F: Endoscopic management of vascular lesions. p. 126. In Silvis SE (ed): Therapeutic Gastrointestinal Endoscopy. Igaku-Shoin, New York, 1984

47. Welch CE, Athanasoulis CA, Gladabini JJ: Hemorrhage from the large bowel with special reference to angiodysplasia and diverticula disease. World J Surg 2:73, 1978

5

Endoscopic Sphincterotomy: Nonsurgical Treatment of Common Bile Duct Stones

With the advent of the duodenoscope, the papilla of Vater and through it the bile and pancreatic ducts became freely accessible for studies, spearheading a remarkable advance in the diagnosis of conditions affecting this anatomic region. Less than 5 years after the first report by McCune in 1968[32] of cannulation of the ampulla of Vater, endoscopic retrograde cholangiopancreatography (ERCP) had already attained the status of an established diagnostic procedure,[21] a testimony of its widespread popularity. Increasing experience of ERCP and the radiographic interpretation soon led to the recognition that certain common pathological anatomy could be mechanically corrected by simple endoscopic electrosurgery. The concept that the sphincter can be divided, the lower end of the bile duct exposed, and the stone in the duct extracted all done endoscopically was shown to be a feasible and practical proposition by both German and Japanese workers[5,24] in 1973. By the 10-year anniversary of the first publication of this technique, more than 50,000 procedures have been done worldwide for the treatment of calculous obstruction of the bile ducts. The technique is within the grasp of most experienced endoscopists, and the results published in large surveys indicate that low complication rate is attainable generally. Today the complications of sphincterotomy have been well studied and the indications well defined.

RATIONALE

The fundamental difference between endoscopic and surgical sphincterotomy deserves emphasis. The basic principle of the endoscopic procedure is division of the intramural segment of the bile duct in the duodenum without extending the cut to outside of the duodenal wall, an event that would constitute perforation. It should be emphasized that dividing the intramural bile duct, but not necessarily complete sphincterotomy, is the primary goal, and if this results in complete sphincterotomy (which it does in many instances) so much the better; but complete sphincterotomy must not be pursued at the expense of violating the basic principle, thereby causing perforation. By contrast, the objective of the surgical operation of sphincteroplasty (Fig. 5-1) is a complete sphincterotomy; sutures are placed as the sphincter is divided. It is no major mishap (indeed, in many cases

A

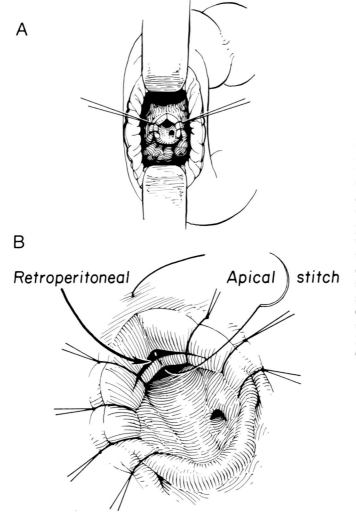

B

Retroperitoneal **Apical** **stitch**

Fig. 5-1 The surgical operation of sphincteroplasty. (A) The general view after traction of the edges of the orifice. (B) Closeup view clearly showing the extramural extension of the incision being repaired by the sutures. The operation differs from sphincterotomy in that the sphincter fibers can be completely divided by extending the incision to outside of the duodenal wall. (Fig. B from Coppe D: Gallbladder and calculous biliary tract disease. P. 739. In Fromm D (ed): Gastrointestinal Surgery. Churchill Livingstone, New York, 1985.)

it is necessary) to extend the cut outside the duodenal wall, since it is immediately converted into a sutureline; the overriding consideration of the opration is to attain as large an opening as possible. Jones[22,23] showed in 50 anatomic dissections that in most cases a complete division of the sphincter cannot be achieved without an extramural component; if the observation is correct then endoscopic sphincterotomy must often be incomplete. Many endoscopists claim that the appearance of a gush of bile indicates the complete division of the sphincter fibers, a convenient clinical end point but unfortunately unsubstantiated by studies. Some favor the term papillotomy to represent incomplete sphincterotomy but there is little virtue to have another name as long as it is recognized that endoscopic sphincterotomy need not be complete. An incomplete sphincterotomy is acceptable and sometimes necessary in endoscopic practice because the segment of intramural duct is short; as long as the resulting opening allows stones to be extracted, the procedure is deemed successful. Most endoscopic sphincterotomies produce an orifice of 1 to 2 cm in diameter, enough to allow the largest stone found in that particular patient to pass. The claim that restenosis would be inevitable following sphincterotomy (complete or partial), but not sphincteroplasty, has not been substantiated by extensive modern data (see Complications, Restenosis).

INDICATIONS AND CONTRAINDICATIONS

In general, endoscopic sphincterotomy is used predominantly for benign biliary conditions affecting the lower common bile duct.

Common Bile Duct Stones

Since the established treatment for common bile duct stones is surgery, therapeutic endoscopy is indicated originally in patients who are poor surgical risks. In good risk patients, surgery is usually indicated because cholecystectomy can be carried out concomitantly.

Recurrent stones in the common duct following previous surgical removal is another indication, since reoperation carries significant morbidity, including recurrence of retained stones.[18,36,43,49] Even if the T-tube tract is usable for percutaneous retrieval (see Chapter 7), a sphincterotomy has the advantage of adding some degree of protection from future recurrence, which has been shown to be higher in those who recurred once.[27,36] It has become the preferred treatment for retained or recurrent stones in at least one surgical group.[4]

Patients who have had a previous cholecystectomy presenting with common duct stones for the first time are indicated for the endoscopic procedure, even though the hazards of an operation on the common bile duct need not be excessively high. The endoscopic procedure takes less time to perform, requires much shorter hospitalization, inflicts little pain, and costs less than surgery.

Endoscopic sphincterotomy for common duct stones in the presence of an intact gallbladder, whether it contains stones or not, is currently controversial. Acute cholecystitis is known to develop in 2 to 3 percent of such patients following sphincterotomy, the vast majority within the first year.[10,14] A further 8 to 10 percent of patients may require elective cholecystectomy for chronic symptoms in the ensuing 5 years.[14] The pathophysiologic basis appears to be that the inflow of bile into the gallbladder, which is dependent on ductal pressure, is significantly disturbed after the ampullary sphincter has been severed, contributing to stasis in a gallbladder that is often already pathologic. In any case, sphincterotomy is still a valuable emergency treatment for poor risk patients, when choledocholithiasis is complicated by cholangitis. Elective cholecystectomy can always be performed when the acute crisis is over.

Emergency endoscopic sphincterotomy is effective in treatment of cholangitis associated with ductal stones.[9,20,40,45] Dramatic improvement occurs within hours of the decompression.

Surgical sphincteroplasty or choledochoduodenostomy is indicated when the stones in the common duct are large: Any stone that exceeds 2.5 cm in diameter should not be removed endoscopically unless the patient would not tolerate an operation. Special endoscopic technique is required to extract large stones, increasing the risks of complications. When the stone is impacted behind a long stricture, it cannot be retrieved endoscopically, as the sphincterotomy may not be safely extended enough to abolish the stricture. Choledochoduodenostomy is indicated for this circumstance.

Stenosis of the Papilla

Although the diagnosis of papillary stenosis can often be made on clinical grounds, such as recurrent jaundice or cholangitis, it should always be confirmed with strict radiologic and manometric criteria in order to avoid unnecessary procedures. The external appearance of the papilla provides little clue. The short stenosis is easily missed on ERCP, since the cannulation bypasses it. Elevated intraductal pressure as measured by ERCP manometry[2,15] and stasis of radiologic contrast are important signs of

much safer in the dilated ducts than in the nondilated duct, as the sphincter appears to be shortened due to ductal dilation, and the duct is closely approximaed to the duodenal wall even in the extramural portion. Furthermore, the dilated bile duct may be entered through this tubular impression via an infundibulotomy (see Techniques).

The endoscopic anatomy of the papilla as seen inside the duodenum is shown in Figure 5-4. The most frequent configuration is for the common bile duct to course almost vertically and the pancreatic duct almost horizontally, the 11:10 position of the hands of the clock. However, as the termination of both ducts runs directly toward the endoscope, the two come together closely for a short distance, in effect separated from each other by a septum. Other anatomic variants are shown in Figure 5-2, with the estimated incidence as indicated. The papilla itself has varied appearance, the commonest of which is a low excrescence or mound. The almost constant hoodlike transverse fold is a useful landmark, since the cut should ordinarily extend up to but not through it. The vertical fold(s) (the frenulum) facilitate the recognition of the ampulla, since it is striking in the midst of transverse folds.

Manometrically the sphincter is, on the average, a 4 to 6-mm-long high-pressure zone, generating a mean of 15 mmHg (about 20 cm bile)

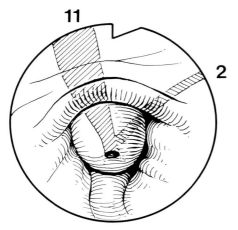

Fig. 5-4 Luminal view of the papilla. A mental picture of 11:10 position of the hands of the clock represents the direction of the bile and pancreatic ducts.

pressure above the intraduodenal pressure, and 4 mm above the intraductal pressure.[2,15] Cyclic pressure peaks of up to 100 mmHg (136 cm bile) are recorded in the normal sphincter, at about 4 per minute. The sphincter pressure is the principal determinant of the resistance of bile flow in the normal subject. The secretory pressure the liver is capable of generating has been measured in cholecystectomized subjects[25] and ranges from 29 to 39 cm of bile. The duct has a sparse coat of longitudinal muscle that does not contribute much to bile flow. No peristaltic function has ever been shown in the bile duct. During the interdigestive period when the liver is not generating much secretory pressure, bile flows into the gallbladder, since the prevailing sphincter tone is higher than the intraductal pressure. Despite such spot pressure measurements, however, bile obviously also enters the duodenum even during fasting, a fact well known to endoscopists; apparently one-half the bile secreted by the liver during fasting leaks pass the ampulla and trickles into the duodenum, probably during the noncotractile phase of sphincteric activity.[35] The rest of the bile flows to the gallbladder, where it is concentrated.[47] After sphincteroplasty, the cyclical high-pressure waves in the normal sphincter are abolished and the tone is lowered.[34] It is likely that in such patients the gallbladder filling is more sluggish, although as yet there is no data to substantiate this suspicion.

The sphincter relaxes in response to cholecystokinin in humans. Neural influences play an as yet unknown physiologic role; the vagus probably modulates a variety of hormonal stimuli and is responsible for the intrinsic rhythmic tone.[44]

TECHNIQUE

Equipment

Figure 5-5 shows the commonly used equipment for sphincteroplasty in the United States. A standard sphincterotome (Fig. 5-5B), modeled after the Erlangen prototype, has a short catheter tip (0.5 cm), behind which is an exposed wire that can bowstring by increasing the tension

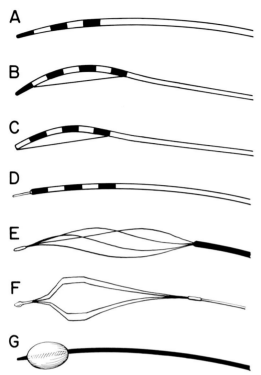

Fig. 5-5 Commonly used instruments in sphincterotomy. (A) ERCP cannula (with tapered tip). (B) The sphincterotome (Erlangen type) has a catheter tip, and the cutting wire begins 5 mm before the tip. (C) The precut sphincterotome with cutting wire running right to the tip. (D) The needle electrode for scalpel cutting. (E) The Dormier stone basket (for smaller stones). (F) The quadrangular basket (for larger stones). (G) The Fogarty biliary balloon catheter.

on the handle. An infrequently used model (Fig. 5-5C) is the precut modification, which resembles the standard model but without the catheter tip; the wire extends right to the tip. It is used when the duct can only be cannulated for a few millimeters, the precut modification enlarges the papilla opening for better exposure of the bile duct.

The preferred duodenoscope is one with a large channel, 2.8 mm or larger (such as the 3.7-mm channel that accepts 7 to 8 Fr. accessories), as considerable suction remains while the instrument is still in the channel. A nasobiliary stent, required to circumvent cholangitis following sphincterotomy is much easier to insert via

a large channel. Other instruments commonly used to extract stones are the Dormier basket (for smaller stones) (Fig. 5-5E), the quadrangular basket (for larger stones) (Fig. 5-5F), the biliary balloon (Fogarty) catheter (Fig. 5-5G), the biliary balloon dilator (Gruntzig not shown), and the lithotripsy basket (not shown). The latter is the same as the stone basket, except that the wires are of high tensile steel and the sheath is made of metal capable of providing the counterpressure necessary for the basket wire to cut through the stones. The biliary balloon catheter has a 1-cm balloon inflatable by a syringe and a central lumen for contrast study. The dilators operate on the same principle as the esophageal and angioplasty dilators, namely, preformed balloons that keep their shape under high pressure, and dilation is effected by radial force on the stricture. A needle electrode (Fig. 5-5D) for making simple cuts is occasionally required. A nasobiliary cathether should also be at hand (see Chapter 6). One or two ERCP cannulae (Fig. 5-5 A) must also be standing by, prefilled with 30 percent diatrizoate connected to smoothly operating glass syringes with air-tight connections.

A dependable electrosurgical unit must be used; the desirable characteristics and the safety precautions of such a unit have been detailed in Chapter 2. The operator must be familiar with the characteristic and power output of the machine, including what setting would give the appropriate effect in a subject of given weight.

First-rate radiologic facilities must be available. The most satisfactory arrangement is to perform the procedure in the radiologic suite itself; the help of a radiologist in positioning either the equipment or the patient to obtain the optimal views and spot films is essential.

Preparation

The patient must be adequately sedated and relaxed for the duration of the procedure. Premedication with diazepam or meperidine is required. If barium studies have been obtained recently, freedom from residual opacities must be verified radiographically before the procedure. Prophylactic antibiotics are used in patients who have had positive blood cultures from biliary sepsis, high grade calculous obstruction, cardiac valvular disease, and previous history of septicemia due to biliary tract manipulations, although a few endoscopists do use antibiotic prophylaxis routinely in all patients. An intravenous line must be in place for medications such as sedatives or smooth muscle relaxants. Although routine antibiotic prophylaxis is controversial, there is a consensus that the endoscopic equipment and instruments must have been thoroughly disinfected. The surgical team must be aware of the procedure being performed, and the patient must be told of the possiblity that emergency surgery may be required either to obtain better drainage when endoscopic procedure has failed, or to deal with complications that may arise.

Endoscopic Technique

THE PRELIMINARY CHOLANGIOGRAPHY

A basic requirement for success is a rapid and smooth ERCP; thus the endoscopist must be conversant with the diagnostic technique, the key steps of which are now reviewed.

With the patient on the left lateral position and the left arm behind the back, the duodenoscope is inserted and passed to beyond 40 cm. The stomach is inflated slightly, the tip is depressed to view the antrum. The endoscope is advanced toward the pylorus until 2 cm before the opening, when the tip is restored to the neutral position. As the tip is straightened, the pylorus disappears from the view like a setting sun. Advancement into the pyloric canal is indicated by an initial red-out, followed by a rush of duodenal mucosal gland pattern. The superior duodenal angle is next negotiated by some clockwise rotation and right lateral flexion of the tip (Fig. 5-6). Depression of the tip will now permit a partial axial view of the second portion of the duodenum. After obtaining a hold by hooking at the angle, the endoscope is withdrawn to reduce the loop accumulated in the

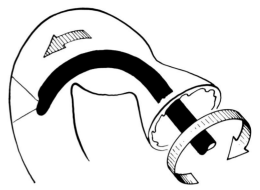

Fig. 5-6 Negotiation of the superior duodenal angle is done by right lateral flexion and some clockwise rotation of the endoscope.

stomach. Withdrawal may continue as long as the view in the duodenum does not change, usually until the 60 to 70 cm mark. The patient is now assisted to the prone position, rotating 90 degrees to the right. The lens now faces the inner wall of the duodenum.

Once resettled, the search of the duodenal papilla is begun. This is also a good time to give intravenous glucagon, 0.2-mg bolus, to obtain relaxation of the duodenum. When the plicae circularis are widely spaced and the movements are minimal, optimal condition for cannulation has been attained. If the papilla is not directly in view, it is looked for more proximally first by withdrawing the endoscope while scanning the medial wall. In the distal half of the second portion of the duodenum, the medial wall is relatively flat and devoid of plicae. In this area, vertical folds may be recognized leading proximally to the papilla, which is a nipple or moundlike structure. Other landmarks are the hooding of the papilla by a transverse fold, the tubular impression of the intramural common bile duct, particularly when dilated. The enlarged papilla behind an obstructed duct may be very striking, sometimes almost polypoid in appearance. When a diverticulum is found, the papilla is usually situated at the rim rather than at the bottom.

Once the papilla is located, the endoscope is brought en face to it, usually by withdrawal of the endoscope, thereby reducing the bends, if this has not been done before—or if more has accumulated. Small moves are essential; the upward swing of the cannula imparted by the elevator while the cannula is advanced must be memorized. The direction of the bile duct is estimated. Aiming passes of the cannula (dry runs) are practiced before cannulation, to gauge visually how the swing of the cannula would coincide with the estimated direction of the bile duct which usually runs almost parallel with the duodenal wall. While the right thumb and index finger advance the cannula, the left thumb controls the elevator and alters the degree of upswing. Cannulation can only be successful if this swing is in the correct axis of the bile duct. A traumatic first attempt often prejudices any subsequent attempts because the resulting edema and sphincter spasm tend to make the orifice even more difficult to recognize.

A preliminary cholangiogram is now done with a standard ERCP cannula. This cannula has a blunt tip and may not be usable for cannulating a tight stenosis, but it causes less trauma. A tapered-tip cannula may be required if the opening is tight, but it can inflict trauma on the papilla and make insertion of the sphincterotome difficult. The cannula must have been primed with contrast and connected to the injection system. A trial of manual injection is monitored under fluoroscopy. If, despite using the technique outlined designed to achieve selective injection, the pancreatic duct is filled, injection is stopped and the cannulation is redirected at an even more cephalad direction and a little to the left until the bile duct is seen to be filled. Dilated ducts may need to be filled slowly. Spot films are taken at several positions. Some endoscopists would use the sphincterotome instead of the cannula for the preliminary cholangiogram if sphincteroplasty is planned and if a high-quality cholangiogram has previously been obtained. The insertion of the sphincterotome is likly to be more difficult than the cannula, since it is less flexible and, when the tip is hung up in a fold of mucosa due to less than ideal alignment, the sphincterotome simply would not advance.

The films are scrutinized for the length of the sphincter (the distance from the tip of the duct to the infundibulum, or the intramural length), the length of stricture if any, the width of the dilated ducts, and the number and size of the stones. When the stricture extends to outside of the wall of the duodenum, or when the stones are larger than 2.5 cm, sphincterotomy should be abandoned. When the duct is packed with stones, extraction of some stones to establish drainage to avoid cholangitis is mandatory even if an adequate sphincterotomy cannot be accomplished.

TECHNIQUE OF SPHINCTEROTOMY

Insertion of the sphincterotome is facilitated by the knowledge gained by the cannulation and radiography (see Fig. 5-7). The first objective is to insert the sphincterotome smoothly and freely into the bile duct with the wire oriented correctly. It is not sufficient just to rely on the feeling that the sphincterotome has gone in exactly as the preceding cannulation, as the pancreatic duct may still be inadvertently cannulated. Radiologic confirmation by injecting a small amount of contrast and monitoring under the fluoroscope is essential, although some experts rely on fluoroscopic observation of the movement of the sphincterotome up and down the duct to differentiate it from pancreatic duct cannulation. The sphincterotome is then withdrawn to expose a length of wire depending on the desired length of cut, which must be adjusted to point at 11 to 12 o'clock position with the duodenal axis being 12 o'clock. The most crucial step of the entire procedure is the positioning of the sphincterotome; it pays to spend most of the procedure time in correct positioning. The position of the wire may be changed by passing the unflexed sphincterotome up the duct, rotated somewhat in the desired direction, and withdrawn while flexing to see whether the desired effect has been achieved. Another tip is to rotate the endoscope slightly to get the wire to the correct orientation while it is unflexed inside the duct. Often it is more

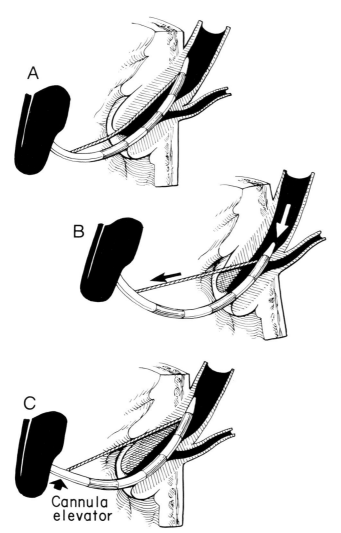

Fig. 5-7 (A) Sphincterotome in position ready for sphincterotomy. (B) Extension of the cut by flexing the sphincterotome (tension along black arrow) alters the angle of the cutting wire, in addition it may permit the sphincterotome to slip either out (usually, white arrow) or in, altering the length of wire inside the duct and therefore the length of cut. (C) Extension of the cut may also be done by using the cannula elevator of the duodenoscope. The sphincterotome is pushed upwards with little change in the angle of the cutting wire as shown by the arrow, which indicates the direction of movement of the cutting wire.

expeditious to pass a new sphincterotome, and so more than one should be on hand. If a shorter cut is desired, more wire should be visible, usually 10 to 15 mm of the 30-mm sphincterotome should be outside the duct. Tension on the wire is increased to form the quarter- or half-bow, visibly tenting the sphincter to form a ridge, which marks the intended incision. When this is judged satisfactory (Fig. 5-7A), short bursts of blended current are passed and the appearance of the mucosa closely scrutinized. The mucosa first blanches, then a split of the sphincter occurs first at the opening expos-

ing the wire. Under clear vision the split is lengthened by increments, extending the cut upward using the cannula elevator, until 10 to 13 mm of incision has been achieved (Fig. 5-7C). An alternative technique is to use more flexing of the bow, but excessive flexing may cause the sphincterotome to slide out, changing the length of the cutting edge (Fig. 5-7B). Much larger volume of tissue is cut toward the last few mm of the incision than in the beginning and therefore takes longer. A gush of bile occurs as the mucosa of the duct is exposed, a mark of adequate sphincterotomy. Most endoscopists assume that this is the sign of complete division of the sphincter fibers, a point many experienced biliary surgeons take exception to. This done, the tensed sphincterotome may be moved back and forth with little resistance across the incised papilla. The transverse fold across the top of the papilla (Fig. 5-2) is used as a landmark; the usual sphincterotomy incision is extended right up to the fold. When longer incisions are required, this fold may be crossed, but the risk of perforation and hemorrhage is considerably increased.

The main difficulty occurs when the papilla cannot be cannulated satisfactorily. The various steps of the cannulation technique must be retraced, including repositioning of the endoscope, using a new sphincterotome, more cephalad swing, and using more glucagon. Sometimes it helps to first cannulate with a tapered cannula and outline the lower duct with some contrast. Patient perseverance is the best advice; it is well to remember that the second-line techniques are also the last resort techniques because they are all high risk options, used mainly by the experts dealing with the exceptional cases.

If cannulation is unsuccessful and it is believed that the ductal lumen is better exposed if the superficial part of the sphincter is cut first, a papillotomy may be undertaken. This is achieved with a precut sphincterotome, where the wire runs right up to the tip, and cutting can be done with the instrument inserted for a few millimeters. The regular sphincterotome can then be used to cannulate the exposed duct. However, not infrequently after the precut, the endoscopist is still unable to see the duct or to insert the sphinctertome and, as edema forms rapidly, the view gets worse. Not only is obstruction unrelieved, but it may actually be aggravated. Precutting is therefore best reserved for special circumstances; it is not a sure rescue for the inexperienced. Even experts resort to it in fewer than 5 percent of cases.

When the papilla is bulging with an impacted stone, the orifice may be visible, but the sphincterotome or cannula may not be admitted for more than 1 or 2 mm. This circumstance is suitable for the cutting-down method, using a needle electrode. The instrument is a fine monopolar electrode, with a 3-mm-long fine wire tip. When used with blended current, the sphincter may be cut on top of the impacted stone. After the stone is removed, the regular sphincterotome may be inserted to complete the sphincterotomy.

When the intramural portion of the bile duct is dilated and appears as a vertical tubular structure, a cut may be made to create a choledochoduodenostomy proximal to the papilla (infundibulotomy), a technique used in Europe[29] but seldom seen in the United States. Needle aspiration is used to confirm that the tabular impression is in fact the bile duct, but when the impression is clear cut even this step may be omitted. A vertical stab wound with the needle electrode, 2 to 4 mm long, is made at the most prominent part of the impression, followed by insertion of either the regular sphincterotome to extend the incision up and down until a 1- to 2-cm incision has been made. This is a high-risk maneuver since; by definition, the infundibulum is the beginning of the extramural bile duct. As pointed out in the discussion of surgical anatomy, only adventitial tissue exists between the duct and the duodenal wall in the region just above the ampulla. When the duct is dilated, this segment of the bile duct is in close contact with the duodenal wall, enabling the procedure to be undertaken. The stones are removed from the duct through this opening.

Often the interventional radiologist is able to pass a guidewire, taking the percutaneous transhepatic route, into the bile duct and advance it through the papilla. The direction of the guidewire protruding from the papilla gives the best guide to position the sphincterotome for cannulation. If sphincterotomy is still not possible, the radiologist may be able to dilate the papilla using Gruntzig balloon dilators over the guidewire. The dilated sphincter should then be much easier to work with.[19]

If none of these options appears attractive, the procedure may either be reattempted on another day, referred to a more experienced colleague, or abandoned altogether, referring the patient for surgery.

STONE EXTRACTION

After sphincterotomy, the available options are (1) to leave the stones to be passed spontaneously, (2) to clear the duct with instrumentation over one or more sessions, the endoscopic equivalent of surgical exploration of the common bile duct, or (3) to leave a nasobiliary drain to circumvent cholangitis for possible stone dissolution therapy and for restudy, the endoscopic equivalent of surgical T-tube drainage. Considerable judgment is required to make a wise decision.

If stones are visible at the orifice after completion of the sphincterotomy, they are helped into the duodenum by any number of instruments. If they are seen high up in the left or right hepatic duct, a general rule is to let them pass spontaneously. Manipulation of these high-lying stones is only indicated when there is significant ductal obstruction behind them, when there is clinical cholangitis, or when there is a high likelihood of a large stone falling into the sphincterotomy precipitating obstruction in the next several days before the edema of the incision subsides. The majority of patients will have extrahepatic stones well inside the bile duct, for which extraction procedure will be necessary.

The simplest technique is to use the biliary balloon catheter. The catheter is inserted into the duct to beyond the stones and the balloon (1-cm diameter) inflated. The principle of using this balloon is the same as the Fogarty embolectomy catheter, and it works only if the duct is not much larger than the stone. Although the balloon is reasonably durable, it may rupture if it strikes against an irregular surface, such as the cannula elevator of the endoscope. Full inflation of the balloon in a small intrahepatic duct may rupture the duct and cause bleeding in the liver parenchyma. When the balloon is properly inflated, traction of the catheter will move the stones toward the sphincterotomy. It should be noted that the direction of traction is markedly altered at cannula elevator of the endoscope, and so a surprisingly large amount of force is needed to pull the balloon toward the endoscope. When the stone is visible through

the orifice, extending the tip of the endoscope with the balloon catheter fixed should deliver the stone into the duodenum, where it is left to be passed (Figs. 5-8 and 5-9B). Multiple passes may be necessary, each pass is aimed at removing the most distal stone. The balloon also serves to calibrate the orifice. Some endoscopists routinely calibrate the orifice before extraction. If a 1-cm balloon catches at the orifice, the opening is just under 1 cm, and stones larger than 1 cm will require enlargement of the orifice.

Another instrument that can be used is the Dormier basket. This instrument is indicated for large ducts—but not for large stones. The basket is passed closed and only opened after reaching a point beyond the stone. Then the

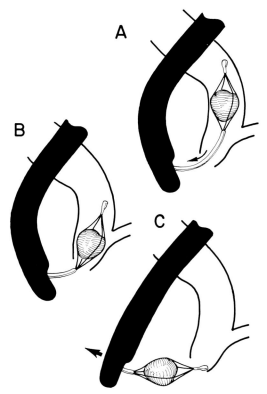

Fig. 5-8 Using the basket for stone extraction. (A) The stone is trapped by the open basket. Traction on the basket brings the stone toward the orifice. (B,C) The final 2 cm of the duct is cleared by extending the tip of the endoscope while maintaining traction of the basket. The identical technique is used for balloon extraction of stones.

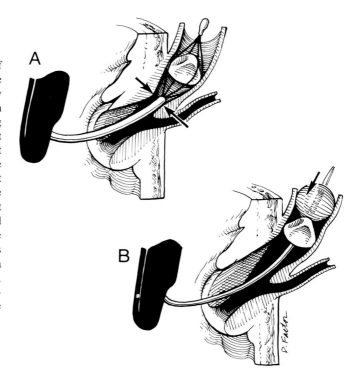

Fig. 5-9 (A) The mechanism of entrapment of basket. If despite some stretching the sphincterotomy is still smaller than the stone, then the basket, prevented from closing by the stone held within it, cannot clear the orifice. The stone cannot be easily discharged back into the duct either. If the duct is large, it is sometimes possible to disengage the stone by moving the basket back and forth in the duct, aided by gravity and positioning of the patient. Surgical disimpaction is necessary in many cases. (B) If a balloon catheter is used instead, the catheter can be removed by deflation of the balloon, even if the stone cannot be extracted.

basket is withdrawn in the open position in order to trap the stone, monitored under fluoroscopy. Even so, it is difficult to appreciate the spatial relationship of the wires of the basket and the stone, and a certain amount of trial and error is still necessary. The basket is withdrawn fully open (with the stone in it) and may only be partially closed at the papilla in order to clear it. As the basket is 2 cm or so from the orifice, the tip of the endoscope is depressed, thereby extricating the basket and stone from the duct (Fig. 5-8). If the sphincterotomy is smaller than the stone, entrapment of the basket may occur. This danger should always be considered before attempting to extract a large stone. Disengagement may not be possible, but it should be attempted by gently pushing back into the duct to give the stone plenty of space to fall out of the basket while it is fully open, followed by a trial of withdrawal (see under Complications). If the lithotripsy basket had been used instead, such difficulty may be overcome by cutting the stone into pieces. As yet, only a few experts have personal experience with this recently introduced instrument.

When the first exploration with the biliary balloon catheter produces no result, it should be repeated under fluoroscopy. Other helpful measures include tilting the table head up and irrigating with saline through either the biliary balloon catheter or an ERCP cannula. A larger balloon may be used if the duct is significantly larger, such as 2 cm or more in diameter, but a basket is generally indicated. A larger sphincterotomy is only indicated when the stone, as judged on radiography, is larger than the existing opening.

Even if it has been decided that the stones are left to be passed, one should still consider whether a nasobiliary drain should be placed at this time. For a solitary stone judged to be smaller than the sphincterotomy and quite out of reach, leaving a drain is meddlesome. A nasobiliary catheter is indicated when (1) there are large stones that cannot be removed after sphincterotomy, (2) there is a risk of cholangitis from the ensuing edema or from the stone falling down and getting impacted at the sphincterotomy, or (3) chemical dissolution is contemplated. Often a cholesterol stone, larger than

2.5 cm and therefore judged unsafe to remove, may be reduced in size by chemical dissolution before extraction. The nasobiliary drain may obviate a second duodenoscopy, as high-quality cholangiograms can be obtained through it. The technique of placing the nasobiliary catheter is described in Chapter 6.

Dissolution of stones with various solutions through the nasobiliary catheter has been summarized.[28] In general, the success rate is mediocre compared with extraction, with response rate no better than 50 to 60 percent when attempted either through a T-tube or nasobiliary drain. It is time consuming, requires prolonged hospitalization, and 60 to 80 percent of patients experience side effects such as vomiting, abdominal cramps, or diarrhea. The agent monooctanoin is the current agent of choice for cholesterol,[48] while a mixture of EDTA and bile acids (such as ursodeoxycholic acid and cholic acid) has been claimed to be effective for calcium bilirubinate stones. A new agent, methyl tert-butyl ether (MTBE), has been shown to have 50-fold activity over monooctanoin[1] in vitro and is being tested clinically. In vitro studies also point out the importance of stone-agent contact, attainable by creating turbulence in the infusion system and by bile exclusion, since the agents often float on bile while the stones sink. Under optimal stone-agent contact the efficacy is much enhanced. Stone dissolution by nasobiliary catheter using more effective agents such as MTBE is likely to have a significant clinical role in the near future.

Special Situations

Increased difficulty comes from unusual anatomy due to the presence of diverticula, previous surgery, or unfavorable anatomical variant.

A SHORT INTRAMURAL SEGMENT

When the choledochoduodenal junction is at more or less right angles, the segment may be very short, just wider than the thickness of the duodenal wall. The sphincterotomy cannot be more than 3 to 4 mm without running the risk of perforation. Surgical sphincteroplasty is indicated.

THE PAPILLA IN A DIVERTICULUM

The diverticulum in this region is usually *pseudodiverticulum,* consisting of mucosa only. If the papilla opens at the bottom of the diverticulum, endoscopic sphincterotomy cannot be safely done in this situation. However, in most cases the diverticulum opens near the papilla, which sits on the rim of the opening, and sphincterotomy can be performed in the usual way. The orientation of the cutting wire becomes crucially important.

PREVIOUS OPERATIONS

Billroth II Gastrectomy

The papilla is approached retrograde from the distal duodenum; the familiar route of the ERCP cannot be used. Many authors find it is simpler to use an end-viewing endoscope with a small turning radius for the control section, such a pediatric panendoscope, with the patient lying supine. The Sohma type of sphincterotome (shark's fin) may be used but the conventional Erlangen type will usually do.

Billroth I Gastrectomy

After a generous resection of the first portion of the duodenum, the ampulla comes to lie very close to the gastroduodenostomy. There may also be varying degrees of rotation of the duodenum upon the stomach. The tip of the duodenoscope may have to ride astride the anastomosis, an unstable position at best. Both searching and cannulation are rendered considerably more difficult.

Previous Choledochoduodenostomy

A forward-viewing panendoscope should be used with the patient on the supine position for cannulation of the anastomosis, but a cholangiogram can only be obtained with a balloon catheter preventing the loss of contrast into the duodenum. The air in the biliary tree in this condition, unlike air bubbles introduced inadvertently during cholangiography, does not interfere with interpretation of the radiographs if the head down position is maintained during exposure, since the air here serves more like double contrasts. Incision to enlarge a strictured choledochoduodenostomy is hazardous, and should only be attempted if the cholangiogram shows a diaphragmlike stenosis at the anastomosis. For all other types of narrowing, balloon dilation should be used instead. Biliary balloon dilators are fashioned after the Gruntzig catheters (see Chapter 6). Infrequently, following stenosis of a choledochodenostomy, stagnation in the distal common bile duct (the sump syndrome) may be treated by drainage by a sphincterotomy at the ampulla with the conventional technique.

Previous Sphincterotomy or Sphincteroplasty

An endoscopic sphincterotomy is simpler to revise than a surgical sphincterotomy. Generally a stenotic endoscopic sphincterotomy results from residual sphincter fibers, although restenosis (estimated to be 6 percent or so) may be due to scarring. The incision can be enlarged with the sphincterotome in the usual manner. A stenotic surgical sphincterotomy or even sphincteroplasty are associated with more scarring. The duodenotomy suture line, opposite the ampulla, appears as either a vertical or oblique or even transverse mucosal ridge, depending on the direction of the duodenotomy. Occasionally it is marked by residual silk sutures. The duodenal loop itself may be altered in shape from the previous mobilization, but does not usually present any major problem. The papilla

is hardly recognizable as such, it is usually flat with the bile duct opening to the upper end of a narrow slit, while the pancreatic duct opens to its lower end. Cannulation is difficult as the axis of the lower duct may be markedly altered. These challenging cases are sometimes approached by combined radiologic–endoscopic techniques, using percutaneous transheptic placement of guidewire which is advanced through the papilla, followed by endoscopic sphincterotomy. Even so, the hazard of perforation is increased as the intramural part of the duct has been previously incised. Revision must be confined to incision on the scar, the extent of which is difficult to appreciate.

COMPLICATIONS

Bleeding

Bleeding is the most common complication in all series. Less than one-half are limited in extent and do not require transfusion. In the more serious bleeders, including delayed bleeding presenting days after the procedure, transfusion and hemodynamic stablization is the first line treatment.

Continued bleeding with circulatory instability requires intervention. Endoscopic option is rarely attempted, mostly because few of the probes available for hemostasis (e.g., heater probe, bipolar probes, laser waveguides, injectors) are designed to be used with the duodenoscope. The exposure is unlikely to be easy; the lesion is often at the end of the cut, where further endoscopic treatment may invite perforation. Radiological methods are worth trying, particularly the vaso-occlusive techniques, but the rich collaterals in the pancreatic arcade may require more than one superselective catheterization. If the bleeding vessel is demonstrated to be a branch of the anterior or posterior superior pancreaticoduodenal artery, usually a transverse branch occurring anywhere from 0.5 to 3 cm above the papilla, embolization with steel coils may be feasible. Whenever possible, the arcade distal to the bleeding branch is embolized first, followed by embolization of the arcade proximal to it. Failure of this modality to arrest bleeding requires emergency surgery. Surgical treatment is the most certain for immediate hemostasis, but delayed rebleeding, often massive, accounts for most of the mortality reported. At operation the second portion of the duodenum is first mobilized by a generous Kocher maneuver. Some retroperitoneal bruising on the inner border of the duodenum marks the site of the lesion, but when extensive, a concomitant perforation must be searched for. Bidigital compression of the pancreaticoduodenal arcade will usually slow down or stop the bleeding as the duodenum is opened opposite the hematoma. The sphincterotomy is identified and converted to a sphincteroplasty, placing serial sutures to approximate the edge of the duodenal mucosa to the ductal mucosa. Sometimes hemostasis is secured upon completion of the sphincteroplasty. If not, the bleeding artery is often identifiable by releasing pressure on the pancreatoduodenal arcade, and is suture ligated. At times the artery may have retracted into the pancreatic head and suture ligation is either ineffective, or that the integrity of the pancreatic duct or lower bile duct cannot be determined with certainty after multiple suture ligations. Ligation of the pancreaticoduodenal artery at its origin from the hepatic artery may be tried, it is unlikely to be effective and a pancreaticoduodenectomy has to be undertaken under those circumstances. A mortality as high as 61 percent has been reported in all bleeding complications requiring surgical intervention.[16,39,42]

Perforation

Retroperitoneal perforation probably occurs more commonly than reported, since it results in few symptoms if minor. A routine contrast study after completion of the sphincteroplasty showing no extravasation does not rule out perforation, since the injection is up the duct; the duodenum may not be completely outlined by the backflow. Air in the retroperitoneal planes is diagnostic. Pneumoperitoneum means perfo-

ration near the anterior pancreatic border with the duodenum. Symptoms of perforation includes persistent and increasing pain, tachycardia, increased fluid requirement, abdominal distension, and signs of peritonitis (for anterior perforation). When no air is demonstrable radiologically, the symptoms can not be clearly differentiated from other related complications such as cholangitis or pancreatitis, as an abscess formed in the head of the pancreas can produce the symptoms and signs of all these.

Initial treatment with rest of the gut by nasogastric decompression, intravenous fluids, broad-spectrum antibiotics, and pain relief is warranted if no free perforation is demonstrable. If symptoms persist or worsen, surgical exploration is indicated. The perforation may be difficult to find even after the duodenum has been mobilized as it is hidden by the head of the pancreas, but tell-tale air bubbles when the part is submerged in saline usually lead to the lesion. Suture repair must be performed from inside the duodenum after exposure by duodenotomy, serosal sutures placed without visualization of the duct runs a high risk of occlusion of the ductal orifice. Conversion into a sphincteroplasty is necessary to ensure adequate pancreatic and bile drainage. Drainage of the retroperitoneal space must be assured.

Pancreatitis

Transient abdominal pain (less than 24 hours) with mild elevation of amylase is not uncommon after the procedure, and does not constitute true pancreatitis. However, if symptoms are severe and persistent, the diagnosis of pancreatitis and or closed perforation must be entertained. The treatment of both is conservative at first. The incidence of true pancreatitis is low in large series, but the mortality of those requiring surgical intervention is 80 to 90 percent,[16,39] suggesting that surgery may be too late in many cases. Since closed perforation may manifest clinically the same way, it is possible that some perforations have been misdiagnosed as pancreatitis, especially in units where a nonoperative policy of treatment of perforation is routinely pursued. Earlier detection of developing complications such as retroperitoneal abscess or pancreatic abscesses with CT scans combined with an aggressive policy of surgical drainage may result in lower mortality.

It is assumed that most pancreatitis is caused by edema of the pancreatic ductal opening. If the pancreatic duct is injured (e.g., partially cut) and recognized during the procedure, early surgical stenting of the duct should be considered although experience is scarce. Some experts claim that using pure cutting current routinely in sphincterotomy reduces or even eliminates the incidence of pancreatitis.

Cholangitis

Cholangitis following sphincterotomy is usually caused by stones becoming impacted at the orifice, which is too small for their free passage. Clinically it manifests as septicemia with jaundice and often pain, arising within a day or two following an apparently uneventful endoscopic procedure. The incidence is between 1 to 2 percent in most series. Endoscopic drainage should be instituted under adequate antibiotic cover. If drainage is unsatisfactory and the stone cannot be disimpacted, surgical intervention should be undertaken without delay. When surgery is required, the surgical mortality is as high as 40 percent. Many endoscopists have adopted the practice of inserting a nasobiliary drain in the duct to circumvent this complication under selected circumstances (Chapter 6). When there are multiple residual stones in the duct, the presence of the drain prevents complete occlusion of the opening, allows infusion for stone dislodgement or chemical dissolution, and permits high-quality follow-up contrast study without endoscopy.

Septicemia

Prophylactic antibiotics is not a routine practice in most centers. However, patients at high risk of septicemia should be placed on antibiotics before undergoing the procedure. Also, the instruments should be thoroughly disinfected before use. Since the clinical manifestation is similar to other complications such as perforation and pancreatitis and cholangitis, these have to be ruled out early in the management.

Entrapment of the Stone Basket

This is likely to happen in the course of extraction of large stones. Figure 5-9A illustrates the mechanics involved. If the stone is larger than the sphincterotomy, the stone prevents the basket from closing and so neither the stone nor the basket can be withdrawn. This complication is identical to that occurring in the radiological technique of percutaneous retrieval of stones through the T-tube tract (see Chapter 7). In fact, the complication may occur even if the stone is just as large as the sphincterotomy, since the basket occupies some space. It may prove impossible to dislodge the stone from the basket in order to disengage the entrapment. Helpful maneuvers include tilting the patient's head down and moving the basket back and forth in the duct under fluoroscopy in the hope of shaking the stone loose. This is unlikely to be successful if the duct is not much larger than the stone. If successful, the basket should be withdrawn open, since in closing it may snare some ductal mucosa and cause ductal injury.

If the stone basket is constructed with a flexible metal sheath capable of withstanding the force necessary to cut through the softer stones (a recently introduced lithotripsy device), the entrapment problem may be solved simply by increasing the force of closure to cut through the stone. If an ordinary basket is used, which has only a polyethylene sheath, the handle should be cut off and endoscope removed. It is then reinserted and the sphincterotomy should be enlarged with a sphincterotome, being careful to avoid unwanted electrical contact with the basket. If it is too risky to enlarge the sphincterotomy further, a catheter may be inserted into the duct to attempt dislodging the stone from the basket. Finally, when every means has failed the cut off basket may be left without tension for spontaneous disimpaction. Surgical removal is undertaken if no progress occurs within a day or two or if symptoms of sepsis occur.

This complication may be avoided if the Dormier basket is not used at all, as a few endoscopists advocate, relying on the biliary balloon for all stone extraction, and resorting to the lithotripsy basket for the largest stones.

Acute Cholecystitis, Empyema of Gallbladder

Acute presentation of this condition may be as soon as 1–2 days following the procedure, but is rare. Gallstone ileus has been reported following a generous sphincterotomy.

LONG-TERM SEQUELAE

Cholecystitis

For patients who have an intact gallbladder, a low incidence of acute cholecystitis (about 2 percent) is observed within 1 year; and perhaps a further 10 percent may require elective cholecystectomy within 2 years for recurrent symptoms of right upper quadrant and epigastric pain typical of chronic cholecystitis.[10,14,29] Considering that the vast majority of these gallbladders already contained stones, sphincterotomy does not seem to have as deleterious an effect on the pathological gallbladder as one would expect from the disturbed pattern of bile flow. Many endoscopists are now routinely performing sphincterotomy for common bile duct stones in patients with intact gallbladders, irrespective of age or surgical risks, a practice bound to impact upon the traditional concept of biliary surgery.

Restenosis With or Without Recurrent Stones

The proponents of surgical sphincterotomy pointed out that the surgical sphincterotomy is likely to result in restenosis since mucosa-to-mucosa suturing is not performed. This created a lingering doubt of the long-term efficacy of the procedure in the early days of endoscopic sphincterotomy. Long term follow-up studies are still limited, since most patients are elderly and do not have a long life expectancy. Several studies, however, are broadly consistent and indicate that 5 to 10 percent may develop restenosis, new stones, or both after 5 years or more.[14,29,37,46] Classen reported 1 to 3-year follow-up of 51 patients with no restenosis.[6] It therefore seems that restenosis has not been a major problem and does not significantly detract from the virtues of the procedure. Stasis from restenosis may generate new stones, and recurrent cholangitis has been reported.

Reflux of Duodenal Content into the Biliary Tree

Air outlining the biliary ducts and reflux of barium occurs in about 60 to 70 percent of patients after endoscopic sphincteroplasty. Almost all postsphincterotomy patients studied in long-term follow-up have chronic bacterial colonization of the biliary tree.[6,46] The clinical significance of these observations is as yet unknown. It is possible that restenosis may lead to cholangitis due to bacterial proliferation in the stagnant bile, leading to stone formation in the obstructed duct.

RESULTS

By 1983, ten years after the introduction of endoscopic sphincterotomy, it was estimated that more than 50,000 procedures were performed, with a generally low mortality and morbidity, a similar tribute to which very few surgical procedures can lay claim. Tables 5-1 and 5-2 summarize the complications and mortalities of several large personal series and surveys. It should be remembered that these are the results obtained by the experts, and do not necessarily represent the results attainable by the not-so-expert practitioners of the art. Even large sur-

Table 5-1. Results of Endoscopic Sphincterotomy: Single-Institution Series

Complication	Hatfield[20] N = 241	Cotton[8] N = 129	Safrany[38] N = 243	Liguory[29] N = 451
Bleeding	2.9%	4.6%	2.8%	4.2%
Cholangitis	2.5%	1.5%	2.0%	1.8%
Pancreatitis	1.7%	0%	1.2%	1.1%
Instrument impaction	1.2%	1.5%	0.4%	—
Retroperitoneal perforation	0%	0%	3.3%	1.6%
Death	0%	1.2%	1.2%	1.1%

veys do not necessarily reflect the true incidence of complications as encountered in daily practice, since it is difficult to standardize the definition of complication among those surveyed.

Despite such reservations, it is clear that the procedure has a low overall mortality and morbidity, considering that most patients belong to the high-risk category. Success in completing sphincterotomy is greater than 95 percent, and of these, 90 percent have successful clearance of stones, so that the total success rate of this procedure for treating choledocholithiasis is about 85 percent.[11,20,29,38,39,41] This success rate is even higher than the overall success rate for ERCP. The reason is that the technique is attempted only by those who are already experts at ERCP, and adjunctive techniques, such as precutting, may aid cannulation. The success rate is unchanged for the subgroup of patients suffering from cholangitis and acute septic complications.[40,45] In these patients, the response to endoscopic sphincterotomy is gratifying, provided decompression has been successful. This is in contrast to surgery, which carries a higher mortality and morbidity in the presence of cholangitis.[13,17,33]

The reverse of success rate, namely, failure to clear the duct of stones, is the equivalent of the oft-quoted surgical complication, retained stones, and is about 10 percent in the hands of those endoscopists who routinely extract stones after sphincterotomy and confirm the clearance with cholangiograms. Therefore, about 15 percent of cases overall the endoscopist is unable to deal successfully with choledocholithiasis, including inability to get to the ampulla, cannulate it, cut it, or retrieve the stones.

The immediate procedure-related complication rate, such as hemorrhage and perforation, is 8 to 10 percent, requiring surgical treatment in only 1 to 2 percent. A mortality of 1 percent is fairly consistent. When deaths from concomitant diseases are included, the mortality figures are somewhat higher, closer to 2 to 3 percent. Considering that most of these patients are elderly poor surgical risks, the endoscopic procedure hardly takes a second seat to surgery.

Many factors are known to influence the development of complications. Seifert[41] showed that sphincterotomy for papillary stenosis doubles the complication rate, as compared with choledocholithiasis. It is not clear why this is

Table 5-2. Results of Endoscopic Sphincterotomy: Multiinstitution Surveys[a]

Complication	U.S.[42] N = 5,790	German[41] N = 7,209	European[39] N = 3,618
Bleeding	1.5 (61%)	1.9 (39%)	2.5 (14%)
Cholangitis	1.3 (8%)	1.1 (39%)	1.4 (22%)
Pancreatitis	2.1 (100%)	1.1 (72%)	1.4 (19%)
Instrument/stone impaction	0.2 (22%)	—	0.7 (11%)
Retroperitoneal perforation	1.0 (4%)	0.7 (31%)	1.1 (35%)
Mortality	0.4%	1.1%	1.4%

[a] All figures are percentages of total number sphinctertomy completed (N). Mortality associated with the complications is in parenthesis.

so; perhaps the lack of fibrosis associated with calculous disease predisposes to perforation. Large stones increase the risk, as do longer sphincterotomies, which are more susceptible to bleeding and perforation. Other known factors are the presence of an intact gallbladder, coagulation abnormalities, and anatomic and surgical deformities that increase the technical difficulties. Age does not seem to influence the endoscopic results.

THE ROLE OF ENDOSCOPIC SPHINCTEROTOMY IN BILIARY SURGERY

Although direct comparison of results of endoscopic sphincterotomy and biliary surgery for calculous disease has been said to be like comparing apples to oranges,[11] the surgical results must nevertheless be surveyed in order to understand the significance of the endoscopic contribution. In a recent international study of more than 1,000 consecutive patients in 21 institutions around the world,[12] the mortality for all primary (first operations) biliary procedures in which the common duct was explored was 4.4 percent, and for all secondary (reoperations) procedures, almost all of which involve the common bile duct, it was 2.3 percent. Both figures agree well with previously published large series from single institutions in the United States.[33] The fact that reoperations carry a lower mortality may reflect the self-selecting nature of the problem; many critically ill patients may not come to a second operation, and more experienced surgeons are usually given to perform the reoperations. It certainly does not mean that they are less technically difficult. Factors contributing to death included advanced age, acute cholecystitis, choledocholithiasis, and concomitant diseases such as ischemic heart disease and cirrhosis of liver. Indeed, in contrast to the endoscopic procedure, the associated conditions rather than the operation itself seem to determine the operative mortality.

In the same worldwide study, the biliary-related complication rate after the primary operations for cholecystectomy with common duct exploration was 19.8 percent, while the complication rate following secondary operations, almost all of which involved the common bile duct, was 40 percent. These figures appear to be higher than previously published results from single institutions, which typically listed complications arising from cholecystectomy with common duct exploration as 14 percent[17] and 16 percent,[4,13] inclusive of nonbiliary complications, such as atelectasis and myocardial infarction. It is difficult to compare different studies, as definition of complications may not be the same. In the international study, the figures for individual U.S. and foreign centers are similar, the consistency lending considerable credence. There was no age specific breakdown in that study, but in all previous studies the mortality and morbidity for the older age group have been much higher than the overall figures.[13,17,33]

The specific complication that measures efficacy of the operative procedure is retained stones. Reliable figures are difficult to come by, but an incidence of 8 percent was reported in those cases where the duct was diligently searched for stones intraoperatively[16,48] and about double that if not. The efficacy of the surgical procedure is thus arguably better than the endoscopic procedure. The overall statistics leave little doubt that surgery for biliary duct is much more invasive than the endoscopic procedure, even though direct comparison can be misleading.

The complications of biliary drainage operations of sphincteroplasty and choledochoduodenostomy are in addition to those already considered for cholecystectomy alone, probably 1 to 5 percent higher.[22,23,30,31] Specific indications for either sphincteroplasty or choledochoduodenostomy are recognized, although there are a large group of patients in whom either operation may be performed. Sphincteroplasty is particularly indicated for stenosis of the papilla with history of pancreatitis, while choledochoduodenostomy is usually chosen for its expediency, and for marked stasis with markedly tortuous and dilated ducts. For all other cases in which drainage is indicated, there has been much argument as to the merit of each drainage procedure: The mortality and operative complication appear to be somewhat higher following sphinctero-plasty,[30,31] a more delicate and time-consuming operation. Pancreatitis and retroperitoneal leak are the specific risks. Choledochoduodenostomy is undeniably easier to do, but it is associated with a specific restenosis rate, and the development of the sump syndrome in the occasional patient.[22,23] As the endoscopic procedure is not designed for a complete sphincterotomy, when the patient has a markedly dilated duct and a long sphincteric segment, endoscopic sphincter-otomy is not likely to provide adequate drainage.

While the complications for endoscopic sphincterotomy are low, the mortality associated with the complication is high, almost 50 percent overall in large surveys (Table 5-2). By contrast, the mortality/morbidity ratio in biliary surgery is between 5 and 10 percent. Such distinct differences are clear even without direct statistical comparison.

How does operating skill influence outcome in endoscopic and surgical procedures? The outcome of endoscopic procedure in general is skill dependent (see Chapter 1), and in sphinctero-tomy, a learning curve may extend to more than 50 procedures for some endoscopists; results are poor during the learning phase.[9] Individual expertise obviously also influences the outcome of biliary surgery, but it is more likely to do so in the area of judgment and the choice of procedures in addition to the actual operating technique, as in many other operations.

With these facts at hand, the role of endoscopic sphincterotomy for choledocholithiasis may be seen in better perspective. First, the endoscopic procedure has a clearly established place for the patient unfit for surgery, including those with cholangitis and septicemia. The presence of the gallbladder influences the choice only in that when acute cholecystitis or empyema coexists with choledocholithiasis, the treatment for stones should be surgical. A gall-bladder that is the seat of chronic symptoms may influence the choice of surgery for the ductal stones, but it can also be argued that endoscopic sphincterotomy should be done first, and

that cholecystectomy can be performed electively with a lower morbidity and mortality. One tends to recommend surgery if the endoscopist is lacking in expertise or if an experienced biliary surgeon is available. Surgery is definitely indicated if the stones are large (over 20 to 25 mm) and multiple, if the patient has had a previous Billroth II gastrectomy, if the papilla is known to be situated at the bottom of a diverticulum, or if stones are impacted above a stricture longer than a sphincterotomy can safely correct. A markedly dilated and tortu-ous duct is best drained by a choledochoduode-nostomy.

These considerations are subject to revision as techniques in endoscopic intervention continue to advance. Already large stones are removable by a lithotripsy basket introduced recently; it remains for experience to accumulate to prove it safe. Clinical tests of more efficacious stone dissolving agents are underway and if successful may have similarly profound effect on the selection of endoscopy versus surgery. Stones found above strictures, now thought to be out of reach to most endoscopists, may not be so if the stricture can be dilated with balloon dilators (see Chapter 6), followed either by crushing of the stones or by dissolution. New endoscopic technology developed for fracturing of stones in the urinary tract may be modified in future for use in the biliary tract. Even more potential exists for the prevention of retained stones by appropriate deployment of preoperative endoscopy (see Chapter 7), such as ERCP. Per papilla choledochoscopy may be possible in the future with development of a daughter biliary endoscope that can be inserted via the duodenoscope for a thorough inspection of the entire biliary tree, a far better method of exploration of the bile ducts than the existing surgical technique.

The rhetorical question often asked by the accomplished young endoscopist is: if the endoscopic technique is safe and efficacious for high-risk patients, why not for low-risk patients? A look at the complication rates suffices to cause most surgeons to pause and think. Although the overall mortality is low, biliary surgery is associated with a significant morbidity, undoubtedly high in the elderly patient with multisystemic disease but still substantial in the younger better-risk patients. The cost, hospital bed utilization, time off work, patient preference, all favor the endoscopic procedure,[11] even in the 20 percent or so where more than one endoscopic session is required. Admittedly surgical sphincteroplasty is superior in attaining a large opening and complete division of the sphincter fibers, but is this routinely necessary for the majority of patients with the uncomplicated stones in the common duct? It is in this area that the impact of endoscopic sphincterotomy is just beginning to be felt. The increasing trend to offer to good-risk patients the less invasive procedure will eventually force a reexamination of the traditional role of surgery in calculous disease of the biliary tract. It is clear to this author that operations other than cholecystectomy will increasingly be looked on as a secondary procedure in the not so distant future. Surgeons will be called upon to operate for common duct stone only after failure of endoscopic sphincterotomy or perhaps for cases anatomically unfavorable for the endoscopic method and for complications secondary to the endoscopic procedure. It is not unreasonable to predict that operation on the common bile duct for stones will eventually be replaced by an endoscopic procedure, just as colotomy for polyps has been replaced by endoscopic polypectomy. Rapid endoscopic technological development is likely to impact most on this area of GI surgery, and in order to use these techniques as well as surgery appropriately, full integration of the surgical and endoscopic skills is essential in any clinical centers caring for such patients. An algorithm for the management of clinical obstructive jaundice is given in Chapter 6.

THERAPEUTIC ENDOSCOPY OF THE PANCREATIC DUCT

Theoretically, much that has been developed to relieve obstruction of the lower end of the bile duct can be applied to the pancreatic duct.

However, there are only a few conditions in which obstruction is confined to the lower end of the duct; much more commonly the obstruction is multiple and diffuse. As a pilot study, Cotton[7] reported relief of chronic pancreatic pain from pancreas divisum by sphincterotomy of the accessory papilla. It is possible to perform a septectomy or open the pancreatic duct with a fine sphincterotome, but the clinical definition of the condition is difficult and no data so far exist to support this application. A few cases of intubation to relieve carcinomatous obstruction of the pancreatic duct has been reported but the efficacy is unclear.

REFERENCES

1. Allen MJ, Borody TJ, Thistle JL: In vitro dissolution of cholesterol gallstone. Gastroenterology 89:1097, 1985
2. Bar-Meir S, Geenen JE, Hogan WJ, et al: Biliary and pancreatic duct pressures measured by ERCP manometry in patients with suspected papillary stenosis. Dig Dis Sci 24:209, 1979
3. Boyden EA: The anatomy of the choledochoduodenal junction in man. Surg Gynecol Obstet 104:641, 1957
4. Broughan TA, Sivak MV, Hermann RE: The management of retained and recurrent bile duct stones. Surgery 98:746, 1985
5. Classen M, Demling L: Endoskopische shpinkterotomie de papilla Vateriund steinextraktion aus dem ductus choledochus. Dtsch Med Wochenschr 99:496, 1974
6. Classen M, Burmeister W, Hagenmuller F, et al: Long term examination after endoscopic papillotomy. Gastrointest Endosc 25:37, 1979
7. Cotton PB: Endoscopic cannulation and sphincterotomy at the accessory papilla in pancreatic divisum. Gastrointest Endosc 25:37, 1979
8. Cotton PB: Non-operative removal of bile duct stones by duodenoscopic sphincterotomy. Br J Surg 67:1, 1980
9. Cotton PB, Vallon AG: British experience with duodenoscopic sphincterotomy for removal of bile duct stones. Br J Surg 68:373, 1981
10. Cotton PB, Vallon AG: Duodenoscopic sphincterotomy for removal of bile duct stones in patients with gallbladders. Surgery 91:628, 1982
11. Cotton PB: Endoscopic management of bile duct stone (apples and oranges).Gut 25:587, 1984

12. DenBesten L, Berci G: The current status of biliary surgery: An international study of 1072 consecutive patients. World J Surg 10:116, 1986

13. Dowdy GS Jr, Waldron GW: Importance of coexistent factors in biliary tract surgery. (An analysis of 2285 operations.) Arch Surg 88:314, 1964

14. Escourrou J, Cordova JA, Lazorthes F, et al: Early and late complications after endoscopic sphincterotomy for biliary lithiasis with and without the gallbladder "in situ." Gut 25:598, 1984

15. Geenen JE, Hogan WJ, Dodds J, et al: Intraluminal pressure recording for the human sphincter of Oddi. Gastroenterology 78:317, 1980

16. Geenen JE, Vennes JA, Silvis SE: Resume of a seminar on endoscopic retrograde sphincterotomy. Gastrointest Endosc 27:31, 1981

17. Glenn F, McSherry CK, Dineen P: Morbidity of surgical treatment for non-malignant biliary tract disease. Surg Gynecol Obstet 126:15, 1968

18. Hampson LG, Petrie EA: The problem of stones in the common bile duct, with particular reference to retained stones. Can J Surg 7:361, 1964

19. Hatfield ARW, Murray AS, Lennard-Jones JE: Periampullary diverticula and common duct calculi: A combined transhepatic and endoscopic technique for difficult cases. Gut 23:889, 1982

20. Hatfield ARW: Endoscopic sphincterotomy and gallstone removal. p. 119. In Motson RW (ed): Retained Common Duct Stones, Prevention and Treatment. Grune & Stratton, New York, 1985

21. Ingelfinger FJ: Endoscopic pancreatocholangiography: Progress and problem. (Editorial.) N Engl J Med 287:879, 1972

22. Jones SA, Smith LL: A reappraisal of sphincteroplasty (not sphincterotomy). Surgery 71:565, 1972

23. Jones SA: The prevention and treatment of recurrent bile duct stones by transduodenal sphincteroplasty. World J Surg 2:473, 1978

24. Kawai K, Akasaka Y, Murakami K, et al: Endoscopic sphincterotomy of the ampulla of Vater. Gastrointest Endosc 20:148, 1974

25. Kjellgren K: Persistent symptoms following biliary surgery. Ann Surg 152:1026, 1960

26. Kune GA: Surgical anatomy of the common bile duct. Arch Surg 89:995, 1964

27. Kune GA: Gallstones. p. 169. In Kune GA, Sali A (eds): The Practice of Biliary Surgery. 2nd Ed. Blackwell, Boston, 1980

28. Leuschner U, Baumgartel H, Klempa J: Chemical treatment of choledocholithiasis. p. 81. In Classen M, Greenen J, Kawai K (eds): Non-surgical Biliary Drainage. Springer-Verlag, New York, 1984

29. Liguory C: Endoscopic sphincterotomy. p. 373. In Kune G, Sali A (eds): The Practice of Biliary Surgery. 2nd ed. Blackwell, Boston, 1980

30. Lygidakis NJ: Choledochoduodenostomy in biliary calculous diseases. Br J Surg 68:762, 1981

31. Lygidakis NJ: A prospective randomized study of recurrent choledocholithiasis. Surg Gynecol Obstet 155:679, 1982

32. McCune WL, Shorb PE, Moscovitz H: Endoscopic cannulation of the ampulla of Vater: A preliminary report. Ann Surg 167:752, 1968

33. McSherry CK, Glenn F: The incidence and causes of death following surgery for non-malignant biliary tract disease. Ann Surg 191:271, 1980

34. Moody FG: Papillary function and physiology. p. 163. In Salmon PR (ed): Gastrointestinal Endoscopy. Advances in Diagnosis and Treatment. Williams & Wilkins, Baltimore, 1984

35. Ono K, Wanatabe N, Suzuki K, et al: Bile flow mechanism in man. Arch Surg 96:869, 1968

36. Orloff MJ: Importance of surgical technique in prevention of retained and recurrent bile duct stones. World J Surg 2:403, 1978

37. Rosch W, Riemann JR, Lux G, et al: Long-term follow-up after endoscopic sphincterotomy. Endoscopy 13:152, 1981

38. Safrany L: Duodenoscopic sphincterotomy and gallstone removal. Gastroenterology 72:338, 1977

39. Safrany L: Endoscopic treatment of biliary-tract diseases. An international study. Lancet 2:893, 1978

40. Safrany L, Cotton PB: A preliminary report: Urgent duodenoscopic sphincterotomy for acute gallstone pancreatitis. Surgery 89:424, 1981

41. Seifert E: Endoscopy and biliary disease. p. 73. In Blumgart LH (ed): Clinical Surgery International. The Biliary Tract. Churchill Livingstone, New York, 1982

42. Silvis SE, Vennes JA: Endoscopic retrograde sphincterotomy. p. 231. In Silvis SE (ed): Therapeutic Gastrointestinal Endoscopy. Igaku-Shoin, New York, 1984

43. Smith SW, Engel C, Averbrook B, et al: Problems of retained and recurrent common bile duct stones. JAMA 164:231, 1957

44. Tansy MF, Kendall FM: Choledochoduodenal junction. p. 93. In Friedman MHF (ed): Functions of the Stomach and Intestine. University Park Press, Baltimore, 1975

45. Vallon AG, Shorvon PJ, Cotton PB: Duodeno-scopic treatment of acute cholangitis. Gut 23:A915, 1982

46. Vallon AG, Cotton PB, Holton J: Clinical and endoscopic follow-up after duodenoscopic sphincterotomy. Gut 22:A889, 1982

47. Van Berge Henegouwen GP, Hofmann AF: Nocturnal gallbladder storage and emptying in gall-stone patients and healthy subjects. Gastroenter-ology 75:879, 1978

48. Venu RP, Geenen JE, Toouli J, et al: Gallstone dissolution using monooctanoin infusion through an endoscopically placed catheter. Am J Gastroenterol 77:227, 1982

49. Way LW, Admirand WH, Dunphy JE: Management of choledocholithiasis. Ann Surg 347:176, 1972

6

Nonsurgical Drainage of the Obstructed Biliary Tract

The first sphincterotomy, performed only 6 years after the first endoscopic cannulation of the ampulla, opened the door to the entire field of per oral therapeutic endoscopy of the biliary tract. In the beginning, therapeutic efforts were directed toward calculous diseases in the patient unfit for surgery, but success soon encouraged the development of techniques for palliation of nonresectable malignant conditions.

As in the evolution of many techniques of nonsurgical intervention, the development of endoscopic drainage of the biliary system was preceded by the percutaneous radiologic method. The disadvantages of the radiologic method, mainly the complications associated with the percutaneous puncture of the liver, simply served to highlight the advantages of the endoscopic approach. Sphincterotomy was the first endoscopic method of drainage of the biliary tract. For lesions higher than the sphincter, drainage by intubation has to be utilized. The nasobiliary drain was used in 1976 by Nagai et al.[35] to prevent cholangitis after sphincterotomy for choledocholithiasis. This technique was subsequently applied to decompress malignant obstruction.[58,59] As a long tube with a fine lumen, high resistance to flow made it unsuitable for long-term use. The endoprosthesis[44,45] was next developed for internal drainage; it was

shorter and therefore had less resistance to flow. Bile was drained internally, obviating the loss of bile and the discomforts of a tube draining to the outside. As the skill progressed, higher and higher obstructive lesions were tackled, and the prostheses were inserted deeper and deeper into the biliary tree. At the same time, to overcome frequent blockage (which invariably leads to cholangitis), larger and larger prostheses were used. Today, multiple prostheses may be inserted, one for each of the major ductal systems for obstruction of the bifurcation; and prostheses as large as 15 Fr. can be inserted by a combination of endoscopic and radiologic methods without surgery.[38] These endoscopic techniques eliminate the disadvantages of radiologic and surgical intubation and have already earned a place in modern biliary surgery. Much research is still needed as many technical problems have remained unsolved.

In this rapidly developing field, it is particularly important for the clinician to retain a sense of perspective as to what therapeutic endoscopy and surgery can achieve in order not to be carried away by undue optimism and enthusiasm for a new technique. Unlike sphincterotomy, insertion of an endoprosthesis involves implantation of a foreign body into the biliary system, where some stasis will always be inevitable due to partial obstruction, even when the endoprosthesis is effective in achieving some degree of decompression. Infection is therefore a main concern. Experience with surgical intubation for benign strictures has taught surgeons that clogging due to debris and sediment is a function of the duration of implantation. Despite glowing reports in the endoscopic literature that accompany the development of each larger prosthesis, clogging will predictably occur no matter the size. Attacks of cholangitis brought on by clogging signal an urgent need to change the endoprosthesis. Particularly in malignant obstruction, the mortality of such attacks, when septicemia is present, is high[24,48] despite antibiotic therapy. Furthermore, *Pseudomonas,* an unusual organism in primary biliary infection, is the predominant organism in such episodes. Camara et al.[13] showed that the endoscope is an important source of *Pseudomonas.* Despite scrupulous antisepsis of the instruments, when cholangitis follows endoscopic manipulations in a previously nonseptic patient, the endoscope must still be suspect. Eradication of the organisms in the presence of a foreign body and partial obstruction is highly unlikely. Therefore, despite the undeniable expediency of the endoscopic methods, this author is convinced that intubation for palliation of malignant obstruction of the biliary tract is conceptually unsound, just as it is for the esophagus (see Chapter 10), although for a different reason. Since the art is still young, all the potential hazards have not been completely described; it is well for endoscopists in nonacademic centers to use this technique with caution and conservatism.

NASOBILIARY DRAINAGE

Indications

Although the nasobiliary drain was originally used for palliation of malignant jaundice, the accepted indications today are confined to short-term or temporary use. This deserves emphasis, since the clinician, on seeing how well it has worked initially in treating acute cholangitis, is tempted to leave it in place for longer than it is intended. Recurrence of cholangitis may be the result (see indications for endoprosthesis). An arbitrary line may be drawn at 2 to 3 weeks.

After sphincterotomy for choledocholithiasis, nasobiliary drainage prevents the residual stones from falling into the lower end of the duct and impacting at the orifice, thereby reducing the hazards of cholangitis. Thus a nasobiliary drain is indicated when residual stones in the duct are not removable at the time of sphincterotomy, when these stones are larger than 2 cm and therefore difficult to remove, and when numerous stones are present. The drain also permits chemical infusion for dissolution of a large stone and for repeat cholangiograms to study the progress of spontaneous passage of stones. Antibiotics can also be instilled, although it is not clear how contributory such a regimen is to combat established infection.

Nasobiliary drainage is an effective nonsurgical temporary decompression of the biliary system in acute suppurative cholangitis.[59] Emergency endoscopic intervention is followed by a gratifying response within hours. The overall mortality, however, is not significantly lower than that of emergency surgery.[59]

Nasobiliary drainage may also be used for preliminary decompression in benign strictures or malignant obstructive jaundice prior to definitive operation. Although a randomized controlled trial of preoperative decompression has failed to show an advantage of such drainage for malignant disease,[23] the data do not apply to nasobiliary drainage as the study was done with external drainage through interventional radiology. Most of the disadvantages of percutaneous drainage are absent in the endoscopic methods such as leakage of infected bile causing peritonitis, bleeding from the punctured liver, hemobilia, and introduction of infection from outside. Several randomized controlled trials are in progress; until supportive data appear preoperative nasobiliary drainage remains an empirical practice.

Technique

THE NASOBILIARY DRAIN

Figure 6-1 shows the configuration of one type of nasobiliary drain equipped with an ingenious self-anchoring device, a preformed loop that anchors it in the duodenum, preventing its displacement in either direction. It is made of polyethylene tubing, 250 cm long, has an internal diameter of 1.4 mm, external diameter of 2.2 mm, and requires an endoscopic channel of 2.8 mm or larger for insertion. Many side holes are provided in the tip segment. For placing larger nasobiliary drains, the large duodenoscopes with a 3.7-mm channel must be used.

For insertion to prevent cholangitis in the presence of an impacted stone, the stone must first be disimpacted by pushing it back into the

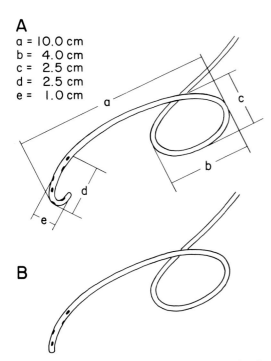

A

a = 10.0 cm
b = 4.0 cm
c = 2.5 cm
d = 2.5 cm
e = 1.0 cm

B

Fig. 6-1 The nasobiliary drain (A, B). Note the dimensions of the preformed loop that forms in the duodenum once the guidewire is removed, a self-anchoring device. Some models (e.g., A) have an additional pigtail in the bile duct for anchorage.

duct. A catheter with some stiffness must be used, such a sphincterotome or a dilating catheter (used for dilating malignant biliary strictures). For bypassing malignant strictures, preliminary dilation with either dilating catheters or balloon dilators is necessary. Some experts advocate using the ERCP cannula with its fine nozzle modified to accommodate a guidewire so that as soon as the preliminary cholangiogram is obtained with this catheter, the guidewire is advanced and the insertion process can begin.

The first step in the actual insertion consists of passing the catheter, be it the ERCP cannula, the balloon dilator, or a sphincterotome with a central lumen, to above the obstruction. A guidewire, 0.9 mm thick, is passed to the proximal duct via the cannula or catheter. Under fluoroscopy, the cannula or catheter is slowly withdrawn: This is done by advancing the guidewire pari passu so that the net result is a stationary guidewire tip.

The nasobiliary catheter is then threaded over the guidewire and advanced under fluoroscopic control to beyond the obstruction. During this process, the endoscope must be placed close to the papilla so as to prevent the guidewire from making a loop prolapsing into the duodenal lumen; when this happens, further pushing may dislodge the tip and allow it to slip out of the bile duct altogether. After the nasobiliary drain is in the correct position, the endoscope is slowly withdrawn while the drain is advanced to keep pace with the withdrawal, the guidewire remaining in place. When the endoscope has been moved into the stomach, the guidewire is withdrawn. As the preformed loop takes shape, the anchoring effect confers some protection from dislodgement. The guidewire is first completely removed; this is followed by removal of the endoscope, which is done as before by advancing the drain at the same rate as the endoscope is withdrawn. As soon as the drain is exposed in the mouth, it is pinched between the fingers and the endoscope completely removed, leaving the nasobiliary drain exiting via the patient's mouth. The drain can be simply rerouted to exit through the nose by inserting a nasogastric tube via one nostril, retrieving it at the oral pharynx. After cutting off the rounded tip of the nasogastric tip, the end of the nasobiliary drain is wedged into the lumen of the nasogastric tube and thus routed through the nostril by pulling on the nasogastric tube. The excess length of the nasobiliary drain is cut off and a Luer lock adaptor applied.

A modification of this nasobiliary drain (Liquory) is the provision of a pigtail for additional anchorage above the obstruction. To place this tube, the guidewire is first withdrawn enough to permit the C to form, which provides some anchorage. The endoscope is then removed. The guidewire is removed last after adjustment of the loop in the duodenum and stomach. Often there is not enough room above the obstruction for complete formation of the C loop, and anchorage cannot be depended on under such circumstance.

A papillotomy (a short sphincterotomy, cutting the superficial fibers of the sphincter) is not necessary unless large-caliber tubes are used. If papillotomy is deemed prudent after the nasobiliary drain is in place, it can still be done by using the needle electrode, cutting down on to the drain at the 10 to 1 o'clock position. Papillotomy facilitates the placement of larger drains, prevents occlusion of the pancreatic duct by the drain, and permits bile to drain around the tube into the duodenum.

POSTPROCEDURE CARE

Decompression is monitored by the amount of the drainage, by changes in liver function, and by nasobiliary cholangiography. Flow rate usually slows down after the first 2 to 3 days. The fall in serum bilirubin with time appears to follow a logarithmic curve, reaching an asymptote at a level depending on the duration of jaundice. Even though drainage tends to decrease, it remains patent for a long time and thus provides continued access to the biliary tree. If the drain is to be used for infusion of agents for dissolution of stones, it may be used as soon as the flow has diminished.

For stone dissolution, the choice of the agent depends on the likely nature of the stone to be dissolved. More than 97 percent of common duct stones have a composition similar to that of gallbladder stones. If guidance is not available, clinical clues have to be relied on. More than 75 percent of stones are predominantly cholesterol; less than 25 percent are pigmented stones, containing calcium bilirubinate.[54] For cholesterol stones, the currently clinically proven agent is monooctanoin (Capmul, glyceryl monooctanoin duoctanoate), but methyl *tert*-butyl ether, shown to have an in vitro activity 50-fold greater than monooctanoin,[3] may be available by the time this book is in print. Monooctanoin is heated in a water bath to 40°C when it changes from gel form to liquid form and then stays liquid at room temperature. It is next sterilized by Micropore (0.22 μm) filtration and is infused via the nasobiliary catheter at 5 to 7 ml/hr using an electronically controlled pump with pressure not to exceed 30 cm water. Cholic acid solution (150 mM) may be used instead of monooctanoin; it has roughly the same clinical success rate despite a lower in vitro potency. Ethylene diamine tetraacetic acid (EDTA) and a bile acid mixture has been shown to be capable of dissolving calcium bilirubinate stones and has been used in Germany.[32] Check cholangiograms should be obtained through the nasobiliary tube weekly. If no change in size is seen after 2 weeks, the therapy is probably ineffective and alternative treatment should be planned. If stones have decreased in size, extraction should be possible; this approach is preferred to waiting for complete dissolution or spontaneous passage, as the nasobiliary drain may also spontaneously dislodge. Diarrhea is a recognized side effect of infusion of either solution. Animal toxicity has been reported for all agents infused into the bile duct; hemorrhagic inflammatory response being the most common. An overall 60 to 65 percent success rate has been the general experience at many centers,[29,32,55] although some investigators are more optimistic.[52,56]

The administration of oral bile salt preparations such as dehydrocholate (Decholin) has the effect of causing increased flow of bile, which becomes light green and much less viscous. However, such bile salts as dehydrocholate are usually metabolized into nonmicelle-forming salts prior to excretion into the bile, thereby lowering the total micellar fraction[47] and increasing the tendency of calcium salts to precipitate, since micelles complex calcium, holding it in solution. The choleresis results from a loss of volume into the ductule lumen by virtue of an osmotic effect. While a thinner bile may be secreted, the increased tendency of calcium precipitation tends to annul the apparent advantage. The clinical efficacy of bile salt feeding to prevent clogging of the drainage tube is unproven despite anecdotal reports.

PLACEMENT OF ENDOPROSTHESIS

The first placement of an endoprosthesis was reported by Soehendra and Reynders-Frederix.[44] The original endoprosthesis was a modified angiography catheter with one pigtail, which served as anchorage above the obstruction. To prevent the prosthesis from migrating farther into the duct, double pigtail catheters were introduced, with one pigtail preventing migration in either direction (Fig. 6-2). The disadvantages of pigtail catheters are that the C requires room to re-form but, even in dilated ducts, especially intrahepatic ducts, there is scarcely enough room for the full loop. Furthermore, they tend to permit only sluggish flow because some degree of taper is needed to form the C, which accelerates clogging by debris and sludge. Most endoscopists now favor the straight tubes (e.g., the straight Amsterdam type), which use side flaps for anchorage (Fig. 6-2). While the side flaps take less room and anchor well, dislodgement is not completely prevented. All endoprostheses are used together with a pusher tubing of same diameter.

The flow rate is related to the fourth power of the radius, according to Poiseuille's law. Thus a 10 Fr. prosthesis would allow over 4 times and 16 times the flow rate as that allowed by 7 Fr. and 5 Fr., respectively, assuming the pres-

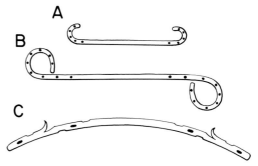

Fig. 6-2 Common endoprostheses (biliary stents). The double pigtails (7 Fr. (A) and 10 Fr. (B), have multiple side holes on both ends. One pigtail is to be placed above the obstruction, while the other stays in the duodenum. The straight types (C) use side flaps for anchorage. They tend to drain better as the pigtails are actually tapers that effectively reduce the internal diameters.

sure fall is not markedly dissimilar across tubes of different diameters. Therefore, the larger the diameter it appears, the better it is for flow. Unfortunately, the problem is not in the limitation of flow, since bile secretion (about 0.5 ml/min) cannot be more rapid than the limiting flow rate of the smallest prosthesis, even allowing increases of an order of magnitude. Mucus, epithelial protein debris, crystals, sediments, and other matter tend to clog even the largest tubes. In drainage of the obstructed biliary system it appears that lessons learned by one specialty are not transmitted to another. Thus surgeons have learned for several decades that the clogging of a U tube for hepatostomy drainage is almost inevitable, due to the inexorable accumulation of mucus and protein debris, irrespective of the size of the tubes and maintenance method. It led to the design of the U tube, so that it can be changed. The interventional radiologist learned this lesson all over; larger tubes worked better but still do not circumvent the need to change them. The high complication rate of endoscopic endoprosthesis insertion in the early years (1979–1983) was attributable to long-term implantation of small tubes. The incidence of cholangitis has been reduced as larger endoprostheses are introduced. The current tendency is to insert larger and larger endoprostheses to provide better decompression and to reduce (although not eliminate) the need to change them. The intrinsic shortcoming in all methods of palliative intubation of the biliary tract is that long-term implantation of a foreign body in a system with some degree of stasis will lead to chronic bacterial colonization and sepsis. Unqualified optimism in this method of treatment is unjustified.

Indications

The placement of an endoprosthesis is indicated mainly for palliation of advanced malignant obstruction of the biliary tract. Before considering palliation, the clinician must first establish that the patient is suffering from a malignancy and that it is incurable by surgery. Resectability varies with location of the tumor; for tumors obstructing the hilum, fewer than 5 to 10 percent are resectable, although many aggressive surgeons claim a much higher resection rate. For tumors located lower in the bile duct, the resectability rate may reach 40 to 50 percent or higher. One major use of the endoprosthesis is to provide preliminary decompression and to help optimize the patient's condition before exploration. If nonresectability is established, the endoprosthesis will then be utilized for palliation.

Less frequently, endoprosthesis has been used to treat benign obstructing lesions when the patient is inoperable because of systemic disease. Fewer than 100 patients were reported in a survey of experienced European centers[46] as of 1985, including those with unextractable stones, postoperative stricture, chronic pancreatitis, sclerosing cholangitis, biliary fistula, and miscellaneous conditions. Siegel[39] reported placing endoprosthesis in 76 patients with stone disease and in 18 patients with benign strictures. The duration of follow-up is not stated, but so far only one patient with sclerosing cholangitis experienced cholangitis. Considering the risk of cholangitis in the presence of a foreign body and suboptimal drainage, these uses must be regarded as experimental at present, even with the scant data available.

Most endoprostheses are inserted for advanced malignant obstruction of the biliary tract. The location of the tumor influences the choice of methods. For high lesions at or proximal to the bifurcation of the hepatic duct, the unaided endoscopic approach is likely to be difficult and a combined radiologic–endoscopic approach should be planned. Double prostheses are indicated for drainage of separate ductal systems and do not prevent clogging. For more proximal locations the 10 Fr. straight endoprosthesis should be used, but the endoscopist must be prepared to follow through with the subsequent management, including changing of the endoprosthesis. It should be remembered that the patient is better off with unrelieved obstructive jaundice without cholangitis, as most of them would be, than with a partially relieved obstruction with repeated attacks of cholangitis due to introduced organisms and the presence of a foreign body. Removal of the endoprosthesis does not restore the original condition.

Techniques

Commercially available endoprosthesis kits are convenient, as they come complete with guidewire, pusher tube, Teflon catheter, and endoprosthesis (see Fig. 6-3). The principle utilized is exchange of catheters passed over a guidewire. The technique described for placing a nasobiliary drain is followed: Each inch of catheter removed must be accompanied by advancement of an inch of the guidewire to keep the position of the guidewire tip constant as monitored under fluoroscopy.

To begin the procedure, a preliminary ERCP is first performed. Some experts use the same ERCP cannula to pass a guidewire, the cannula having first been prepared to accept the guidewire. Others are content simply to remove the cannula after obtaining satisfactory cholangiogram and to proceed to insert a sphincterotome to perform a small sphincterotomy (1 cm or less). A sphincterotomy (or papillotomy) facili-

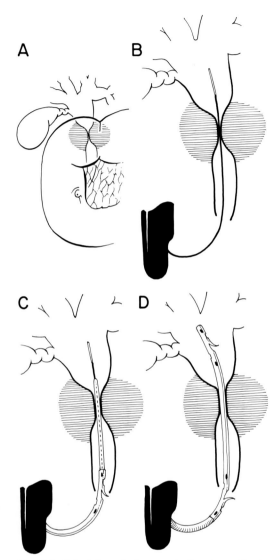

Fig. 6-3 Principles of placement of endoprosthesis. Modified Seldinger technique (A-D). The guidewire is first placed across the stricture (B). A Teflon catheter (acting as a dilator) is then pushed over the guidewire (C). The endoprosthesis, with a pusher tube behind it, is mounted over the catheter and pushed into position under fluoroscopy (D).

tates the passage of the endoprosthesis, and it decreases the risk of inadvertent blockage of the orifice of the pancreatic duct.

Depending on the diameter of the stricture demonstrated on the cholangiogram, a Teflon catheter of appropriate size is selected. This catheter is loaded with the guidewire inside and is passed to above the stricture. If the combination cannot be advanced into the duct due to relative stiffness, the guidewire alone is advanced; the Teflon catheter is then passed over it in order to dilate the stricture. Next the catheter is removed, leaving the guidewire in position. The double pigtail endoprosthesis of correct length is then loaded over the guidewire, followed by the pusher tube of the same diameter. The endoprosthesis is pushed into position. Once position is judged to be satisfactory under fluoroscopy, the guidewire is removed, followed by the pusher tube and finally the endoscope.

The larger endoprostheses, such as the straight Amsterdam type, are actually in many ways easier to pass, work better, and are hence more popular. The initial step is placement of a guidewire above the stenosis, after a preliminary cholangiogram and a short sphincterotomy. A large Teflon catheter (6 Fr. catheter for 10 Fr. endoprosthesis) that fits smoothly inside the endoprosthesis is then threaded over the guidewire with the endoprosthesis loaded over it. The friction of the endoprosthesis over the Teflon catheter is much less than the friction of the pigtail over the guidewire. There is no risk of looping into the duodenum before entering the ductal orifice, since the stiffness permits only a smooth curve. The assembly also has enough body to be used effectively for dilating the stricture on its way to the final position, eliminating any need for separate preliminary dilation. Considerable force can be transmitted by using the endoscopic angulation mechanism in positioning the last few centimeters of the endoprosthesis. When a check cholangiogram shows a satisfactory position, the Teflon catheter is removed, then the guidewire, and finally the pusher tube and the endoscope. When the Teflon catheter is removed, pressure on the pusher tube tends to counteract any tendency to dislodge the endoprosthesis by friction. If deeper placement is needed, the pusher tube is used before removal; if the endoprosthesis seats too deep, a snare should be inserted to apply traction to its lower end. Since the self-retaining mechanism is a side flap, once the endoprosthesis is out of the endoscope, it cannot go back into the endoscope but has to be reloaded, requiring withdrawal of the endoscope. In view of this, some experts advocate using the Teflon catheter alone over the guidewire until the stenosis has been cannulated; the endoprosthesis can then be pushed over it with the pusher tube; otherwise simply failure to cannulate or difficulty in advancing the guidewire up the common duct would entail removal of the duodenoscope to reload the endoprosthesis. The pusher tube is colored differently from the endoprosthesis to facilitate judgment of the length to be left protruding into the duodenum.

When the tumor is obstructing the bifurcation of the hepatic duct, insertion of multiple endoprostheses is indicated, usually one for each ductal system. The technique is identical, but in order to avoid dislodging the first endoprosthesis during placement of the second one, preliminary dilation of the stenosis is often necessary. A steerable catheter inserted through the endoscope is helpful in placing the guidewire into the desired duct, monitored under fluoroscopy. Even so, many time-consuming trials are necessary for correct positioning of the guidewire. The upper reaches of the bile duct do not lend themselves well to forcible dilation because of the long distance from the endoscope to the stenosis.

COMBINED APPROACH: ENDOSCOPIC–RADIOLOGIC PLACEMENT

For difficult cases such as tumors situated high in the duct at the bifurcation and above, the combined endoscopic-radiologic approach is attractive. By a percutaneous transhepatic route, a guidewire is inserted into the bile duct and then orthograde across the stricture, exiting via the papilla into the duodenum. The endoscopist first performs a sphincterotomy, the cannulation being aided by the direction of the guidewire. The tip of the guidewire is next picked up by the endoscopist with grasping forceps and brought out from the mouth. The endo-

scope, the pusher tube–endoprosthesis–Teflon catheter assembly can then be threaded over the oral end of the guidewire and advanced into position under fluoroscopy control. Furthermore, if the assembly of tubes is fixed manually to the guidewire on the endoscopist's end, the radiologist may aid final positioning by traction of the guidewire at the cutaneous end.

POSTPROCEDURE MANAGEMENT

The function of the endoprosthesis is followed clinically and by liver function tests. When occlusion is suspected, a radionuclide scan is first used for confirmation. Duodenoscopy is indicated only if further therapeutic intervention is contemplated. An endoscopic cholangiogram done by cannulating the endoprosthesis is a necessary first step.

Immediately after placement of the endoprosthesis, bilirubin and alkaline phosphatase decrease rapidly but slow down progressively until a low level is reached, depending on the duration of jaundice. For prolonged deep jaundice of several months' duration, the bilirubin may never reach normal despite patency of the endoprosthesis. The trend of change is more significant than any absolute level. Alkaline phosphatase decrease is much slower than bilirubin.

Whenever there is clinical evidence of onset of cholangitis, including fever and other signs of sepsis, increasing jaundice, and often abdominal pain, a radionuclide (e.g., HIDA) scintiscan should be obtained. Blockage of the endoprosthesis is diagnosed by failure of radioactivity to be detected in the intestines within the normal time frame, suggesting that jaundice is due to renewed obstruction. To define the problem further, a preliminary cholangiogram with contrast injected up the endoprosthesis is necessary. Intensive antibiotic treatment for the attendant cholangitis is mandatory. If there is no blockage, the diagnosis should be cholestasis due to sepsis or to diffuse infiltration of the hepatic parenchyma.

If blockage is diagnosed, an attempt to reopen

it should be made. Blockage within weeks of insertion may be due to a blood clot, which may be amenable to clearance either mechanically or by irrigation. Late blockage is generally due to irremovable clogging or tumor overgrowth, necessitating changing the endoprosthesis. The blocked stent is usually easily removed, using a snare for traction. Reinsertion is also uncomplicated; the most problematic area is bypassing the new tumor growth. Forcible dilation is not always possible, as it is difficult to transmit the pressure to the upper reaches of the ductal system. Another difficulty is in directing the guidewire into the correct duct for bifurcation tumors. A combined approach with radiology using a percutaneous guidewire is often helpful.

COMPLICATIONS

Both nasobiliary drainage and endoprosthesis share similar complications.

Cholangitis

Cholangitis remains the most common complication in most series.[22,28,31] Despite antibiotic cover and vigorous disinfection measures for the endoscopes and ancillary equipment, cholangitis often follows the procedure if satisfactory drainage has not been established. For example, if the left hepatic duct remains occluded after drainage of the right duct, cholangitis during the postprocedure period is highly likely. Sometimes endoscopic intubation is simply impossible. Percutaneous radiologic or surgical drainage is indicated for emergency treatment of this serious complication.

Septic episodes following endoscopic biliary procedures are polymicrobial in almost one-half the cases. *Pseudomonas* is the most common isolate from blood or bile in both poly- and monomicrobial infections, *Escherichia coli* is the next most common, followed by other enteric organisms.[24] *Pseudomonas* septicemia is the rule when sepsis occurs in the patients with endoprosthesis[24] and malignant obstruction.

This complication has nearly a 30 percent fatal outcome, with all deaths occurring in cancer patients. Endoscopic manipulation as an etiologic factor is strongly supported by both bacteriologic and epidemiologic evidence.

Complications Due to Sphincterotomy

This is unusual as only a small cut is made. Bleeding, pancreatitis, and failure to cannulate are occasionally encountered due to difficulties in cannulating the empty duct.

Erosions

If too long a segment is protruding into the duodenum, erosions may occur. This is more apt to happen with the larger-caliber prosthesis. Most are asymptomatic and are discovered at endoscopy. They rarely bleed.

Dislodgement

Despite the self-anchoring device in all makes, migration of the endoprosthesis has not been entirely eliminated. Spontaneous passing of endoprosthesis has been noted, probably due to necrosis of tumor tissue supporting the tube.

Acute Cholecystitis

Acute cholecystitis has been reported due to obstruction of the cystic duct by the endoprosthesis, which may have migrated from its original position.

Hemobilia

Rarely, bleeding into the GI tract may be severe enough to require transfusion. It is possible for the hemorrhage to come from common sources, but sloughing of tumor and erosion by the foreign body should be considered as a possible source.

Pancreatitis

This complication has been seen only once by the author, but as the use of endoprostheses becomes more widespread, the complication may be seen more often. The surgical lesson learned with the long-armed T-tube should be heeded. An old practice was to insert one arm of the T-tube through the papilla into the duodenum to permit unimpeded drainage of bile. This was found to be associated with a high incidence of pancreatitis, so the method was abandoned.[21] Apparently the long arm was impeding the pancreatic drainage in its transpapillary position, quite similar to the endoprosthesis being used today, sphincterotomy notwithstanding.

CAUSES OF FAILURE

The major cause of failure is technical difficulty encountered in cannulation of the empty duct. In expert hands this constitutes about 10 to 15 percent of all attempts. In contrast to choledocholithiasis, the common bile duct distal to a malignant obstruction is collapsed and more difficult to work with. The absence of bile makes it much more difficult to determine when the ductal lumen has been entered.

In total obstruction by tumor, irrespective of location, it may not be possible to pass even a guidewire through the malignant tissue. For proximal lesions, the difficulty with selective cannulation of the hepatic ducts has been cited. Furthermore, traversing such obstruction is difficult, as the tumor is quite a distance away from the endoscope.

In case of extreme difficulty, hybrid approaches should be considered. Radiologic placement of the guidewire followed by endoscopic insertion of endoprosthesis has been mentioned previously. Radiologic placement of guidewire may also be combined with operative placement of endoprosthesis. The radiologist first places a guidewire through the malignant

stricture into the distal bile duct and out into the duodenum. Laparotomy is then performed. After duodenotomy exposure of the ampulla, a formal sphincteroplasty is done. Using the preplaced guidewire, Teflon catheters may be passed to dilate the tumor until it accepts a 16 to 18 Fr. endoprosthesis, which is inserted over the guidewire; the final position is adjusted under a C-arm image intensifier. Both dilation and intubation are done through the tumor via the ampulla. The tumor is supported manually by the surgeon. In a single case, this author has found the technique to be a vast improvement over the conventional U-tube technique performed through choledochotomy. The patient's tumor was at the mid-bile duct, 1.5 cm below the bifurcation; satisfactory palliation was achieved with this hybrid technique. The patient expired of metastatic disease after 3 months, before the endoprosthesis required changing.

RESULTS

In interpreting the published results, one must realize that the chance of clogging and of cholangitis is a function of the duration of drainage and that advanced lesions are not compatible with long-term follow-up. The best results therefore tend to come from judiciously selected series. The lowest complication rates are encountered in series in which the median survival is less than 3 to 4 months.

Short-Term Drainage (Nasobiliary Drainage)

Technically, nasobiliary drainage is not a difficult procedure, and the success rate of initial placement approaches 100 percent in most series reported. The main complication is dislodgement of the catheter, which, depending on the model used, varies from 10 to 15 percent, the higher rates in tubes without the self-anchoring device.

When used as an emergency procedure to treat acute suppurative cholangitis, Wurbs et al.[59] reported a mortality of 21 percent in a series of 19 patients (mean age 81) so treated. This was not significantly different compared with 28 percent mortality for 67 patients (mean age 70) treated by surgery. Placement was successful in all 19 patients without technical complications. When used for stone dissolution therapy, placement was regularly successful, but the stone dissolution was only successful in about 60 percent of cases.[17,29,32,55]

Long-Term Bypass (Endoprosthesis)

For malignant obstruction, the Amsterdam group[28] classified their results by the location of the tumor in the biliary system. Placement was successful in 89 percent of 336 patients treated from 1980 to 1982; most failures were in the hilar lesions and in total obstructions. The 30-day mortality for distal common duct tumor was 12 percent, and the corresponding figures were 22 percent and 24 percent for mid-common duct and hilar lesions, respectively. There are no significant differences in 2-year survival by tumor location, averaging 50 percent. In terms of complications, however, the higher the tumor, the more frequent the complications, since high tumors are technically more difficult to obtain the adequate drainage. Early cholangitis was reported in only 8 percent of patients with distal common duct tumors, but in more than 40 percent in the hilar group. Similarly, bilirubin declined in 95 percent of patients with distal common duct tumors but only in 70 percent in proximal lesions. These results were obtained with the straight 10 Fr. endoprosthesis (3.2 mm external diameter and 2.4 mm internal diameter). Results with the 7 Fr. size have been unsatisfactory, owing to the high incidence of severe early cholangitis.

In a 1982 survey of European endoscopists covering 454 patients,[22] similar results were reported. About one-half of the patients had lower bile duct obstruction from carcinoma of the pancreas; the rest consisted of bile duct, gallbladder, and hilar metastatic cancers and a few carcinomas of the ampulla. Successful placement was 84 percent, most failures quoted were due to inaccessibility of the ampulla, including previ-

ous gastric operations, and pyloric or duodenal stenosis. A total of 26.3 percent of patients experienced complications, 77 percent of which were cholangitis. The total mortality was 7.9 percent, but the mortality due to cholangitis was 55.6 percent. Since the introduction of the 3.7-mm duodenoscope and the use of the 10 Fr. endoprosthesis, all endoscopists claim a greatly reduced incidence of cholangitis. The overall complication rate using the large endoprosthesis is about 10 percent, with a mortality of 5 percent, at experienced centers.[22] The bilirubin decreased to one-half the original value in 86 percent of patients. The median survival time was about 2.5 months, no different from the figures reported for surgical or radiologic techniques of palliation. The mean duration of good drainage varied widely, since different materials were used for the endoprosthesis, and ranged from 10 to 90 days, clogging being reported as invariable if the patient was followed long enough. Survival may be prolonged after endoscopic palliation, but there are no objective data.

In 1983 Soehendra et al.[46] surveyed the world experience for the use of endoprosthesis in benign conditions, and reported a lower complication rate compared with intubation for malignancies. The technical success rate was 95 percent, with a 10 percent overall complication rate, without mortality. The most common complication was clogging (6 percent), giving rise to cholangitis (3 percent) in one-half these patients. Dislodgement was reported at about 1 percent of cases. Although the early results appear encouraging, these patients are likely to live longer than those with advanced tumor and, since the complication rate is a function of the duration of implantation, early results may be too optimistic.

BALLOON DILATION OF BILIARY STRICTURES

The Gruntzig balloon catheter has been used for dilation of strictures of the biliary tract, drawing upon the experience with these dilators in the treatment of fibrous strictures elsewhere in the alimentary canal. The most rational use is for stenosis of choledochoenterostomy and for traumatic strictures or recurrent strictures following surgical repair. The duration of efficacy is as yet unknown, although the stenosis can be dilated and clinical improvement observed. Preliminary work investigating the efficacy of dilation for treatment of strictures elsewhere in the biliary system, including sclerosing cholangitis, is in progress,[39] but details are sketchy. It appears that the major advantage of balloon dilation is that no foreign bodies are implanted; how long the beneficial effect will last depends on the nature of the stricture being treated. The experience of dilation for carcinoma of the esophagus suggests that dilation for malignant biliary stricture is likely to be short lived; it therefore cannot be advocated at present. If dilation is followed by endoprosthesis or stenting, the result will depend on the duration the stent has been in place.

Technique

The balloons are handled exactly like any other Gruntzig dilators. The appropriate size balloon is selected (e.g., length 2 cm, diameter 4, 6, or 8 mm). The lumen must be filled with dilute contrast material, such as 30 percent diatrizoate, in order to transmit pressure evenly. Air must first be bled from the line by repeated filling and aspirating, holding the syringe vertically to let air rise to the top. After priming in this manner, the balloon is completely aspirated and folded as two wings, wrapping around the catheter with each wing facing away from the other (in the same closewise or counterclockwise direction), using a twisting motion to slip the balloon folding sheath over the balloon to assist folding. The folded balloon is then immersed into a water bath at 65°C for 1 minute to impart to it a memory; thus, when aspirated to empty at the end of dilation, the collapsed balloon will fold in the predetermined manner, facilitating withdrawal up the instrument channel. After cooling in a cold water bath for 10 seconds, it is ready for use.

A large-channel (3.7-mm) duodenoscope is desirable, as some larger balloons cannot be passed without considerable friction in the channel, despite generous silicone spraying. A guidewire is first passed through the stricture at duodenoscopy. The prepared balloon is now threaded over the guidewire, down the instrument channel, and up the bile duct, until under fluoroscopy the markers of the balloon ride just astride the stenosis. Using a 20-cc syringe containing 30 percent diatrizoate, the balloon is inflated to its predetermined diameter by observation under fluoroscopy. The correct pressure should be monitored by a pressure gauge and should be held at 4 atm for 1 minute. The patient may experience discomfort as the stricture is being dilated, but the symptom should subside promptly as the procedure is terminated. The balloon is collapsed and, since it assumes its prefolded shape, it is readily withdrawn. Dilation may be repeated with a large balloon if indicated by a check cholangiogram.

Because infection and clogging are the major problems in the implantation of an endoprosthesis, the concept of palliating obstruction by laser ablation, as exemplified in esophageal cancer, is particularly attractive for biliary tumors. With the advance of technology in construction of biliary endoscopes and medical lasers, it is likely that the current techniques for laser treatment of esophageal cancer will be extended to biliary tumors in the near future.

OTHER TECHNIQUES OF NONSURGICAL DRAINAGE

External percutaneous drainage under radiological control has been practiced since 1952, and various modifications, such as external–internal drainage or percutaneous implantation of a prosthesis, have since been introduced. The techniques and results are briefly reviewed here in order to gain a perspective of the roles of various methods in the treatment of malignant obstructive jaundice.

Percutaneous drainage is usually performed with two punctures. The first puncture is made with the fine-needle technique, solely for opacification of the intrahepatic biliary tree in order to facilitate the second definitive drainage puncture. The second puncture is performed at the right midaxillary line with a sheathed needle under biplane fluoroscopic control, aiming at a peripheral bile duct (Fig. 6-4). The peripheral location avoids risking injury to major vessels and minimizes dislodgement of the catheter from the ductal system. However, some experts prefer a central perihilar duct for a shorter intrahepatic course and a thicker liver to seal the puncture. The entry of the needle into the opacified duct can be visually recognized: The duct is dented a little before the needle breaks into it. Once entry is confirmed by free bile aspiration, the needle is removed and a guidewire (0.9 mm) is inserted into the sheath and manipulated toward the obstruction, followed by advancing the sheath to the same position. The pigtail drainage cannula, usually 2.5 mm in external diameter (8 Fr.) and approximately 1.4 mm in internal diameter, equipped with multiple side holes, is exchanged for the sheath and advanced to just above the obstruction. The drainage catheter is secured to the skin and connected to a

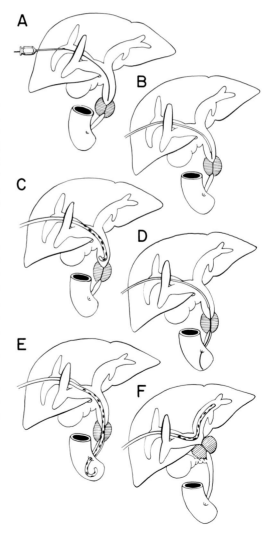

Fig. 6-4 Steps in radiologic placement of endoprosthesis; external drainage and external–internal drainage. (A) Through a needle introduced percutaneously into the dilated bile duct, the guidewire is advanced toward the obstruction. (B) The guidewire cannot be advanced past the obstruction; a Teflon catheter is used to dilate the tract. (C) External drainage is established by loading the drainage catheter over the Teflon dilating catheter. As the guidewire and Teflon catheter are withdrawn, the ''C'' of the pigtail forms, providing anchorage for the drainage catheter. This accomplishes external drainage. (D) If the guidewire can be advanced past the obstruction into the duodenum, the Teflon catheter is advanced over it into the duodenum. (E) The drainage catheter is loaded over the Teflon catheter and advanced into the duodenum. After withdrawal of the guidewire and Teflon catheter, the C of the pigtail forms in the duodenum. Since the catheter has perforations above and below the obstruction, internal drainage is accomplished. The cutaneous end of the catheter is cut short and capped. (F) External drainage of both the left and right duct is accomplished by the use of one drainage catheter (as shown), or multiple catheters.

closed system of drainage, preferably with a small trap containing povodone-iodine[6] to discourage rapid bacterial colonization.

Combined external and internal drainage is the preferred method in the United States; it is done if the guidewire can be manipulated through the obstruction into the distal bile duct, hence into the duodenum (Fig. 6-4). The drainage catheter is pushed over the guidewire so that the pigtail sits in the duodenum. Side holes span the distance of the obstruction, permitting bile drainage into the gut. The external end is spigoted and secured with sutures or tape. The catheter requires diligent maintenance irrigations.

If the guidewire cannot be manipulated across the obstruction, the attempt can be repeated after external decompression has been established for several days; it is then usually possible to convert the system to external–internal drainage. Approximately 80 percent of cases can be drained by the external–internal technique.

Percutaneous placement of the endoprosthesis, popular in Europe, is performed by manipulating a guidewire through the malignant stricture, followed by passage of the largest introducer admissible by the stricture. The introducer is then removed; the endoprosthesis of the same size is passed over the wire and pushed into position by the introducer, which is mounted behind it. The endoprosthesis, usually 6 to 12 Fr. (2 to 4 mm), should be protruding into the duodenum to facilitate future removal in case of blockage, when a new one can be inserted percutaneously. The introducer is left to drain externally for a few days and is then progressively removed.

The technique-related complications reported in large series[11,12,37] were due to hepatic puncture (bile leakage with biliary peritonitis, septicemia, hemobilia, and intraperitoneal hemorrhage); the incidence of each was 1.6 to 2 percent. In addition, subphrenic abscess, hypotension, and renal failure were reported (0.1 to 4 percent). Less serious complications, such as catheter displacement (7 percent), cholangitis (without septicemia) (6 percent), leakage of ascites, and local infection at the catheter site,

occurred more frequently. The total complication rate was more than 20 percent. Twenty-five percent of the serious complications required emergency surgery, with one-half of these ending in death. Overall procedure-related mortality was 1.4 percent. In advanced malignancies, the 30-day mortality after drainage is about 27 percent;[48] these patients are also much more susceptible to major complications.

In postprocedure management, the major difficulty is clogging of the catheter, which should be changed every 2 to 3 months, even for the external–internal systems, where it can be irrigated regularly. Late cholangitis (as distinct from cholangitis during the immediate postprocedure period) is almost always related to malfunction of the drainage system and is as high as 20 percent, depending on the duration of survival, the longer the higher the risk.[19,26] Polymicrobial colonization of the biliary tree occurs in 80 percent of cases within 20 days,[34] often giving rise to septicemia, especially when the catheter is dislodged. In those with external drainage only, bile loss can pose a significant problem, which should be prevented by refeeding the bile, such as through an endoscopic gastrostomy (see Chapter 12). Bacterial contamination of the bile, however, can also trigger off secondary problems. For the internal drainage, changing of the prosthesis is probably required every 2 to 3 months; the advantage of the closed system is offset by the disadvantage of inaccessibility of the system for irrigation.

In expert hands, endoprosthesis placement by radiologic technique is successful in about 88 percent of cases. Significant relief of jaundice has been observed in more than two-thirds of cases, while at least 17 percent experienced no improvement.

The major disadvantage of the radiologic method is the puncture of the liver with its associated risks, such as bile leak, peritonitis, hemorrhage, and intrahepatic injury, resulting in hematoma, hemobilia, arteriovenous malformations, and rarely abscess formation. These complications, about 6 percent total, are avoided by the transpapillary endoscopic approach. The mortality, success rate, and quality of palliation are otherwise about the same in both modalities.

One potential use of percutaneous drainage was for preliminary biliary decompression prior to surgical operation. Retrospective studies indicated that operative mortality is related to hyperbilirubinemia. It therefore appeared a rational approach to drain an obstructed biliary system before surgical resection in the hope of a better outcome. A well-controlled trial[23] using preoperative radiologic percutaneous drainage showed that such use conferred no advantage in lowering mortality but the morbidity was increased due to the technique of drainage. Also, increased infective complications were found in the group drained preoperatively. Most surgeons do not use preliminary drainage in current practice.

RESULTS OF SURGICAL TREATMENT OF MALIGNANT OBSTRUCTION

Curative Resection

For carcinoma of the head of pancreas, the chance of cure after pancreaticoduodenectomy is so remote that many question whether the operation is ever justifiable. Nonsurgeons often quote a prohibitive operative mortality of 50 percent as the argument against resection but, despite widely varying earlier results, data in the 1970s indicate a consistent operative mortality rate of 8 to 16 percent[10,49,57] in major series, and in selected personal series the figure is even lower, less than 6 percent.[27,33] The practical difficulty is that, even at operation it is impossible to be certain, frozen section notwithstanding, that the tumor originates in the pancreas as distinct from the ampulla, or in the intrapancreatic portion of the bile duct, which carries a better prognosis if the tumor is completely resectable. The procedure is therefore performed, when the tumor is deemed resectable, on the basis of such uncertainty, allowing the patient the benefit of the doubt, particularly because the operative mortality in competent hands need not be high.

For carcinoma of the bile duct, resection is the only treatment that offers cure. For the purpose of surgical treatment, the tumor is classified as upper third (to cystic duct), middle (cystic duct to upper border of duodenum), and lower third. The cure rate is substantial with a reasonable operative mortality for tumors in the middle and lower third of the bile duct. Tompkins et al.[53] reported an 8 percent mortality for pancreatoduodenectomy for lower bile duct cancer and no mortality for tumors of the middle third, in the UCLA experience of 95 patients. A 24 percent in survival was recorded from a total of 42 patients with tumor of the middle and lower third of the bile duct. A 25 percent 5-year survival for 32 patients with bile duct cancer treated by resection has been reported by Warren et al.[57] The Toronto experience of the past 15 years, reported by Langer et al.,[30] is quite similar.

Carcinoma arising at the hilar area is a different situation. Resection rate is generally low, since the tumor is thought to involve the portal vein or hepatic artery early. Operative mortality, with rare exceptions,[1,2] is 23 to 50 percent.[20,53] The survival after palliative surgery is no different from that after intubation drainage. Palliative resection for tumor in this region is much harder to justify; resection is only undertaken if it can be complete. Recently Adkins et al.[1] reviewed the experience at Vanderbilt and suggested that with an aggressive approach, long-term survival can be attained even with hilar lesions. Seven patients with upper third lesions underwent resections without a death in the last 8 years, compared with a mortality of 33 percent during the two preceding decades. Resection of the hilum of the liver is sometimes possible with preservation of the portal vein and hepatic artery (skeletonization resection); in other instances, hepatic lobectomy may be necessary. Reconstruction by Roux-en-Y hepaticojejunostomy has been found satisfactory. The mean survival of these seven patients was 2 years. Blumgart[9] also has seven surviving patients (out of 17), some for as long as 4 years after resection of hilar tumors. The point that deserves emphasis is that complete excision can be curative, but there is no way to tell except by meticulous exploration. Often the clinician simply gets discouraged by the location and radiologic appearance and pronounces the lesion incurable. With new endoscopic palliative techniques freely available, the temptation to undertake palliation right away is strong unless there is a firm policy to explore meticulously all patients with this lesion, as long as there are no preoperative indications of nonresectability.

Surgical intubation was described by Smith[40] and more recently by Terblanche.[50,51] The U-tube is inserted operatively after a choledochotomy which enables the malignant stricture to be traversed bluntly by a metal sound (e.g., Bakes dilators), routing the tube to the surface of the liver and to the skin. Depending on the ease of dilation, tubes of up to 18 Fr. (5.7-mm) external diameter may be inserted. The procedure is far less accurate or elegant than the percutaneous radiologic counterpart, and the advantage of the larger-diameter tubes is only marginal in view of the disadvantages of an open operation. The results for cancer are not superior to those attained nonsurgically. The endoscopic method of intubation carries less morbidity not only because it avoids an open operation, but because the liver is not punctured. A hybrid approach, combining either endoscopic or radiologic insertion of a guidewire followed by surgical intubation through the ampulla, is worth future research and development to be considered in the most difficult cases after failure of pure nonsurgical techniques.

In view of the disadvantage of the foreign body and the generally unsatisfactory results of intubation, biliary-enteric anastomosis has been proposed as a palliative procedure. Employing the approach to the left hepatic duct for biliary benign strictures, good results have been obtained in 45 patients[5] in one series with a mean survival of 13 months. The procedure involves little blood loss and provides satisfactory drainage via the left duct, with a much-reduced incidence of cholangitis and satisfactory palliation for longer periods than possible with tubes.[9] This left hepato-enteric anastomosis as a palliative measure is under investigation in many centers, and data may be forthcoming in a few years.

RESULTS OF SURGICAL TREATMENT OF BENIGN BILIARY STRICTURE

Iatrogenic or traumatic strictures of the biliary tract are known for their technical challenges in surgical repairs, often requiring repeated attempts; many patients eventually die from complications of biliary cirrhosis. Recent developments in techniques, utilizing the mucosa-to-mucosa hepaticojejunostomy of either the sutured[4] or sutureless[41] methods, have largely overcome the problem and modern results of surgical repair indicate a much better prognosis.[4,8,18,41–43] Thus in experienced hands, the operative mortality can be under 1 percent, with complications of 9 percent, most of which were wound and intraperitoneal infections.[4] The techniques used by Bismuth et al.,[4] Hepp and Couinaud,[25] and Blumgart and Kelley[7] are based on the anatomic studies of Couinaud[16] and utilize the left hepatic duct at the confluence with the right duct to create a 3 to 4-cm long hepaticojejunostomy. The transverse segment of the left hepatic duct is actually extrahepatic (although sometimes hidden by the overhanging quadrate lobe) and is easily exposed at the base of the quadrate lobe by division of the fusion line of the lesser omentum and the Glisson's capsule. In Bismuth's hands, at least 88 percent have excellent long-term (10 to 20 year) results, and only 7 percent required reoperation because of restenosis. The shorter-term results obtained by Blumgart are equally encouraging,[8] with 90 percent excellent results at a mean follow-up of 3.3 years. The operative mortality is dependent on the liver function and the degree of portal hypertension;[8] very low mortality can be attained if the liver function is relatively intact. Good results are also reported by the sutureless mucosal graft method of Smith,[43] but these are shorter-term follow-up studies.

Surgical intubation with the U-tube has been reported for benign strictures,[14,36] but the results are much less satisfactory compared with the direct repair method, mainly due to the problems of chronic stenting. The diameters of the tubes used ranged from 16 Fr. (5 mm)[36] and 19 Fr. (6 mm) through 31 Fr. (10 mm).[14] From such long-term studies as that of Cameron et al.,[14] is derived our knowledge of the natural history of chronic biliary intubations. In the Johns Hopkins series of 25 patients followed for 1 to 6 years, the transhepatic stent was placed across a hepaticojejunostomy after excision of the original stricture. Bile leak occurred around the hepatic exit site in all cases initially, taking 2 to 3 weeks to close. Clogging from sludge was invariable in chronic implantation; a regimen of changing the tube every 3 months or so was needed to circumvent leakage around it in the event of clogging. Subphrenic abscesses, sepsis from early bile leak, and wound infections were early complications. Late deaths from sepsis occurred when the tube was irrigated or manipulated. It would appear that the endoscopic stenting technique may eliminate the complications associated with the hepatic puncture and bile leak, but the basic inherent problems of endoprosthesis, namely, clogging and infection, would not be substantially different. If clogging were to occur with the large tubes used in the surgical technique, the same would happen to the much smaller ones used in the endoscopic technique.

THE ROLE OF ENDOSCOPIC DRAINAGE IN BILIARY SURGERY: AN INTEGRATED APPROACH TO OBSTRUCTIVE JAUNDICE

The algorithm (Fig. 6-5) summarizes the pertinent discussion in Chapters 5 and 6 of the therapeutic armamentarium for obstructive jaundice, assuming the availability of expertise but emphasizing the minimal reduplication of tests.

Obstructive jaundice is first investigated with either ERCP or percutaneous cholangiography. ERCP is preferred if the history is suggestive of stone disease. Subsequent management depends on whether benign or malignant disease is established. For common bile duct stones, an endoscopic sphincterotomy can be performed and stones extracted for all patients. All but the highest-risk patients should then undergo an elective cholecystectomy if the gallbladder

has not yet been removed. When stones cannot be extracted because of size or location, a trial of stone dissolution can be instituted by nasobiliary catheter, followed by repeat of endoscopic extraction if necessary. Residual stones in the upper reaches of the biliary tree not causing symptoms may be left to be passed through the sphincterotomy. For traumatic strictures, balloon dilation may be tried, but surgical resection and repair with hepatojejunostomy should be performed whenever feasible.

For cancerous obstruction, resectability must first be determined at surgical exploration, provided that no evidence of nonresectability, such as metastasis, has been found by noninvasive means. For completely resectable lesions in the middle and lower third of the bile duct, the appropriate resection operation (usually a pancreatoduodenectomy) is performed unless a positive diagnosis of pancreatic carcinoma can be established at surgical exploration. Surgical bypass, such as cholecystojejunostomy or choledochojejunostomy, combined with bypass of intestinal obstruction, if indicated, is used for carcinoma of the head of the pancreas and for nonresectable lower bile duct tumors.

For resectable hilar tumors, appropriate resection of the entire lesion is indicated, resecting the bile ducts with or without hepatic lobectomy, using hepaticojejunostomy for reconstruction. For most hilar tumors and all nonresectable tumors of the bile duct, palliation by cholangioenteric anastomosis now under investigation, appears to be promising. If technically feasible, it should be attempted; otherwise, per papillary placement of endoprosthesis is performed endoscopically or by a combined radiologic–endoscopic approach for difficult lesions. Endoscopic endoprosthesis may also be used for both benign and malignant conditions in patients expected to live only a short time because of the late stage of the natural history.

Great strides have been made not only in nonsurgical, but also in surgical, treatment of biliary disease. The advance in surgical treatment of difficult traumatic strictures and bile duct carcinoma is particularly noteworthy. Endoscopic treatment should not be selected for these conditions without consideration of what

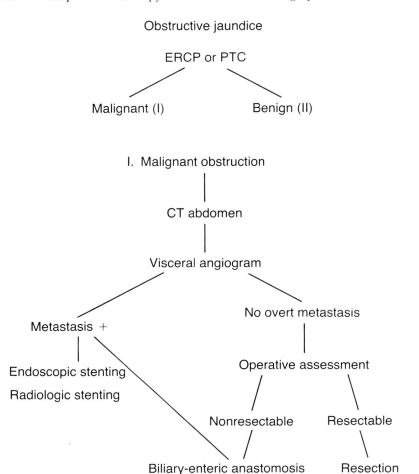

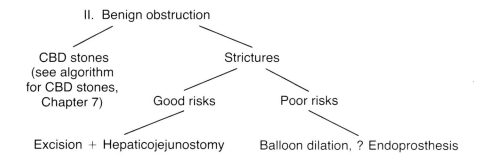

Fig. 6-5 Algorithm. Approach to obstructive jaundice dice (see text).

modern surgery can offer, as indicated by the recent data.

REFERENCES

1. Adkins RB Jr, Dunbar LL, McKnight WG, et al: An aggressive surgical approach to bile duct cancer. Am Surg 52:134, 1986
2. Akwari OE, Kelly KA: Surgical treatment of adenocarcinoma—Location: Junction of the right, left and common heptic biliary ducts. Arch Surg 114:22, 1979
3. Allen MJ, Borody TJ, Thistle JL: In vitro dissolution of cholesterol gallstones. Gastroenterology 89:1097, 1985
4. Bismuth H, Franco D, Corlette MB, et al: Long term results of Roux-en-Y hepaticojejunostomy. Surg Gynecol Obstet 146:161, 1978
5. Bismuth H, Corlette MB: Intrahepatic cholangioenteric anastomosis in carcinoma of the hilus of the liver. Surg Gynecol Obstet 140:170, 1975
6. Blenkharn JI, MacPherson GAD: An improved system for external biliary drainage. Lancet 2:781, 1981
7. Blumgart LH, Kelley CJ: Hepaticojejunostomy in benign and malignant high bile duct strictures: Approaches to the left hepatic ducts. Br J Surg 71:257, 1984
8. Blumgart LH, Kelley CJ, Benjamin IS: Benign bile duct strictures following cholecystectomy, critical factors in management. Br J Surg 71:836, 1984
9. Blumgart LH: Bile duct strictures. p. 796. In Fromm D (ed): Gastrointestinal Surgery. Churchill Livingstone, New York, 1985
10. Braasch JW, Gray BN: Considerations that lower pancreatoduodenectomy mortality. Am J Surg 133:480, 1977
11. Burcharth F, Jensen LI, Olesen K: Endoprosthesis for internal drainage of the biliary tract. Gastroenterology 77:133, 1979
12. Burcharth F, Efsen F, Christiansen LA, et al: Nonsurgical internal biliary drainage by endoprosthesis. Surg Gynecol Obstet 153:857, 1981
13. Camara DS, Gruber M, Barde CJ, et al: Transient bacteremia following endoscopic injection sclerotherapy of esophageal varices. Arch Intern Med 143:1350, 1983
14. Cameron JL, Gayler BW, Zuidema GD: The use of silastic transhepatic stents in benign and malignant strictures. Ann Surg 188:552, 1978
15. Cotton PB, Burney PG, Mason RR: Transnasal bile duct catheterization after endoscopic sphincterotomy: Method for biliary drainage, perfusion and sequential cholangiography. Gut 20:285, 1979
16. Couinaud C: Recherches sur la chirurgie du confluent biliaire supérieur et des canaux hépatiques. Presse Med 63:669, 1955
17. Dawson J, Cockel R: Retained common bile duct stones: Mono-octanoin or endoscopic sphincterotomy? Gut 23:906, 1982
18. Fernandez M: Treatment of benign strictures of the bile ducts. World J Surg 4:479, 1980
19. Ferrucci JT Jr, Mueller PR, Harbin WP: Percutaneous transheptic biliary drainage. Radiology 135:1, 1980
20. Fortner, JG, Kallum BO, Kim DK: Surgical management of carcinoma of the junction of the main hepatic ducts. Ann Surg 184:68, 1976
21. Glenn F, Cameron JL, Complications following operations upon the biliary tract and their management. p. 527. In Hardy JD (ed): Complications of Surgery and Their Management. WB Saunders, Philadelphia, 1981
22. Hagenmuller F: Results of endoscopic bilioduodenal drainage in malignant bile duct stenoses. p. 93. In Classen M, Geenen J, Kawai K (eds): Nonsurgical Biliary Drainage. Springer-Verlag, New York, 1985
23. Hatfield ARW, Tobias R, Terblanche J, et al: Pre-operative external biliary drainage in obstructive jaundice, a prospective controlled clinical trial. Lancet 2:896, 1982
24. Helm EB, Stille W: Infective complications. p. 113. In Classen M, Geenen J, Kawai K (eds): Nonsurgical Biliary Drainage. Springer-Verlag, New York, 1984
25. Hepp J, Couinaud C: L'abord et l'utilisation du canal hépatique gauche dans les réparations de la voie biliaire principale. Presse Med 64:947, 1956
26. Hoevels J, Ihse I: Percutaneous transhepatic insertion of a permanent endoprosthesis in obstructive lesions of the extrahepatic bile ducts. Gastrointest Radiol 4:367, 1979
27. Howard JM: Pancreatico-duodenectomy. Forty-one consecutive Whipple resections without an operative mortality. Ann Surg 168:629, 1968
28. Huibregtse K, Tytgat GN: Palliative treatment of obstructive jaundice by transpapillary introduction of large bore bile duct endoprothesis. Gut 23:371, 1982

29. Jarrett LN, Bell GD, Balfour TW, et al: Intraductal infusion of mono-octanoin: Experience in 24 patients with retained common duct stones. Lancet 1:68, 1981

30. Langer JC, Langer B, Taylor BR, et al: Carcinoma of the extrahepatic bile ducts: Results of an aggressive surgical approach. Surgery 98:752, 1985

31. Laurence BH, Cotton PB: Decompression of malignant biliary obstruction by duodenoscopic intubation of the bile ducts. Br Med J 280:522, 1980

32. Leuschner U, Wurbs D, Baumgartel H, et al: Alternating treatment of common bile duct stones with a modified glyceryl-1-mono-octanoate preparation and a bile acid-EDTA solution by nasobiliary tube. Scand J Gastroenterol 16:497, 1981

33. Longmire WP, Shaffy OA: Certain factors influencing survival after pancreatico-duodenal resection for carcinoma. Am J Surg 111:8, 1966

34. McPherson GAD, Blenkharn JI, Nathanson B, et al: Significance of bacteria in external biliary drainage systems: A possible role for antisepsis. J Clin Surg 1:22, 1982

35. Nagai N, Toki F, Oi J, et al: Continuous endoscopic pancreato-choledochal catheterization. Gastrointest Endosc 23:78, 1976

36. Praderi R: Twelve years experience of transhepatic intubation. Ann Surg 179:937, 1974

37. Riemann JF, Lux G, Roesch W, et al: Nonsurgical biliary drainage—Technique, indications and results. Endoscopy 13:157, 1981

38. Seigel JH, Daniel SJ: Endoscopic and fluoroscopic transpapillary placement of a large caliber biliary endoprosthesis. Am J Gastroenterol 79:461, 1984

39. Siegel J: Endoscopic decompression of the biliary tree. p. 263. In Silvis SE (ed): Therapeutic Gastrointestinal Endoscopy. Igaku-Shoin, New York, 1984

40. Smith R: Hepaticojejunostomy: Choledochojejunostomy. Br J Surg 51:183, 1964

41. Smith R: Strictures of the bile ducts. Proc R Soc Med 62:131, 1969

42. Smith R: Obstructions of the bile duct. Br J Surg 66:69, 1979

43. Smith R: Le traitement chirurgical des stenoses de voies biliaires. Chirurgie 106:318, 1980

44. Soehendra N, Reynders-Frederix V: Palliative Gallengangdrainage. Dtsch Med Wochenschr 104:206, 1979

45. Soehendra N, Reynders-Frederix V: Palliative bile duct drainage: A new endoscopic method of introducing a transpapillary drain. Endoscopy 12:8, 1980

46. Soehendra N, de Heer K, Kempeneers J: Endoscopic implantation of bilioduodenal endoprostheses in benign bile duct stenoses. p. 90. In Classen M, Geenen J, Kawai K (eds): Nonsurgical Biliary Drainage. Springer-Verlag, New York, 1985

47. Soloway RD, Hofman AF, Prensky AL, et al: Triketocholanoic acid: Hepatic metabolism and effect on bile flow and biliary lipid secretion in man. J Clin Invest 52:715, 1973

48. Stambuk EC, Pitt HA, Pais OS, et al: Percutaneous transhepatic drainage, risks and benefits. Arch Surg 118:1388, 1983

49. Tepper J, Nardi G, Suit H: Carcinoma of the pancreas: Review of MGH experience from 1963 to 1973—Analysis of surgical failures and implications for radiotherapy. Cancer 37:1519, 1976

50. Terblanche J, Louw JH: U tube drainage in the palliative therapy of carcinoma of the main heptic duct junction. Surg Clin North Am 53:1245, 1973

51. Terblanche J: Carcinoma of the proximal extrahepatic biliary tree—Definitive and palliative treatment. Surg Annu 11:249, 1979

52. Thistle JL, Carlson GL, Hoffmann AF, et al: Mono-octanoin, a dissolution agent for retained cholesterol bile duct stones, physical properties and clinical application. Gastroenterology 78:1016, 1980

53. Tompkins RK, Thomas D, Wile A, et al: Prognostic factors in the bile duct carcinoma. Ann Surg 194:447, 1981

54. Trotman BW, Ostrow JD, Soloway RD: Pigment vs cholesterol cholelithiasis: A composition of stone and bile composition. Am J Dig Dis 19:585, 1974

55. Velasco N, Braghetto J, Csendes A: Treatment of retained commonbile duct stones: A prospective controlled study comparing mono-octanoin and heparin. World J Surg 7:266, 1983

56. Venu RP, Geenen JE, Toouli, et al: Gallstone dissolution using monooctanoin infusion through an endoscopically placed nasobiliary catheter. Am J Gastroenterol 77:227, 1982

57. Warren KW, Choe DS, Plaza J, et al: Results of radical resection for periampullary cancer. Ann Surg 181:534, 1975

58. Wurbs D, Classen M: Transpapillary longstanding tube for hepatobiliary drainage. Endoscopy 9:192, 1977

59. Wurbs D, Phillip J, Classen M: Experiences with long standing nasobiliary tube in biliary disease. Endoscopy 12:219, 1980

60. Wurbs D: Endoscopic papillotomy. Scand J Gastroenterol 77(suppl):107, 1982

7

Operative and Postoperative Endoscopy of the Biliary Tract: Options in Management of the Retained Stone

The clinical problem of retained common duct stone is a complex one. The true incidence is difficult to ascertain due to difficulty in data gathering. For example, if the duct was never studied, how is one to know whether there were stones or not? Many different incidences are quoted, depending on which denominators are used. It has been estimated that a 5 percent incidence of overlooking stones exists if one considers all patients in whom there is an indication for exploring the common duct, but this incidence increases to 10 percent when stones had actually been recovered during the exploration.[23] For those patients requiring reexplorations, the incidence of overlooked stones is even higher, as much as 20 percent if there had been two previous explorations.[13,18] A 5 to 25 percent estimate has generally been quoted in the United States.[23] Ensuring complete removal of stones in the common bile duct still eludes the modern surgeon. The term *retained common duct stone* is applied to three possible situations: (1) The stone was not detected (or "overlooked," if one assumes it is always detectable) at the time of surgical exploration; (2)

the stone was left behind by the surgeon, as it cannot be removed due to difficult locations, technical hazards, or the patient's condition; and (3) stones re-formed in the duct since exploration. The predominant cause of recurrent stone in the common duct is poor detection,[23] and improvement in this area of the surgical technique would theoretically reduce the incidence. Advance in biliary endoscopy provides help not only in preoperative and intraoperative detection but also a means of retrieval by either endoscopic per-papillary or percutaneous route utilizing the T-tube tract.

The surgical operation of exploration of the common bile duct is conceptually an unsatisfactory procedure because the anatomy precludes direct examination of much of the territory. It is traditionally a blind procedure, heavily dependent on palpation, indirect tactile sensation through the use of sounds, and the retrieval of stones and sludge through forceps, scoops, and irrigation. Since the duct courses within the pancreas in its lower end and receives branches from within the liver, such technique has severe limitations. Operative cholangiography has significantly reduced the incidence of retained stones, but it is not perfect, and its routine use is still a matter of controversy. By and large, it is extolled by surgeons who use it routinely and are skilled at its performance and interpretation, while others point out that unless it is expertly performed the procedure is time consuming, full of pitfalls, and may lead to unnecessary exploration of the common duct. Prejudices aside, it is technically difficult to decide what is a blood clot, air bubble, sphincter spasm, or stone from shadows alone. More importantly, routine search with operative choledochoscopy after a negative cholangiogram turns up more stones in 14 to 24 percent of cases.[5,11,24] It is thus clear that operative cholangiography alone will not completely solve the technical challenge of exploration of the common duct. It is against this background that operative choledochoscopy was introduced: It is thought that direct and complete visualization of the ductal lumen should solve the technical difficulties of common duct exploration.

The original choledochoscope, modified from the cystoscope, was developed by Wildegans in 1953;[27] the same operative principles are still used in the modern rigid choledochoscopes. The first-generation fiberoptic choledochoscope was introduced in the early 1970s. The optics were no match for that of the rigid instrument, the controls were cumbersome, and the instrument remained unpopular until recently when the second-generation fiberoptic choledochoscope appeared, which eliminated most of the design imperfections of the earlier models. In current practice, both the rigid and flexible instruments are widely used. When properly performed, operative choledochoscopy takes less than 10 minutes, including setting up of the instrument, certainly taking less time to do than an operative cholangiogram.

It should be pointed out that operative choledochoscopy does not replace operative cholangiography for two reasons: (1) the upper reaches of the biliary system are not accessible to the choledochoscopes, and (2) the status of the ampulla of Vater before manipulation can only be assessed radiologically by a preexploration cystic duct cholangiogram.

Indications and Contraindications

Operative choledochoscopy is designed to be an integral part of the operation of exploration of the common bile duct and therefore has the same indications. It is particularly useful when exploring for small stones, for distal ductal pathology, and for biopsy of ductal neoplasms. Direct biopsy or cytology under vision on suspicious lesions can only be done through choledochoscopy. Retrieval of stones via the choledochoscope is much more certain than irrigation or blind instrumentation.

The only common contraindication is when the duct is too small for safe insertion of the instrument: any duct smaller than 5-mm diameter excludes the use of this modality. When blind manipulation of the ampulla of Vater is contraindicated, as in acute pancreatitis, choledochoscopy can still be carried out safely provided dilation of the ampulla is avoided.

Equipment

All rigid choledochoscopes are usable for nephroscopy, hence the term choledochoscope/nephroscope. The rigid instrument is a right-angled endoscope with a 4- or 6-cm horizontal arm and a 25-cm vertical limb, with a cross section of 5×3 mm (Fig. 7-1). The optics, typically the Hopkins rod–lens system, are superior to fiberoptics of the same cross section. Because of the rigidity, the instrument is easy to control with one hand. A detachable instrument guide allows the choledochoscope to direct an operating instrument to the desired location. A built-in irrigation channel affords infusion of saline to distend the ductal system, since viewing is underwater, just as in cystoscopy. The commonly used accessories are the balloon catheter, the stone basket and the biopsy forceps. A pressure system of infusion is preferred, using the blood transfusion pressure cuff.

The fiberoptic version (e.g., the Olympus CHF 4B) has a rigid section (34 cm) and a flexible section (33 cm), which has a diameter of 5 mm (Fig. 7-1). The claimed superiority over the rigid endoscope is its ability to conform

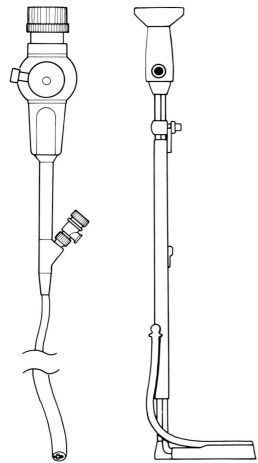

Fig. 7-1 The rigid and flexible choledochoscopes. The rigid instrument has a snap-on instrument guide attached, through which a flexible stone forceps or balloon can be directed to the target. The flexible instrument has the advantage of a longer working length.

to the curvature of the common bile duct and to turn corners, since it has a directable tip. The latter advantage is only realized in viewing the tertiary ducts in the liver, hardly a common use. The directional control is operated by the same hand that holds the endoscope, making it a more maneuverable instrument than the older version. However, the hand then becomes too close to the eye of the endoscopist, risking contamination. An instrument channel, 2-mm diameter, accepts the commonly used accessories, such as the biopsy forceps, the stone basket,

and the balloon catheter. To distend the duct, saline is infused via the same channel.

As in all operative endoscopy, aseptic technique dictates that the face and mask be kept as far away from the field as possible. For this reason the use of a miniature television camera coupled to the endoscope greatly facilitates all operative endoscopy, particularly for therapeutic endoscopy. Coordinated maneuvers by the assistant are much more successful by observing the action displayed on the monitor; at the same time, the risk of breaks in the aseptic technique are reduced, as are the physical strains on the operators.

Technique

In the opinion of this author, all operative choledochoscopy should be performed after a preliminary cystic duct cholangiogram. The procedure should be used to replace all the blind maneuvers of the traditional exploration, such as grasping with the stone forceps, and sounding with various dilators.

The exposure of the common duct must include a generous Kocher maneuver, mobilizing the second portion of the duodenum and the head of the pancreas to permit bidigital palpation of the ampulla. The supraduodenal segment of the duct is carefully palpated between finger and thumb. The intrapancreatic segment is then palpated for stones, but the duct itself cannot be felt. Finally the sphincter mechanism is palpated.

The technique for cystic duct cholangiography has been standardized, and excellent descriptions have been published.[4] The purpose of the cholangiogram is to visualize the ductal anatomy, the intrahepatic ductal lesions if any, the emptying into the duodenum, the length of the sphincteric segment, the size of the opening of the ampulla of Vater, and the size and lesions in the common duct itself. Briefly, the first cystic duct cholangiogram is taken with a small amount of dilute contrast (3 ml of 25 percent Hypaque) in order to outline the ampulla in the undisturbed state and to observe the early emptying into the duodenum. A second exposure is then obtained with larger volume of contrast (e.g., 6–12 ml) in order to see the intrahepatic branches, the ductal anatomy, and the size and number of stones. A third exposure is sometimes used with more contrast for the same purpose.

An oblique 2-cm incision is made on the anterior wall of the duct immediately above the duodenum. This is the author's routine incision for ductal exploration. Should the findings of the exploration indicate, this incision can be converted into a choledochoduodenostomy readily by making a mirror-image incision on the duodenum (Fig. 7-2), the resulting anastomosis is thus free of tension. Stay sutures are placed on the edges of the incision, and the rigid choledochoscope is inserted toward the ampulla after retracting the right lobe of the liver. By crossing the stay sutures while the saline infusion is in progress, leakage from the incision is reduced

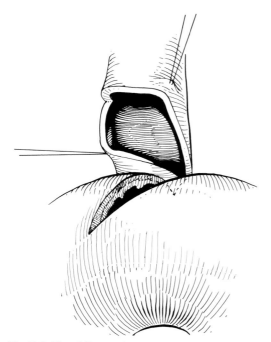

Fig. 7-2 The oblique supraduodenal choledochotomy on a dilated duct is readily converted to a choledochoduodenostomy. The incision on the duodenum is a mirror image of that on the bile duct as the duodenum is to be "rolled" onto the duct by completing this procedure.

and satisfactory ductal distention is obtained for examination (Fig. 7-3). To permit inspection of the entire lower duct, the right hand of the operator must align the ampulla in a straight line with the horizontal arm, while the left hand controls the shaft of the endoscope (Fig. 7-3). If the straightline view is not obtained, it is usually because the duodenum has not been adequately mobilized. A red-out will be seen if the tip is in contact with the wall. Backing off or withdrawing will restore the luminal view. To ensure that the entire lower segment of the common duct has been examined, the ampulla must be visualized though not cannulated. Failure to see the ampulla means that the ductal examination is incomplete, and stones hidden in the nonvisualized segment cannot be excluded. The ampulla is usually star shaped, with mucosal folds radiating from it, the dark void of the duodenum being visible at the center. It can also be round and patulous, triangular, pinpoint, or fish mouthed. The pancreatic ductal orifice is rarely visible with this instrument. It is unnecessary to advance the instrument for more than 1 to 2 cm downward once the horizontal arm has been completely introduced.

Exploration of the distal duct is done under vision using the balloon catheter. The catheter is first advanced into the duodenum. The balloon is then partially inflated (0.5 ml) and brought into the duct. As the ampulla yields, the balloon is seen springing into the duct. It is then completely inflated (1 ml) before further withdrawing toward the endoscope. Both endoscope and catheter are withdrawn slowly to bring any debris out of the ductal system. To extract a loose stone, the basket is preferred, although the balloon at times suffices. The basket is inserted until the tip has passed the stone. Once the stone is trapped, the basket is tightened and the entire ensemble withdrawn out of the duct. For an impacted stone, or a stone growing in a diverticulum of the duct so that only the tip is visible, the stone forceps must be used. The first step is to pry loose the stone, followed by retrieval. Berci et al.[5] recommended catheterization of the cystic duct remnant before extracting small stones in a dilated duct, as such stones

Fig. 7-3 Technique of operative choledochoscopy. The liver edge is retracted to permit insertion. The traction sutures on the common bile duct are crossed to reduce leakage of saline. The right hand of the surgeon straightens the bile duct (traction in the direction of the arrow) while the left hand controls the endoscope.

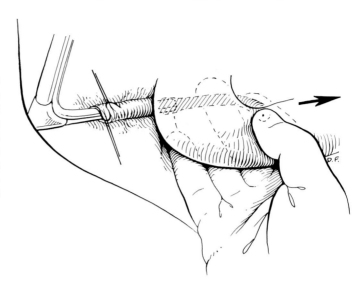

may be lost into this hidden space, and then migrate back into the common duct after the operation.

To inspect the upper portion of the duct, the endoscope is reinserted and aimed toward the hilum of the liver. The carina, the bifurcation into the right and left hepatic duct, is first identified. The right hepatic duct is distinguished by many orifices of the tertiary ducts visible a short distance beyond the carina. The left duct is usually without branches for some distance, but one orifice may be visible to the endoscope in the dilated system, sometimes so close to the carina that it simulates a trifurcation. Occasionally the left duct courses rather horizontally to the patient's left, making insertion of the rigid endoscope impossible. Any stones that are found are extracted by a similar technique. Stones visible in the origin of the tertiary system may sometimes be dislodged by applying suction to the irrigation channel. Reinfusion and suction may have to be done several times. Dislodged stones are much more readily retrievable in the secondary ducts.

Extrinsic compression appears as a smooth slit obstructing the progress of the endoscope without an intraluminal mass. For intraluminal neoplasms, targeted biopsy, directed brush cytology are obtained under vision as in any endoscopic procedure.

Endoscopic procedures are limited to extraction of stones and biopsy in general. Sometimes anastomotic strictures may be dilated with the Gruntzig balloon catheters (see Chapter 11) but not with the fragile biliary Fogarty catheter. If feasible, however, many surgeons would elect to perform surgical procedures on the stenosis, since the most difficult part of the operation, namely, exposing the ductal anatomy, is nearly accomplished by the time exploration of the duct is undertaken. By the same token, stenosis of the ampulla, when diagnosed by choledochoscopy, should be treated with transduodenal sphincteroplasty rather than endoscopic sphincterotomy.

The flexible endoscope is used somewhat differently. Insertion is easier and a smaller ductal incision (0.5 cm) may be used. Stay sutures are still essential, but leakage of saline is minimal. The modern fiberoptic choledochoscope has a rigid section, greatly stabilizing the instrument to permit a one-hand operation. Kockerization of the duodenum is not eliminated, since the duct still should be palpated. However, because the flexible shaft conforms to the curvature of the duct easily, the ampulla of Vater is visualized without the need to straighten the duct. The other hand of the operator is then available to operate the accessories, such as the basket, a minor advantage over the rigid endoscope.

The directional controls should be left neutral and unlocked. As the endoscope is advanced gradually, the lumen is automatically displayed, and the ampulla comes into view. After visual inspection of the lower duct, the balloon catheter is passed into the duodenum and the balloon partially inflated, brought into the duct, and then fully inflated, all under visual control as described with rigid endoscopy. Similarly, stones are extractable by passing the basket via the instrument channel.

It is in the examination of the upper ducts that the flexible endoscope is clearly superior. Here the directional controls may be used wtih advantage to enter the first 1 or 2 cm of the tertiary ducts in a dilated system. The horizontal left duct is entered easily. In the opinion of this author, the greatest advantage of the flexible endoscope is its longer usable length, which makes it the instrument of choice in exploring a duct from the duodenum through a sphincteroplasty, or after a previous enterobiliary anastomosis. For exploring the duct via the chole-choenterostomy, for example, the stab incision is made on the intestinal loop at a convenient site close to the anastomosis, and endoscopy of the ductal system is accomplished by cannulation of the choledochoenterostomy. Many operative procedures can be performed endoscopically, such as dilation or electrosurgical incision of strictures, including that of the anastomosis, balloon extraction of sludge and debris, and basket extraction of stones, avoiding much tedious and hazardous dissection at the porta hepatis.

The fiberoptic choledochoscope may also be used per papilla via a duodenostomy after sphincteroplasty. The usual clinical circumstances are as follows: There is clinical evidence of common duct stasis, including the clinical history and appearance of the duct at laparotomy. A cystic duct cholangiogram then delineates the anatomy, showing the location of stones and the length of stenosis, if any, at the ampulla. If there is no contraindication for sphincteroplasty, the duodenum is opened, and a sphincteroplasty is performed. Common duct exploration is done last, utilizing solely per papilla operative choledochoscopy without choledochotomy. The fiberoptic choledochoscope is inserted into the lower bile duct via the wide-open sphincteroplasty. Distention of the bile duct with saline infusion is easily attainable without the need to modify the standard technique. Retrieval of stones is under vision, using either the balloon, the basket, or the four-prong stone grasper. Even stones above the bifurcation are easily within reach of the fiberoptic choledochoscope. The main advantage of this technique is elimination of a choledochotomy and T-tube drainage, both of which contribute significantly to complications. This author has performed this procedure in five patients to date without complications other than transient hyperamylasemia in one patient.

POSTPROCEDURE MANAGEMENT

There is some debate as to the need for routine T-tube drainage following ductal exploration. Certainly the safety of primary closure of the common bile duct without a T-tube has been well shown. Also, the morbidity associated with T-tube drainage is not inconsequential, including leakage, displacement, and colonization of the common bile duct with bacteria[26] due to prolonged foreign body implantation. Some surgeons therefore advocate a primary closure, especially in patients in whom choledochoscopy has exonerated all possible causes of postexploration problems. However, a small incidence of overlooked stones (3 percent) is still possible under such ideal circumstances.[5,12] If the T-tube has been inserted, these stones can be retrieved nonoperatively in the vast majority of cases through the T-tube track. Routine T-tube insertion is therefore recommended on this basis.

The success rate of endoscopic extraction of overlooked stone is enhanced if the correct T-tube had been used at the time of exploration. Such a tube should have a large diameter of the long limb, typically 16 to 20 Fr. to facilitate the percutaneous endoscopy. The short T-limb for insertion into the duct need not be large;

12 to 16 Fr. suffices for most ducts. This bidiameter T-tube is produced commercially (Wheelan-Moss T-tubes, Davol, Inc., Cranston, RI). If such tubes are not available, the long limb of the regular 16 Fr. T-tube may be enclosed in a 20 Fr. catheter slit open longitudinally. The practice of coiling the long limb of the T-tube before routing it through the abdominal wall makes the extraction procedure difficult and hazardous, while conferring no safeguard to accidental dislodgement. It should be discouraged. The straight matured fibrous tract of 16 Fr. or larger admits the fiberoptic choledochoscope (or bronchoscope) without the need for preliminary dilation.

Complications

It is difficult to attribute common postoperative complications such as atelectasis, wound infection, or subphrenic abscess specifically to operative choledochoscopy. The following mechanical problems, however, are more specific.

LACERATIONS OF THE BILE DUCT

Theoretically, lacerations of the bile duct are possible with the rigid endoscope, but it really takes some rough handling for this complication to occur. Most often this involves tearing of the ductal incision, which can be repaired with fine absorbable sutures. Perforation is also possible; this can also be repaired after adequate exposure. T-tube drainage should be instituted as for all ductal repairs.

DAMAGE OF AMPULLA OF VATER

Passing the endoscope through the ampulla may traumatize it sufficiently to result in tearing or edema. The effect is like passing a large sound through the ampulla. The most feared immediate sequela is pancreatitis. It carries a 30 percent mortality, extrapolating from the data of postoperative pancreatitis following ampul-

lary procedures. The remote effect may well be stenosis of the sphincter of Oddi.

LOSS OF THE STONE

A stone in the bile duct may be displaced, in the process of extraction with the balloon, into the cystic duct remnant, remaining hidden during the subsequent search. The follow-up T-tube cholangiogram, however, would show the stone which has returned to the common duct after it has been closed. A stone may also be lost in the subhepatic space after it has been extracted from the duct. Chronic suppuration may result if the stone is heavily infected.

SEPTICEMIA

Excessive infusion pressure when the bile is infected may trigger septicemia, with intraoperative hypotension as the sole manifestation. It is always important to have the anesthesiologist on the lookout for unexplained hypotension during the procedure.

HEMORRHAGE

Hemorrhage may follow biopsy, but bleeding from the incision is the more likely. The choledochal plexus of vessels can be prominent if inflammation is acute. Electrocoagulation of the duct should be avoided, as a bile fistula may result. Bleeding is often observed after blind sounding, especially when cholangitis is present.

LEAKAGE

Bile may leak from the choledochotomy suture line, or from the cystic duct stump, manifested as excessive drainage of bile from either the drain or simply around the T-tube. The patency of the T-tube and its position in the duct must be ascertained by contrast study and appropriate action taken. One common cause is displacement of one limb of the T-tube outside the bile duct, diverting bile to the peritoneal cavity or to form a collection that then drains to the outside around the T-tube. If this occurs early, or if the signs and symptoms of biliary peritonitis are prominent, reoperation to reposition the tube and establish adequate drainage is necessary. If contrast study shows the T-tube in good position, the fistula is managed by continued drainage, as spontaneous closure can be expected.

STENOSIS

Stenosis of the bile duct at the site of choledochotomy can only be partially attributed to operative choledochoscopy. Improper closure of the incision is the most likely cause of stenosis.

Results

The efficacy of operative choledochoscopy is measured by the incidence of overlooked and irremovable stones. The results were reviewed by Shore and Berci[25] in 1976; newer data show similar results.[1,10,12] Overall, it varies between 0 and 16 percent, obviously dependent on the skill of the operator. The real incidence is impossible to estimate, as some of these findings are based on small series, some without postexploration T-tube drainage and cholangiograms, and a few include irremovable stones. An incidence of 1 to 2 percent of overlooked stones and 1 percent irremovable stones can be expected when this technique has been employed under optimal conditions.[1,10,12,25]

Routine deployment of operative choledochoscopy has advantages other than reducing the incidence of overlooked stones. Much time is saved once the surgeon is confident of the findings so he can proceed to the next logical operative step. If one accepts the premise that visual inspection is less traumatic and more accurate than blind instrumentation, the appeal to the surgeon's instincts alone would assure

it a permanent place in the armamentarium of surgery of the bile ducts.

PERCUTANEOUS CHOLEDOCHOSCOPY (VIA T-TUBE TRACT)

Retained common duct stone diagnosed by T-tube cholangiography in the postoperative period can be treated nonoperatively. In 1973 Burhenne described a method of basket extraction via the steerable catheter under fluoroscopic control[8] that quickly gained popularity. Since 1975, however, many groups have had success with percutaneous choledochoscopy.[2,6,7,14,15,22,28] The endoscopic method enjoys at least four advantages over the radiologic technique. First, visualization of the "filling defect" affords a surer diagnosis of retained stone, since at times the "stone" turned out to be a blood clot, a papilloma, or other lesion. Second, once the endoscope is in the common duct, the stone is trapped under visual control, a much more expedient technique than the hit-or-miss attempt under fluroscopy, where the precise spatial relationship between the basket and the stone is never clear. Third, radiation exposure to both the patient and the operator is decreased. Finally, the ampulla is not unknowingly violated, as may occur under fluoroscopy.

Equipment

The fiberoptic choledochoscope or bronchoscope meets the requirements of small-diameter, short bending section and appropriate optics. Both instruments come with their basket accessories usable via the instrument channel. A set of plastic tubes of increasing diameter (12 to 24 Fr.) with a blunt round tip are used as dilators over a guidewire. Fluoroscopy must be available. Videoendoscopy (using a television camera attachment) makes it easy for assistants to coordinate their efforts with the procedure.

Technique

The procedure should not be performed sooner than 6 weeks after T-tube drainage to allow time for the tract to mature. In stable patients it may be scheduled as an ambulatory procedure to be performed in the endoscopy room equipped with fluoroscopy; otherwise, it should be done in the radiology suite. The patient is administered appropriate prophylactic antibiotics if a bile culture has been positive the day before. Premedication with diazepam or Demeral is desirable.

After verification of the location of the stone by preliminary cholangiography, a guidewire is inserted via the tube into the segment of the bile duct where the stone resides (either above or below the T) under fluoroscopy. The T-tube is then removed over the wire. If the stone is large (6 to 10 mm), the tract may need to be further dilated to 22 to 24 Fr size.

The fiberoptic choledochoscope (or broncho-scope) is then threaded over the guidewire and advanced through the tract into the common duct under fluoroscopy. Some endosopists dispense with the guidewire. The endoscopic view shows only the guidewire in a fibrous tunnel. Once in the common duct, however, fluoroscopy can be stopped and endoscopy can begin. The guidewire is removed. The ductal system should be generously irrigated to aid visualization. When the stone is observed, the endoscope should be positioned at an ideal distance, about 2 cm from the stone; any closer than this may distend the duct and cause it to migrate farther distally. The basket is advanced until the stone is trapped within it. With the stone secured, the endoscope and basket combination is withdrawn together.

Alternatively, a Fogarty catheter may be passed beyond the stone and the balloon then inflated. By bringing the balloon toward the endoscope, the stone may be held against the lens and removed in this manner with the endoscope.

Whether stones can be safely pushed through the ampulla into the duodenum is a question that cannot be answered with available data.

Many factors have to be considered. For a loose small stone and a patulous ampulla, extraction is likely to be simple. For a stone impacted at the ampulla, retrieval is probably easier, certainly more controlled. Since stricture of the sphincter of Oddi has been associated with spontaneous passage of stones, it is unwise to court this complication by pushing the stone through the ampulla.

As soon as the endoscope is removed, a catheter is advanced into the duct for drainage. The catheter is removed only after a final negative check cholangiogram. If residual stones are still present, a second session is scheduled. As many as 50 percent of patients require more than one session to clear the biliary system completely of stones.

Complications

DISRUPTION OF THE T-TUBE TRACT

This complication is usually signaled by an undue amount of pain during the phase of dilation of the tract or during insertion of the choledochoscope. Shoulder pain suggestive of diaphragmatic irritation due to bile or pneumoperitoneum is accompanied by right-sided or generalized abdominal pain. The diagnosis is confirmed by demonstrating extravasation of contrast. If a guidewire had been used and is still in place, a catheter (e.g. 18 to 20 Fr.) can be passed over it to drain the duct. Stone extraction may be attempted again in several weeks. Operative treatment is required if the tract is lost, if no guidewire has been used, or if the patient has developed continued peritoneal irritation or deterioration.

SEPTICEMIA

Instrumentation of a chronically infected ductal system is likely to result in fever, chills, and leukocytosis even when prophylactic antibiotics have been administered. The severity of the episode is greatly reduced, however, with such prophylaxis.

NAUSEA AND VOMITING

Berci[3] noted that in about 20 percent of patients nausea and sometimes vomiting developed after the procedure on the first day. The etiology is unknown but is probably not related to premedication.

FAILURE TO RETRIEVE THE STONE

A tortuous T-tube track, a stone firmly impacted, and a stone in a diverticulum or upper reaches of the undilated biliary tree are factors that, singly or combined, may make it impossible to gain access to either the bile duct or stone.

STENOSIS

Stricture of the T-tube site may theoretically occur from excessive trauma due to instrumentation, but this has not been reported in large series. A case of stricture at the ampulla was reported in one series,[3] but it is unclear what role is played by percutaneous choledochoscopy.

IMPACTION OF THE BASKET

The endoscopist should be aware of this trap if the stone is larger than the T-tube tract. After the stone has been trapped in the basket, it is difficult to untrap it. If the trapped stone cannot be removed because the tract is too small, and the basket cannot be closed because of the stone, then the basket is trapped in the duct, a most disconcerting situation. Forceful retrieval risks disruptions of the tract. Operative removal may be necessary. If a lithotripsy basket has been used instead, the stone can be cut into small pieces by tightening the basket, the fragments are then removed individually.

Results

In Berci's series[3] of 55 patients, complete clearance of retained stones was accomplished in 95 percent of cases, although more than one session was required in 28 patients. There was no mortality. Only one patient required operative reexploration of the common bile duct. There were two instances of disruption of the T-tube tract during the process of dilation of a fine and tortuous tract. There were three failures, all due to an impassable tract. Burkitt,[6,7] Moss,[21,22] and a number of other investigators[14,15] have reported success rates of 95 to 100 percent clearance of all stones.

RADIOLOGIC RETRIEVAL OF RETAINED STONE

With the advent of the steerable catheter, the T-tube tract was used for stone retrieval under fluoroscopic control.[25] Some disadvantages of the endoscopic method over the radiologic method were discussed in the previous section. The radiologist's hands are usually in the fluoroscopic field during manipulation of the catheter; during a prolonged procedure, the radiation exposure can be substantial. The limit of resolution of the TV monitor is about 3 to 4 mm; stones smaller than this size may not be visible on the fluoroscopy but will be visible in the spot films. However, the major advantage of the radiologic technique is that the steerable catheter has a smaller diameter, is more flexible, and has a smaller turning radius than the choledochoscope, although this difference has practically disappeared with introduction of the new generation of choledochoscopes or bronchoscopes due to improved instrument design. When the stone is out of reach of the endoscope, such as in the peripheral ducts or in major undilated hepatic ducts that do not admit the endoscope, the steerable catheter must be used. The catheter is also advantageous in situations in which multiple smaller stones are present, as these can be removed with multiple passes of the basket through a stationary catheter, which serves for all intents and purposes as a large instrument channel.

Technique

The procedure is performed under fluoroscopy on an outpatient basis, with optional premedication such as diazepam. As in percutaneous choledochoscopy, after a preliminary cholangiogram, a guidewire is inserted into the duct via the T-tube, which is then removed (Fig. 7-4). The guidewire is not considered necessary by many experienced radiologists, but if the guidewire can first be placed at or beyond the stone, the subsequent manipulation is facilitated. The steerable catheter, which has cables built into the wall to enable the tip to be directable, is essentially a "flexible endoscope without the optical system." It is 30 cm long, 13 Fr. (4.3 mm) in diameter, and has a 3-mm lumen, capable of accepting many instruments

such as the Dormia basket. The steerable catheter is then threaded over the guidewire and passed into the bile duct toward and then beyond the stone. The guidewire is removed, and the Dormier basket is introduced closed until it just protrudes from the tip of the steerable catheter. It is opened until it fills the duct, moved back and forth, or rotated one way or another to trap the stone. Once trapped, the stone is seen to move with the basket; it is held by drawing the open basket into the steerable catheter. The stone, basket, and catheter are then withdrawn together (Fig. 7-4 D) through the T-tube tract. For multiple stones the procedure is repeated. More than one session may be required for many stones or fragments.

Stones larger than 10 mm may create a problem in their journey through the tract. They should only be fragmented by firm, steady pressure of the lithotripsy basket when it cannot be moved into the tract. Most stones are usually

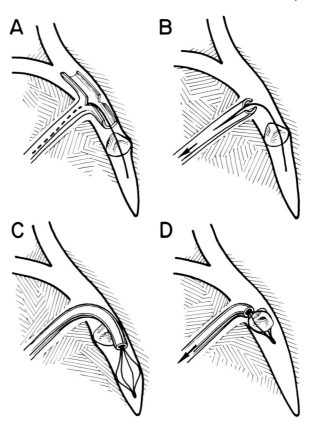

Fig. 7- 4 Steps in percutaneous radiologic removal of retained stones. (A) Guidewire introduced to the stone through the T-tube. (B) T-tube removed. (C) Steerable catheter is first introduced to just beyond the stone; basket in its sheath is next inserted inside the steerable catheter. The basket is opened beyond the stone. (D) Stone trapped in basket. Steerable catheter, basket, and stone removed together.

soft; cutting them into smaller pieces is not difficult. If a hard stone is encountered, considerable force may be required. The major fragments are then removed by multiple passes of the basket through the steerable catheter. Small fragments inside the duct may be left to be passed, monitored by follow-up studies. Fragments left in the tract must be removed. Because the lumen of the steerable catheter is considerably larger than the instrument channel of the choledochoscope, stone fragments or smaller stones can be removed without the need to move the steerable catheter, a significant advantage over the choledochoscope.

Distal impaction of the stone in the ampulla is almost never complete, as contrast can be seen passing into the duodenum. Positioning the steerable catheter to the stone and applying strong suction may serve to dislodge it, which may then be retrieved in mid-duct by the usual maneuver. If suction fails, a Fogarty catheter should be inserted beside the stone, through the ampulla, and into the duodenum. The balloon is inflated and brought back into the duct, moving the stone towards the steerable catheter. Once the stone is in optimal position, it can be removed with the basket.

Following extraction, a simple catheter (14 Fr.) is left in the duct for drainage and subsequent study, but it also serves to keep the tract open for further sessions, if needed. It is removed only after the check cholangiogram showed the ducts to be completely cleared of stones.

If a large stone is to be removed, the tract must be appropriately dilated in a preliminary session. The tract is dilated with progressively larger plastic blunt-tipped catheters threaded over the guidewire; it is possible to attain 20 Fr. (6.4 mm) during the first session and to 28 Fr. (9 mm) several days later. A catheter of the same size is left for a few days for the tract to mature after each session of dilation.

Complications

Burhenne[9] collected the results of the radiologic technique of retrieval in 38 institutions in 1976, 3 years after the introduction of the technique. The total morbidity was 5 percent, and no mortality occurred in more than 600 patients. More recent update by others[20] indicated two deaths in more than 1,000 extractions, for a mortality of less than 0.2 percent. This is thus the safest procedure for extraction of retained stones.

DISRUPTION OF T-TUBE TRACT

This can be caused by the steerable catheter but more often occurs as a result of dragging a large stone through a narrow tract. Contrast leakage may show free communication with the peritoneal cavity or simple loculation. Whenever possible the tract should be intubated so bile can drain to the exterior. Antibiotic treatment alone sufficed in all reported cases, although the patient should be evaluated by a surgeon in the early post procedure period to monitor the onset of signs of peritonitis or sepsis. If the tract cannot be found and the patient continues to have pain and peritonitis, surgical exploration is indicated. The disrupted tract is found operatively and the common duct is drained by intubating the tract, which is almost always identifiable.

PERFORATION OF THE BILE DUCT

This is a possibility, as tenting under fluoroscopy is frequently observed, but no cases occurred in the collected report.

SEPTICEMIA/BACTEREMIA

Transient fever without other manifestation occurred in 2 percent of cases. In a few of these patients, positive blood cultures, usually of the same organisms cultured from the T-tube, were obtained. A direct relationship with the duration and the complexity of the procedure appeared likely. As in choledochoscopic extraction, all patients should be put on prophylactic antibiotics as guided by preliminary bile culture.

SUBHEPATIC BILE COLLECTION

Leakage of bile may collect in the tract transiently and be reabsorbed later. If there is disruption of the tract, the collection may be anywhere, such as in the subhepatic space. The condition is usually first treated expectantly with antibiotics. If signs of sepsis develop or if the collection compresses on the ductal system, operative drainage is indicated. Subphrenic abscesses were not reported in that series, although this author has drained two patients for subphrenic abscess following this procedure. A fragment of stone was found associated with such an abscess.

LOSS OF STONE FRAGMENTS IN THE TRACT

This is usually easily recoverable; when they fragment, however, some may be lost, since they are not radiopaque. An occasional abscess may result.

IMPACTION OF THE BASKET

This is the identical trap discussed under percutaneous choledochoscopic retrieval of a large stone. If the stone is larger than the tract, the basket will not clear the T-tube tract. It will be trapped inside the duct, since the stone cannot be easily disengaged from the basket. Many instances of tract disruption are caused by forcibly dragging the stone in an effort to avoid this difficult situation. Disimpaction actually requires cutting the stone by forcible closure of the basket; fortunately many stones are soft enough to permit this, but surgical disimpaction may be necessary for hard stones.

HEMORRHAGE

Rarely hemorrhage occurs when preliminary dilation of the tract has been necessary. Although this complication is usually minor and of little consequence, the procedure should be terminated, especially in a patient with abnormal coagulation; the condition should be observed and treated conservatively.

VASOVAGAL REACTION

The incidence of this complication is under 0.5 percent. It is readily correctable by cessation of manipulation.

PANCREATITIS

The incidence was 0.3 percent in Burhenne's collected series, a much lower rate than that following common duct exploration.

OTHER COMPLICATIONS

When the filling defect is a papilloma rather than a stone, bleeding may result from attempted removal. The basket may be caught by the papilloma and cannot be retrieved. Operative removal will then be necessary.

The success rate is dependent on the skill of the radiologist; in experienced hands, it is over 95 percent. The major cause of failure is inability to traverse a tortuous and tenuous T-tube tract.

CHOICE OF OPTIONS

With the proliferation of new techniques, the surgeon must ask how all of these are going to affect the results of the treatment of common duct stones. As yet, there are no controlled data to permit dogmatic statements, but specific options can be discussed by considering what is already known about these techniques.

Operative Cholangiograms Versus ERCP

It is a provocative thought that an adequate preoperative ERCP may conceivably eliminate the need for operative cholangiograms in many situations. If ERCP can be performed reliably and more expeditiously than an operative cholangiogram, this may well be a viable option. Certainly a good negative ERCP eliminates the need for routine operative cholangiograms. The disadvantages of operative cholangiography are well known: (1) it takes up valuable operating time, (2) it is done without fluoroscopy and the filling is not monitored, (3) the patient cannot be moved into different positions, and (4) unlike ERCP, the duodenal aspect of the ampulla is not visualized or "felt" by cannulating under direct vision. The advantages of ERCP over operative cholangiography are many: When indicated, manometry can be performed at ERCP, allowing the diagnosis of stenosis of papilla to be established objectively. If stones are found on ERCP, endoscopic sphincterotomy and stone retrieval may be done, thereby avoiding a choledochotomy and its associated morbidity (see Chapter 10). If ERCP shows the duct is very large and indicative of marked stasis, if endoscopic stone retrieval is unsuccessful, or if other abnormality is discovered, such as tumor or stricture, then an operative exploration, especially in the form of operative choledochoscopy, is strongly indicated. Operative cholangiography remains indispensible, however if unexpected findings at cholecystectomy demand clear elucidation of the ductal anatomy or pathology.

Surgical Exploration of the Common Duct Versus Endoscopic Sphincterotomy

Surgical exploration using choledochoscopy has the best result of all methods in assuring clearance of stones (1 to 2 percent).[1,10,12,25] Endoscopic sphincterotomy followed by stone extraction may not clear the duct in at least 10 percent of cases but has the advantage of a lower mortality and morbidity. The two procedures complement each other. Perhaps if surgical exploration with choledochoscopy is reserved as a secondary procedure after failure of endoscopic sphincterotomy, the overall morbidity of common duct stones may be reduced.

Choledochoduodenostomy or Sphincteroplasty, Versus Endoscopic Sphincterotomy

Arguments have continued among surgical proponents of sphincteroplasty versus choledochoduodenostomy for many years. Sphincteroplasty is said to be more direct, avoids the sump syndrome which develops when the accumulated vegetable debris blocks the duct distal to the choledochoduodenostomy, and affords direct removal of impacted stones at the ampulla with the pancreatic duct in clear view.[17] The ampulla can be opened as wide as the duct.

The proponents of choledochoduodenostomy point out that the procedure tends to afford better drainage when the duct is markedly tortuous[16,19] and can be accomplished expeditiously in the elderly or obese patient. It is the only suitable drainage procedure in the presence of a lower bile duct stricture longer than 2.5 cm. The procedures are not mutually exclusive and are indicated by the particular circumstance of the case.

Endoscopic sphincterotomy is completely different from the open operations; it involves a cut that will permit extraction of a stone no larger than 2 cm, its chief virtue being a nonoperative procedure. Endoscopic sphincterotomy is unsuitable in the presence of marked stasis and tortuously dilated ducts or when the stone is so large as to demand a dangerous endoscopic sphincterotomy. It is therefore the procedure of choice for the severely ill patient but not for the severely ill bile duct.

Retrieval of Retained Stones: T-Tube Tract Versus Endoscopic Sphincterotomy

Both the radiologic and endoscopic techniques of percutaneous retrieval by means of the T-tube tract have a lower morbidity and mortality, and a better success rate for stone clearance than endoscopic sphincterotomy (95 percent vs 90 percent). (See Chapter 5.) In practice it depends on the availability of expertise, as well as local preference, in any particular institution, there being little choice between the

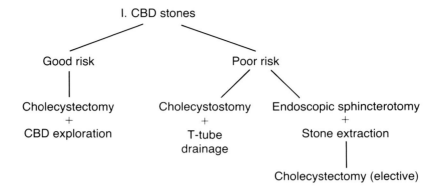

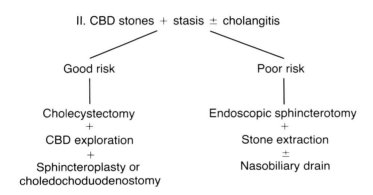

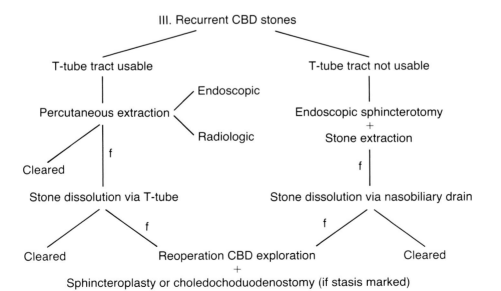

Fig. 7-5 Algorithm for management of common bile duct (CBD) stones. f = failed.

two. The endoscopic approach is definitely indicated when the T-tube tract is not usable (i.e., no T-tube, small T-tube, or tortuous tract) or when larger stones have to be extracted. By contrast, if the patient has had a Billroth II procedure, the T-tube approach is preferable. Endoscopic sphincterotomy adds some degree of protection against future recurrence by providing some form of drainage.

Stone Dissolution: T-Tube Tract Versus Nasobiliary Drain

Stone dissolution has a much lower success rate than mechanical extraction but is indicated for irremovable stones such as those impacted in a diverticulum or very large stones (over 2.5 cm) in cases unsuitable for surgery. For large stones, the procedures may be combined: Extraction should be reattempted after partial dissolution. Dissolution of large stones is time consuming and poorly tolerated due to many side effects.

When a T-tube is present, it should be used. High concentration of solvent can be delivered to the stone if a fine catheter with a small balloon is inserted via the T-tube and directed to the region of the stone. The T-tube drains the bile away from the infused solvent. Solvent contact with the stone is the most critical factor for success. If the stone is in the intrahepatic ducts, T-tube infusion is useless. Nasobiliary tube infusion may be attempted, provided the drain can be positioned near the intrahepatic calculus. A sphincterotomy is not necessary, although if dissolution is unsuccessful, one may be performed for drainage and the anticipation of spontaneous passage.

AN INTEGRATED TREATMENT PLAN FOR COMMON BILE DUCT STONES

The algorithm (Fig. 7-5) summarizes the roles of endoscopy and surgery in the treatment of common duct stones. For the ordinary case of primary stones, an initial per-oral endoscopic

approach by sphincterotomy followed by retrieval is reasonable, especially in patients unfit for surgery. When this is contraindicated because of the difficulty of local anatomy (e.g., Billroth II gastrectomy) or because of the presence of large stones, choledochotomy and operative choledochoscopy are indicated. Cholecystectomy should be done electively in those who had been treated with only the endoscopic procedure. For the complicated case with either acute cholecystitis or empyema of gallbladder, or both, surgery is the obvious choice.

A surgical drainage procedure (choledochoduodenostomy, sphincteroplasty) should be considered in addition when there is evidence of long-standing stasis such as a markedly dilated duct and considerable sludge and mud in the biliary tree. This author believes that surgical sphincteroplasty is a more satisfactory procedure for papillary stenosis, the objective documentation of which is elevated intraductal pressure (opening pressure above 16 cm H_2O) and a low flow rate (10 ml/min at 30 cm H_2O pressure) on manometry. Sphincteroplasty is indicated particularly when there is a history of associated pancreatitis. Choledochoduodenostomy is preferred when an expeditious procedure is desirable.

For secondary or recurrent (retained) stones, much depends on the previous operation. If the patient has a usable T-tube tract, percutaneous extraction (radiologic or endoscopic) should be performed. If no T-tube tract is usable, or if stones are large (but under 2.0 cm), they should be extracted by the papilla route after endoscopic sphincterotomy. For even larger stones, dissolution methods may be combined with extraction: Dissolution technique is used primarily for reduction of the size of stones, if achievable. Reoperation is indicated when these procedures have failed.

REFERENCES

1. Bauer JJ, Salky BA, Gelerant IM, et al: Experience with the fiberoptic choledochoscope. Ann Surg 196:161, 1982.

2. Berci G, Hamlin JA: A combined fluoroscopic and endoscopic approach for retrieval of retained stones through the T-tube tract. Surg Gynecol Obstet 153:237, 1981

3. Berci G, Hamlin JA, Grundfest WS: Combined fluoroendoscopic removal of retained biliary stones. Arch Surg 118:1395, 1983

4. Berci G, Hamlin JA: Operative cholangiography. p. 19. In Cuschieri A, Berci G (eds): Common Bile Duct Exploration. Martinus-Nijhoff, Boston, 1984

5. Berci G: Choledochoscopy. p. 359. In Dent TL, Strodel WE, Turcotte JG (eds): Surgical Endoscopy. Year Book, Chicago, 1985

6. Birkett DH, Williams LF: Choledochoscopic removal of retained stones via a T-tube tract. Am J Surg 139:531, 1980

7. Birkett DH, Williams LF Jr: Postoperative fiberoptic choledoschoscopy, a useful surgical adjunct. Ann Surg 194:630, 1981

8. Burhenne HJ: Nonoperative retained biliary tract stone extraction: A new roentgenologic technique. AJR 117:388, 1973

9. Burhenne HJ: Complications of nonoperative extraction of retained common duct stones. Am J Surg 131:260, 1976

10. Chen MF, Jan YY, Chou FF, et al: Use of fiberoptic choledochoscope in common bile duct and intrahepatic duct exploration. Gastrointest Endosc 29:276, 1983

11. Feliciano DV, Mattox KL, Jordan GL: The value of choledochoscopy in exploration of the common bile duct. Ann Surg 191:649, 1980

12. Finnis D, Rowntree T: Choledochoscopy in exploration of the common bile duct. Br J Surg 64:661, 1977

13. Glenn F: Retained calculi within the biliary ductal system. Ann Surg 179:528, 1974

14. Hwang MH, Yang JC, Lee SA: Choledochofiberoscopy in the postoperative management of intrahepatic stones. Am J Surg 139:860, 1980

15. Jakimowicz JJ, Mak B, Carol EJ, et al: Postoperative choledochoscopy. A five year experience. Arch Surg 118:810, 1983

16. Johnson AG, Rains AJH: Prevention and treatment of recurrent bile duct stones by choledochoduodenostomy. World J Surg 2:487, 1978

17. Jones SA: The prevention and treatment of recurrent bile duct stones by transduodenal sphincteroplasty. World J Surg 2:473, 1978

18. Lygidakis NJ: Early re-operation after surgery for calculous biliary tract disease. Br J Clin Pract 36:127, 1982

19. Lygidakis NJ: A prospective randomized study of recurrent choledocholithiasis. Surg Gynecol Obstet 155:679, 1982

20. Mason RR: Percutaneous extraction of retained gall stones. p. 77. In Motson RW (ed): Retained Common Duct Stones, Prevention and Treatment. Grune & Stratton, New York, 1985

21. Moss JP, Whelan JG Jr, Powell RW, et al: Postoperative choledochoscopy via the T-tube tract. JAMA 236:2781, 1976

22. Moss JP, Whelan JG Jr, Dedman TC III, et al: Postoperative choledochoscopy through the T-tube tract. Surg Gynecol Obstet 151:807, 1980

23. Orloff MJ: Importance of surgical technique in prevention of retained and recurrent bile duct stones. World J Surg 2:403, 1978

24. Rattner DW, Warshaw AL: Impact of choledochoscopy on the management of choledocholithiasis. Ann Surg 194:76, 1981

25. Shore JM, Berci G: Choledochoscopy. p. 291. In Berci G (ed): Endoscopy. Appleton-Century-Crofts, New York, 1976

26. Silen W, Wertheimer M, Kirshenbaum G: Bacterial contamination of the biliary tree after choledochostomy. Am J Surg 135:325, 1978

27. Wildegans H: Endoskopie der tiefen gallenwege. Arch Klin Chir 276:652, 1953

28. Yamakawa T, Komaki F, Shikata J: Experience with routine postoperative choledochoscopy via the T-tube sinus tract. World J Surg 2:379, 1978

8

Polypectomy

COLONIC POLYPECTOMY: RATIONALE

Polyps in the GI tract have a varied natural history, depending on location and histology. Polypectomy through the rigid sigmoidoscope was practiced for many years prior to the fiberoptic era. A mechanical strangulating snare was also used with the early fiberoptic gastroscope for gastric polyps, but the procedure often produced bleeding, as electrocoagulation was not used with it. The technique of colonic polypectomy was developed by Shinya in 1969, which soon revolutionized the treatment of colonic polyps. Before the advent of the endoscopic technique, colonic polypectomy, other than for polyps in the distal sigmoid and rectum with long stalks, was an open operation, carrying a significant morbidity.[26] Today polypectomy by colotomy is obsolete, a classic example of how therapeutic endoscopy has come to replace an open surgical operation and illustrates well the logic of the intraluminal approach for an intraluminal lesion. The greatly reduced mortality and morbidity of the endoscopic procedure quickly established itself as the procedure of choice for colonic and other polyps accessible to the endoscope.

One would have thought that so simple and effective a procedure for so common a condition would have provided the final solution of the clinical problem posed by the colonic polyp. As polyps in the colon are exceedingly common, it promises to threaten the national endoscopic resources just to survey and treat millions of colonic polyps and polyp-prone patients. To state the problem it is essential to review the current knowledge and belief of the fate of colonic polyps. Table 8-1 lists the histologic varieties of colonic polyps. The variety with the most clinical significance is the adenomas, a true neoplasm of epithelial origin. About 80 percent of all polyps are adenomas, which have a potential, now established beyond doubt, for malignant change.[6,19,36] The issue of malignant change was controversial 20 years ago,[8,46] but the evidence of a cancer-polyp sequence, accumulated particularly since the widespread deployment of colonoscopy, is quite overwhelming.[34,35] With the exception of malignancy complicating long-standing ulcerative colitis, the vast majority of adenocarcinoma are now thought to arise from a preexisting adenoma.[21,33,36,48] Factors particularly linked to malignant change have been identified: These include increasing size, increasing degree of epithelial dysplasia, and a villous growth pattern. The time it takes for an adenoma to develop into cancer is unknown; most evidence indicates that it is an extremely slow process, invariably over 5 years and averaging 10 to 15 years or even a lifetime. The clinical prevalence of co-

Table 8-1. Polypoid Lesions of the Colon and Rectum

Neoplastic
   Adenomas
      Tubular adenomas
      Villous adenomas
      Tubulovillous adenomas
   Carcinoma
Hamartomatous (Peutz-Jeghers)
   Juvenile
   Hemangiomas
Inflammatory
   Ulcerative colitis
   Lymphoid polyps
Unclassified
   Metaplastic (hyperplastic)

lonic polyp is also not precisely known, although it is estimated that about 10 percent of the Western population may be expected to harbor one or more adenomas in their lifetime.[14,42] Of all the adenomas removed from the colon, 5 to 10 percent may already be the seat of invasive carcinoma.[45] It is considered unethical to conduct a controlled trial to ascertain the value of polypectomy, since indirect evidence clearly shows that the incidence of carcinoma can be reduced by removal of all polyps. A frequently quoted study is Gilbertsen's[19] massive survey showing that with diligent proctosigmoidoscopic removal of all accessible polyps, the incidence of rectal cancer in that population was reduced. Shinya reported an 11-year experience with 712 patients who, after colonoscopic polypectomy, self-selected into two groups: those who returned for regular follow-up evaluation and those who did not. Sixty-four percent of the group followed up with colonoscopy developed polyps, of whom 8 percent had severe dysplasia and 7 percent carcinoma in situ. All polyps were removed when found, no invasive carcinoma developed, and no one died from colon cancer. By contrast, in the group who did not return for colonoscopy, metachronous carcinoma occurred in at least 8.9 percent of patients.[45] Bussey[7] further showed that in familial polyposis following subtotal colectomy, the development of rectal cancer can be prevented by proctoscopic removal of polyps as they arise. Thus 95 percent of all polyps removed are in a sense ''prophylactic'' for cancer. Furthermore, in the population that had a previous polypectomy, the yield of polyps in the future has

been shown to be much higher, as high as 30 to 40 percent over a 10-year period of follow-up.[45] It is the sheer magnitude of the clinical burden that poses a major logistic problem if one considers the recurrent nature of the condition and the need for lifelong follow-up evaluation of such a large segment of the population. Should all patients over a certain age be screened for polyps? Should all polyps incidentally discovered by radiography be removed? How frequently should these patients be colonoscoped for the rest of their lives? There are no easy answers to these questions, which arose only following the general availability of colonoscopic polypectomy.

Indications and Contraindications

If colonoscopy is performed for an indication other than polyps, all polyps discovered incidentally should be removed and submitted for histologic examination unless it is not safe to do so. If a polyp is discovered on barium enema examination, the following factors may strengthen or weaken the case for colonoscopic polypectomy.

SIZE OF THE POLYP

Before the advent of colonoscopy, surgical removal was justified only when the polyp was 1 cm or larger, since the incidence of invasive carcinoma in smaller polyps is too low[21] for an operative procedure to be deemed cost effective. Although the cost and risks of endoscopic polypectomy are much reduced, they would still be substantial if looked at cumulatively over a number of years. This author personally favors retaining a somewhat arbitrary size criterion for the endoscopic procedure and does not feel compelled to remove an asymptomatic polyp smaller than 0.5 cm, as detected radiographically, a position not necessarily endorsed by all. The author also does not consider any polyps too large to resect without colonoscopic evaluation of appearance, stalk, and other aspects (see under Technique). The truly large polyps may actually be polypoid carcinoma, which would contraindicate polypectomy; however, that should be clear on colonoscopy.

NUMBER OF POLYPS

When the polyps are so numerous as to merit the diagnosis of familial polyposis, polypectomy is clearly contraindicated; the appropriate procedure in that case is colectomy. Resection need not include the distal rectum, where polyps are easily accessible to the endoscope, making it possible to preserve sphincter function in these patients. When multiple adenomatous polyps are dispersed throughout the colon, the indication for polypectomy is strengthened even if none of the polyps are large enough to qualify under the arbitrary size criterion. By contrast, when the polyps are most likely inflammatory in nature (e.g., histologic proof of at least a few of them), complete removal of all such polyps is unnecessary.

THE STALK

A sessile polyp is difficult but not impossible to resect endoscopically. When it is large and sessile, the risk of injury is increased, as is the chance of incomplete removal. For very large sessile growths, such as a villous adenoma covering more than one-half the circumference of the colonic mucosa, endoscopic polypectomy is contraindicated, as 30 percent of these lesions harbor malignancy. When the polyp is obviously malignant on closer inspection, polypectomy is contraindicated (see under Technique). Endoscopic ablation of villous adenoma by laser photocoagulation is considered in the last section of this chapter.

THE CLINICAL SETTING

For patients with a history of colon cancer in the immediate family, previous cancer of the colon, and familial history of any of the precancerous syndromes, colonoscopic removal of new polyps is indicated.

In general the procedure is contraindicated if the risk and discomfort to the patient outweigh the potential benefit. Severe diverticular disease; previous pelvic surgery with marked adhesions; redundant, tortuous, or spastic colon; or cardiac dysrhythmia significantly add risk and discomfort to colonoscopy, which should not be done for trivial reasons such as a small round shadow in the cecum. For such a patient, annual double-contrast enema may be used to follow any growth, resorting to colonoscopy only if the indication is stronger. Colonoscopy is contraindicated for women in the first and third trimester of pregnancy with previous history of miscarriage. Any acute colitis may increase the likelihood of injury; both colonoscopy and polypectomy should be delayed until the inflammatory process has subsided. Other notable conditions that contraindicate colonoscopy are anticoagulant therapy, recent myocardial infarction, recent colonic anastomosis (1 to 2 weeks), intraabdominal abscess, and suspected colonic perforation.

Technique

EQUIPMENT

In addition to an adequate endoscopic room or suite with an area for preparation of the patient, a good endoscopic electrosurgical generator is essential. The characteristics and property of the electrosurgical current are discussed in Chapter 2. Although CO_2 is not regularly used, a low-pressure source should be available in the room, as an occasionally poorly prepared patient may require CO_2 for electrosurgery.

In selecting the numerous snares available, the only important requirement is that the loop element not be easily deformed. The depth of wire retraction into the sheath, usually adjustable, should be more than 10 mm; 12 to 20 mm is satisfactory. If the last 3 cm of the sheath is graduated, the size of the polyps may be measured accurately. The handle should have a provision to measure the thickness of the enclosed stalk. A rotatable snare is unnecessary, but it is useful for the technique whereby the polyp lassoed by loop rotation (see endoscopic techniques). Most "truly rotatable" snares will not rotate in a controlled manner if the snare is coiled. One must not depend on rotation to open the snare in the plane of the polyp, (a frustrating experience, as it either does not rotate or rotates excessively). A special right-angled snare is useful for the polyp situated behind a flexure or fold and is modified from an existing snare by constructing a short metal sheath to be slipped over the tip of a regular snare and glued in place (refer to Fig. 11-10). The loop then opens and closes at almost right angles to the body of the snare. A "home-made" snare is also useful: The loop element is formed by a single wire looped on itself. It has no handle and is operated by pulling one end of the wire while the other end is held stationary. It requires two hands to operate; but if the polypectomy snare is operated by an assistant this is not much of a disadvantage. The advantages of the "home-made" snares include positive sensation of catching the stalk, a good feel of cutting, easy disassembly and removal should snare entrapment occur (see Complications). The shape of the loop is unimportant; the hexagon loops demonstrate marginally improved resistance to deformity. More than one snare should be available for any one procedure, should the two-snare technique be called for.

Fluoroscopy is contributory only in the complicated case. In general, the need for it can be anticipated in situations such as an excessively tortuous colon, multiple previous abdominal and pelvic surgery, or difficult location of polyps. If the endoscopy room is not equipped with fluoroscopy facilities, advanced arrangement should be made.

The choice of colonoscope is mostly a matter of personal preference. The author prefers a single channel instrument for its greater flexibility. A double-channel endoscope is less flexible and is only occasionally needed. It is useful for lower GI bleeding, for multiple polyps requiring multiple retrievals, and for cases in which double snaring may be needed. Some experts use a dedicated upper GI endoscope for most routine colonoscopy and claim that they regularly reach the cecum with 100 cm of available shaft for insertion; the better flexibility more than makes up for the shorter length. Obviously, this is not for every endoscopist. All modern colonoscopes are fully insulated for electrosurgical work without exposed metal parts and equipped with a grounding button for the S cord, in case the instrument functions as a capacitor during electrosurgery (see Chapter 6).

PREPARATION OF THE PATIENT

A clean colon facilitates localization of the polyp, discovery of coexisting polyps or other diseases (e.g., angiodysplasia patches) not diagnosed by previous radiology, and greatly decreases the risks of complications such as explosion, current leakage into fecal fluid and electrical and mechanical injury of the colon (see Pitfalls in Technique). In the event of a perforation, fecal contamination of the peritoneal cavity is curtailed and, with the colon empty and the injury fresh, primary operative repair may be feasible.

Elective polypectomy is performed as ambulatory surgery except for patients with special complicating medical conditions requiring in-hospital treatment, such as control of congestive heart failure. For rectal and sigmoid polypectomy without the intention to perform total colonoscopy (e.g., when radiologic examination of the proximal colon has been perfectly satisfactory), evacuation of the distal colon with two Fleet enemas 1 to 2 hours before examination is usually satisfactory. Polypectomy is safe provided CO_2 insufflation is used, as the proximal bowel may contain feces, and there may be enough methane or hydrogen to reach explosive concentrations.

For cleansing of the entire colon, two general methods are available. The first is the traditional 2-day preparation with a combined regimen of laxatives and enema such as the following, written in simple instructions given to the patient.

Day 1 Clear liquid diet; cessation of all oral iron preparations.
Day 2 Clear liquid diet; 10 ounces of magnesium citrate at 4 PM
Day 3 Warm tap water enema until return is clear 2 hours before procedure

The above regimen must be modified for patients with inflammatory bowel disease or other diarrheal disorders. The cathartic is omitted on day 2. On day 3 after the first tap water enema administered at 8 AM, a second is given at 12 noon. The procedure is then performed at 2 PM. For the hospitalized patient for whom either enema or purgation is contraindicated for any reason, a 3-day zero-residue liquid diet such as Flexical or Vivonex will produce good results. For habitually constipated patients, their usual aperient should be continued, in addition to 10 ounces of magnesium citrate b.i.d for both day 1 and day 2. Good results are obtained with little discomfort.

The second method, preferred by many endoscopists, is whole gut lavage. This can be done with or without a nasogastric tube. After an overnight fast, at 8 AM on the day of the procedure, warm Ringer's lactated solution may be given by a small nasogastric tube at a rate of 2 L/hr for 3 hours, but a sulfate-containing solution has the advantage of minimizing fluid absorption. The solution (e.g., Colyte) may also be given orally, and the patient should be instructed to drink steadily at a rate of 250 ml/ 10 min. In the event of nausea, an injection of 10 mg of metoclopramide usually resolves the symptoms. Within 1 hour after beginning of the lavage, bowel movements begin. Clear effluent is usually observed 3 to 4 hours later. A total of 6 to 8 L of fluids must be ingested. Colonoscopy, scheduled at 2 PM, may be done sooner when the movement ceases, but some fluid may need to be aspirated. This is a well-tolerated method, and the result is often the best that can be attained. There is no need for prolonged fasting, and the short duration of the regimen is welcomed by most patients.

PREMEDICATION

Antibiotic prophylaxis is used only in the patient with cardiac valvular disease, or those with marked immunosuppression. In particular, antibiotics are not used in the manner of bowel preparation for colonic operations; neither luminal antibiotics (such as neomycin) nor systemic antibiotics are used for the routine polypectomy. When prophylaxis is indicated, this author favors a single dose of metronidazole combined with an aminoglycoside, given intravenously a half-hour before the procedure, at the same time as other premedication. Other regimens used include a combination of ampicillin and gentamicin.

This author routinely uses meperidine intramuscularly in a dose commensurate with the physical status of the patient, given 15 minutes before the procedure. Diazepam is used only occasionally if the patient is particularly nervous and anxious. Some means of IV access, such as a heparin lock, is set up before the procedure for further IV medications, when needed. Glucagon is used only when troublesome spasm is encountered, and preferably at the later stages of the procedure since a floppy colon is difficult to intubate. With air distention, tortuosity worsens and length increases in a toneless colon. However, during the withdrawal phase, a relaxed colon is easier to inspect. General anesthesia impedes the procedure, as the colon is more flaccid and harder to intubate, and the endoscopist is much less aware of overstretching. Despite a higher risk, it is indicated in children, in psychotic patients, and rarely in those with severe and painful anal disease.

For the patient with myocardial disease, an ECG monitor with audible signal is a must to warn the endoscopist of arrhythmia, which frequently occurs with rectal and sigmoid manipulations. Stretching of the sigmoid mesentery is particularly prone to bring on arrhythmia.

Respiratory rate and blood pressure are measured periodically during the procedure by the endoscopy nurse in all patients, but in the cardiac patient the procedure should be terminated if troublesome arrhythmia or hypotension is induced.

Finally, with the patient on the table, a visual inspection of the current pathway is undertaken. The steel grounding plate is not a satisfactory ground for colonoscopic electrosurgery; this author prefers the disposable variety that can be applied with firm adhesion to the skin. With spontaneous movement the patient may be out of electrical contact with the stainless steel grounding plate at any time during the procedure without being noticed as the room is darkened. Modern electrosurgical generators have built-in warning circuits to prevent burns, but it still wastes time.

ENDOSCOPIC TECHNIQUES

The technical details of colonoscopy are well described in many good endoscopy manuals, but some key points deserve emphasis. Since the patient's back faces the endoscopist, it is important for the patient to be forewarned every time a new move is made. Thus the patient should be told as the instrument is inserted, air insufflated, a loop being reduced, and so on; otherwise, sudden moves will only produce apprehension and loss of cooperation.

For smooth and rapid intubation of the entire colon, the configuration of the endoscope, when reaching to the cecum, must be close to a three-quarter circle. Most endoscopists rely almost solely on frequent withdrawals to straighten out the loops, especially the sigmoid loop. Every time a sharp corner has been negotiated, the shaft can be withdrawn without losing ground as the tip is anchored by the turn. Only rarely is the α-loop maneuver used, since no loop is allowed to be formed. Advancing the instrument should almost always produce advance in the endoscopic view (the 1:1 advance); if not, the loop accumulated must be reduced by withdrawal at the first opportunity, that is, after turning the next corner.

In theory it would be desirable to complete the colonoscopy before commencing polypectomy. This is the general plan followed by the author for polyps in the right colon. Polyps in the left colon are removed as they are encountered. This is because of expediency; distances are deceptive as markers; and more time may have to be spent to find the polyps again on the way out. If the polyp is small, it can be retrieved by suction into a trap inserted in the suction line, after which colonoscopy is continued. If the polyp is large, there is little risk of losing it in the lumen, retrieval is left until after completion of the examination. For polyps in the right colon, total colonoscopy is accomplished first, and the polyps are resected during the phase of withdrawal. The reason is to get over the uncomfortable portion of the procedure as fast as possible, since withdrawal and deflation make the patient more comfortable. When there are multiple polyps dispersed on both the right and left colon, a good plan is to first complete the examination of the entire colon, scrutinizing every polyp, as there is a substantial chance that one of them may appear grossly malignant. If there are no suspicious-looking polyps, this author would commence removing the polyps in the right colon first, using a splinting device (see Technique) to facilitate repeated insertion and retrieval of the polyps when they are too large to be recovered via the instrument channel. The specimens must be numbered and put in separate bottles and a map of their location provided to the pathologist. At a second session several weeks later, the polyps in the left colon are resected. In this way invasive carcinoma discovered on histologic sectioning can be traced with certainty to the part of the colon from which the polyp originated.

Numerous tricks are used by various endoscopists to facilitate placing a snare around the target polyp, but the principle is the same. The polyp is first centered in the endoscopic view. The unopened snare is passed down the instrument channel until the tip of the sheath is just visible. The loop is opened under vision. The polyp is lassoed by using the endoscopic directional controls. The tip of the sheath is then placed at the intended site of transection, midway in the stalk if possible. With the tip in this position, the snare is slowly closed. As the tip of the sheath indicates the closed position of the snare, it is most important to place it at the location of intended transection prior to closure of the snare.

One method of facilitating the procedure is to advance the tip of the unopened snare to the site of intended transection. The snare is now opened. It does not matter in what plane the snare opens; the loop element can be completely behind or in front of the stalk. Rotation of the snare (assuming a rotatable snare is used) by rotating the handle will place the loop over the polyp (Fig. 8-1). It should be noted that the rotatable snare gives only uncontrollable rotation at best and is frequently looked upon as

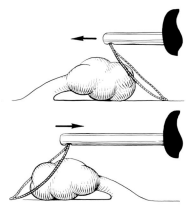

Fig. 8-2 The right-angled snare is useful for some polyps.

a useless function. It is indeed clumsy to use if one relies on this function to give the loop a more workable plane. Used in the way described, however, it does not matter if it overrotates, as the polyp will be snared by the turning-over movement of the loop.

Another method is to use an angled snare. It is unfortunate that a polyp is always depicted in textbook diagrams like a sunflower rising straight from the soil. To lasso this polyp, the conventional snare may well be the instrument of choice. In practice the stalk is usually axial with the endoscope, with the polyp either closer or farther away than the stalk. An angled snare saves much maneuvering. The tip of the unopened snare is first placed at the head of the polyp, the loop opened and simply slipped over the head to reach the stalk (Fig. 8-2). An angled snare is easily improvised from existing snares (see Chapter 11, Fig. 11-10).

Yet another method is to advance the endoscope to beyond the polyp. The closed snare is passed until 2 cm of it is visible. The loop is opened. The endoscope is withdrawn slowly to drag the opened loop over the polyp. If the loop is in the correct plane, the polyp will catch. If it is not, rotation of the snare at the right moment will bring the loop over the polyp (Fig. 8-3).

A fourth method is the reverse of the above: The endoscope is first positioned several centimeters from the polyp. The loop is opened and

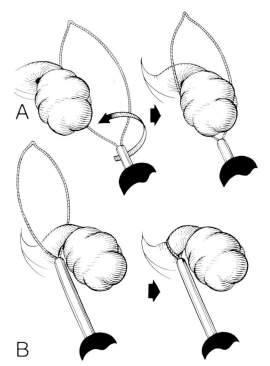

Fig. 8-1 (A) The opened snare, when placed next to the polyp, may lasso the head by rotating the snare. (B) The line of transection is determined by the position of the tip of the snare-sheath.

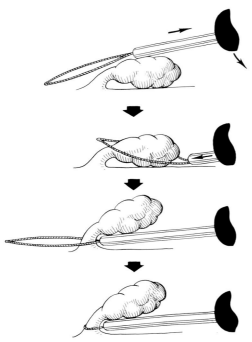

Fig. 8-3 Polyp snaring by dragging the opened snare toward the endoscope.

and the loop must be released and tightened again when only the stalk is seen to be enclosed. The tightened snare is moved to and fro; if the colonic wall moves with it, part of the wall is snared and the loop must be released. A correctly snared polyp turns to a dusky hue within a minute. For a thin stalk, caution must be exercised in tightening or severance may occur before the current is passed. Fortunately a small stalk does not give rise to too much bleeding. This is not the case with the larger stalk, where severance can produce brisk bleeding.

The principles and safety precautions of electrosurgery are discussed in Chapter 2. Before passing the current, the snare should be judi-

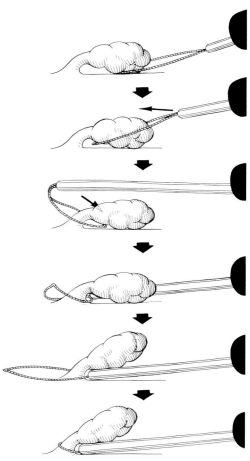

Fig. 8-4 Polyp snaring by pushing the opened snare under the head and then bringing the tip of the sheath to the base.

the snare advanced, dragging the loop behind it (Fig. 8-4). The snare now functions for all intents and purposes as a right-angled snare, and the polyp can thus be lassoed by simply slipping the loop over it. One runs the risk of permanently deforming the loop if the polypectomy is completed in this position. It would be more advisable, once the stalk is encircled but before closure is completed, to swing the snare around by withdrawing the snare so the tip is nearest the lens; the loop is thus reduced (Fig. 8-4).

Often it is not possible to have the entire loop within view, and sometimes the polyp may not be seen during the actual lassoing. However, it is crucial that the entire loop be kept in full view, including the tissue it encloses during closing. It is possible to estimate the size of the stalk by the resistance of the closed loop and the marking on the handle. If the resistance is too great and the reading on the handle indicates a wider stalk than the visual estimation, snaring of the colonic wall must be suspected cially tightened to reduce the cross section of the tissue held by it so as to increase the heat generated by the passage of the current, especially critical in resection of large stalks. Blended current (coagulation with cutting) is commonly used. It is not a good practice to use coagulation followed by cutting as it is impossible to judge when the central arteriole has been coagulated in a large stalk. By contrast, pure coagulation current takes a long time, if ever, to transect a large stalk, risking transmural coagulation. Blended current avoids these difficulties. As the stalk is severed, the stump turns whitish. In a thick stalk where the volume of tissue to be coagulated is large, the central arteriole may still be patent when transection occurs. This is one of the most frequent cause of bleeding. The stump should therefore be inspected routinely: If only an amorphous whitish mass is left, nothing further needs to be done, but if a recognizable vessel is detected, such as a blood-staining or red thrombus, it must be coagulated again with a monopolar coagulating probe or forceps.

Since a variable amount of tissue is snared from polypectomy to polypectomy, it is difficult to know how high a power should be used. The best guide is to begin coagulating with a low power and to slowly turn up the dial while watching for the whitening, smoking, and bubbling effect. Once that is detected, the dial is turned back just a little and coagulation is continued until transection occurs. This procedure ordinarily should not take more than a few seconds. If no coagulating effect is seen after several bursts at a high-power setting (e.g., 75 to 100 watts, totaling 15 to 20 seconds), the entire situation must be reviewed. Beginning with the electrosurgical generator connections, the grounding pathways, the electrical leads of the snare, and finally the volume of tissue ensnared must be checked. All traces of fluid in the lumen must be removed. The loop is released, the tissue within the circular mark examined, and, when necessary, the stalk is resnared, and the maneuver to rule out ensnaring of the colonic wall is repeated.

Lack of coagulation when the generator is functioning indicates current leak, which occurs under several conditions. A common cause is a large floppy head which comes into contact with the wall in several places. Fluid in the lumen bathing the head is another source (Fig. 8-5). When a serious leak is present, even many seconds of high-power coagulation produce no visible effect, a most upsetting experience. For large polyps, distention of the bowel temporarily may prevent the undesirable contacts and current leakage; but in even larger polyps that fill the entire view, the size of the head must be first reduced by piecemeal resection as shown in Figure 8-6. The snare is looped on an upper portion of the head and current applied as the snare is moved to and fro to diminish the risk of mucosal burn in one small area. Higher power and longer application may be required. When the head has been reduced (sometimes after several cuts) the stalk can be seen better for safer electrocoagulation.

A very short stalk is dealt with by lifting the ensnared polyp to create a pseudostalk (Fig. 8-7). Most medium-sized sessile polyps, up to

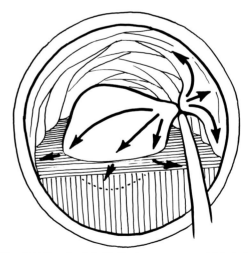

Fig. 8-5 Luminal fluid dissipates current. If it is in contact with the cutting wire, electrosurgery may not be successful. The principle, however, may be used for protecting the colonic wall from burn injuries by injecting saline to bathe only the head. (Chung, RS: Diagnostic endoscopy indications and technique. In Fromm, D Gastrointestinal Surgery, p. 28. Churchill Livingstone, New York, 1985.)

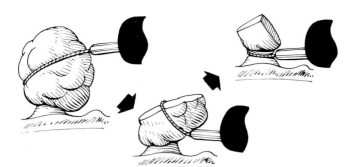

Fig. 8-6 Piecemeal resection of large polyps.

2 cm in diameter, can be resected successfully in this way. Current is not applied until a pseudostalk has been formed. Even so, as low a power setting as will produce a visible effect must be used, as current is being applied to the naked colonic wall proper. More often the polyp is judged as sessile on radiologic appearance alone when in fact it has a stalk that can be snared on colonoscopy examination. This is especially likely if the head is large, hiding the stalk. For truly sessile polyps larger than 2 cm, piecemeal resection should be considered. When the base cannot be safely removed, 0.2 ml of India ink can be injected submucosally, using a flexible injector similar to that used for sclerotherapy to mark the base, pending histologic examination of the resected specimen. If the tissue is benign, a repeat colonoscopy in 4 weeks should be performed for resection of the base. At this time the necrotic area would have separated and epithelialization would have been complete. If only a scar remains but no

base is left, there is nothing to resect; if a small base is left, it can be easily dealt with using hot biopsy forceps or snare, since the exposure is good and there is no polyp to contend with. If malignancy is found in the resected tissue, the patient's treatment should be decided by whether the submucosa of the colonic wall is free of invasion or not (see Malignant Polyp), and whether there has been complete resection.

Bipolar snaring of a polyp has been described[1,10] using two snares (Fig. 8-8), and also using a specially designed bipolar snare.[49] The technique is suitable for the polyp with a large stalk. For the two-snare method, a home-made snare is first passed and the stalk snared and tightened without strangulation. Since the home-made snare has no handle, the colonoscope can be removed leaving the snare held tightened

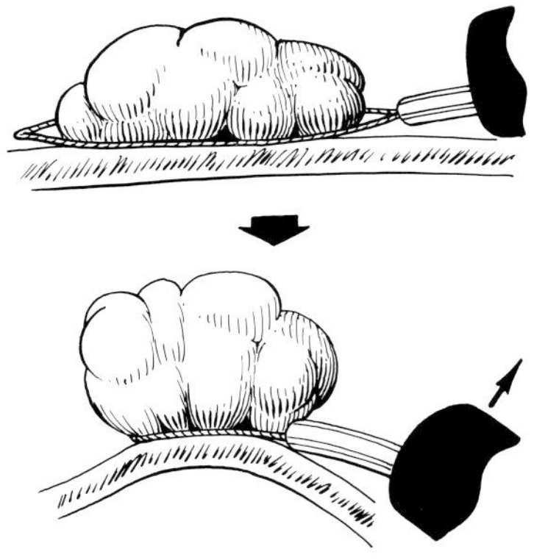

Fig. 8-7 Sessile polyp excision by first creating a pseudostalk.

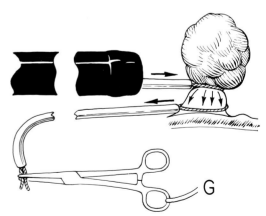

Fig. 8-8 Polypectomy using the double-snare method. If a double channel endoscope is used, both snares can be placed with only one pass of the endoscope. The lower snare is for grounding (G). The tissue between the snares is coagulated.

with a hemostat. The colonoscope is passed again and a conventional snare is used to snare the stalk nearer the head. If a double-channel colonoscope is used, two conventional snares can be placed one after another without the need to withdraw the endoscope. In the bipolar mode, the current is passed from the snare near the head of the polyp and conducted away by the snare near the base without the need for a patient plate. Transection occurs at the higher snare. If bleeding follows transection, the lower snare can be tightened, and bipolar electrocoagulation can be applied to the bleeder with a probe or forcep, utilizing the lower snare as a ground. The bipolar snare simplifies the procedure even further; one element of the snare wire supplies the current, while the other element returns the current to the machine, the two being separated at the tip of the loop by insulated material. The instrument is simply connected to the bipolar outlet of the electrosurgical generator with no need for a grounding plate.

Small polyps, up to 5 to 6 mm in diameter, may be removed by the hot biopsy technique (Fig. 8-9). For this purpose the insulated hot biopsy forceps, a monopolar electrocoagulating forceps with usually 6-mm opened jaws, is used to enclose the entire polyp and traction exerted to lift up the polyp to form a pseudostalk. Current is passed as the forceps are completely closed, the narrow pseudostalk gets most of the heat and separation frequently (although not invariably) occur at that level. The residual of the polyp will be coagulated but the enclosed tissue, being separated from the rest of the colon, does not conduct electricity. If the process of coagulation is quickly over with, heat conduction is not enough to affect the histologic study of the tissue enclosed in the cups of the forceps.

Atypical polyps always raise the suspicion of malignancy. Especially suspicious are irregularity of the head and a non-spherical shape, ulcerations, and a short, wide irregular stalk, which is really the base of a carcinoma. Other signs include a concave surface, nodular periphery with asymmetry, and a stalk that feels unusually firm or hard as judged by closing the snare. When the lassoed polyp is moved and the colonic

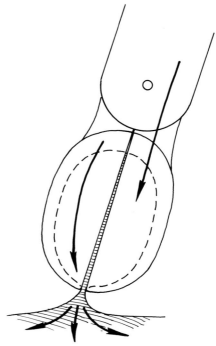

Fig. 8-9 The hot biopsy principle. The enclosed tissue is relatively unaffected by electrocautery while the narrowed base reaches a high temperature and becomes coagulated. (Chung RS: Diagnostic endoscopy: indications and technique. In Fromm D. Gastrointestinal Surgery, Vol. 1. p. 30. Churchill Livingstone, New York, 1985.)

wall is seen to move with it, invasive carcinoma beyond the submucosa is likely. The endoscopist should reconsider the plan of management. If the polyp can be completely excised, careful excision is performed, and the site of the polyp marked with submucosal India ink injection. If it has so broad a base that total excision may be technically difficult, or that incomplete excison will result anyway, a generous biopsy either using the snare as in partial polypectomy, or preferably biopsy forceps without electrocautery should be done. Cytology brushings should also be obtained. The specimen must be palpated for hardness and frozen section requested. When the diagnosis is invasive carcinoma to the submucosa the subsequent management will be clear. The site of the lesion can be identified easily at operation from the serosal aspect because of the India ink injection.

Palpation is the best means of gross detection of malignant tissue; any hardness or induration localized to one area of the polyp should be so described in the pathology requisition form. The tissue is also examined by a hand lens and oriented. There are quite a few different ways of doing this: The principle, however, is to identify the transection line so that the depth of invasion can be determined with certainty. This is important in large polyps excised by several cuts. The author's method is to draw a diagram to identify the cuts in the pathology consultation form, and put the tissue yielded from each cut into a separate bottle (Fig. 8-10). Thus, cut 1 has one transection margin and does not require special marking, but cut 2 has two and cut 3 has three transection margins. A pin may be inserted into one margin to distinguish it from the other, clearly labelled in the diagram. The importance of such specimen handling will be driven home if the endoscopist were involved in a case where the resection margin cannot be read with certainty due to poor labeling.

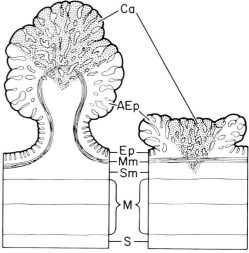

Fig. 8-11 When malignancy is found in the submucosa in the sessile polyp, surgical resection is indicated; this is not necessarily so in the pedunculated polyp, since invasion of the submucosa in the stalk does not have the same clinical significance as invasive of the submucosa of the colonic wall itself (see text). Ca, carcinoma; AEp, adenomatous epithelium; Ep, epithelium; MN, muscularis mucosae; Sm, submucosa; M, muscularis; S, serosa.

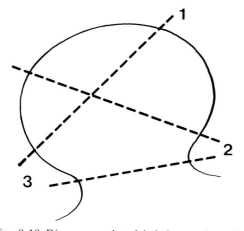

Fig. 8-10 Diagram used to label the specimen for the pathologist when the polyp has been removed piecemeal. The line of transaction of the stalk must be clearly indicated with a pin. (Chung RS: Diagnostic endoscopy: indications and technique. In Fromm D, Gastrointestinal Surgery, Vol. 1, p. 29. Churchill Livingstone, New York, 1985.)

THE MALIGNANT POLYP

When the removed polyp is found to contain malignant tissue, the management decision is based on a careful consideration of the adequacy of the excision, the expected risk–benefit ratio of surgical treatment, and to a lesser extent the degree of invasiveness as judged by histologic appearance.[11,16,22,28,29,39,50]

For carcinoma in situ, defined as malignancy confined to the mucosa without involvement of the submucosa, polypectomy is, by general consensus, a curative treatment for the lesion.[35,50] The patient must be advised to be followed up regularly for future development of similar lesions, with the hope of dealing with them at an equally early stage.

For carcinoma involving the submucosa in the stalk (Fig. 8-11), but not to the resection margin, management is more controversial. Most data support no further surgical treatment if the submucosa of the colonic wall level is not involved, as the pathologic report of the excised colon and lymphatics is always negative of malignancy in most studies.[16,22,35,37,50] Colectomy is not indicated in this situation, particularly when the patient is not a good operative risk.

Polypectomy should be regarded as no more curative than a simple biopsy if (1) the line of transection is not free of cancer, (2) incomplete excision was recognized by the endoscopist at the time of polypectomy, (3) there is no stalk and the submucosa of the colonic wall is invaded (Fig. 8-11), or (4) the invasion of the stalk extends to the level of the general submucosa of the colon. The definitive treatment should be colectomy as for any early carcinoma of the colon, unless the patient is suffering from severe medical illnesses greatly increasing the risk of operation. Under such circumstances, the treatment plan must be individualized as demanded by a careful consideration of the relative risks. Local endoscopic procedures such as laser photoablation may have a role as definitive treatment for selected patients (see Chapter 10, under Rectal Carcinoma).

Just as the general medical condition of the patient influences the decision, so does consideration of certain histologic features of the specimen. Anaplastic appearance (very rare) and lymphatic and perivascular or perineural invasion are considered indicators of high potential for lymphatic spread, tending to tip the balance in favor of surgery even if the stalk margins are free.

Recent analyses of many large series of malignant polyps emphasize the scrutiny of line of transection[11,16,22,28,29,39] and support the approach outlined above. The critical factor influencing nodal metastasis appears to be invasion of the submucosa of the colonic wall, not so much the stalk of the polyp even though it consists of submucosa.[35,37] It should also be realized that a stalk is sometimes created by the endoscopist or surgeon, consisting of submucosa of the colon drawn up by traction on the polyp before transection, a possible cause of confusion in interpretation of the published data. Figure

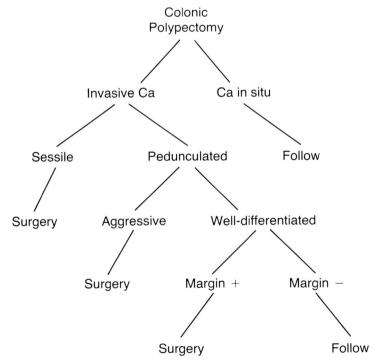

Fig. 8-12 An algorithm for management of the malignant colonic polyp.

8-12 is an algorithm that summarizes the discussion of this section.

Complications

All complications of diagnostic colonoscopy can occur, including reaction of premedications, vasovagal reactions, and postcolonoscopy distention. The following complications are specifically related to polypectomy.

HEMORRHAGE

The incidence varied between 1 and 3 percent[2,32,43,45] in large surveys and is the most common complication of polypectomy. When fragile the stalk may have been transected mechanically before current was applied. Using pure cutting current is another cause. Using too high a power setting, even when it is a blended current, may result in too fast a cutting, severing the vessel before it has been coagulated. When the stalk is large, failure to reduce the cross section by strangulation before passing current may result in inadequate coagulation of the central arteriole. Excessive bleeding may also result when the colon has been injured, but this is likely to be accompanied by other symptoms of perforation.

When spurting bleeding occurs immediately after polypectomy, the endoscopist must act quickly or the view will be lost. The polyp is relinquished and the opened snare is looped over the stump for mechanical strangulation. This will stop the bleeding and remove the threat of loss of view. The length of the stump is then inspected. If it is longer than it is broad, it is safe to apply coagulation current (not blended) until the entire stump turns white. If the stump is short, further coagulation runs a risk of causing a transmural burn; while mechanical strangulation alone would risk delayed recurrent bleeding. A compromise is to maintain mechanical strangulation for 5 to 10 minutes, and then apply electrocautery with a coagulating probe, coagulating forceps, heater probe, or laser photocoagulation to the transection surface.

When the patient presents with passage of much blood per rectum, usually within 24 hours after polypectomy, colonoscopy should be undertaken while bleeding is still active (see Chapter 4), and the bleeding stump identified and appropriately dealt with by resnaring or coagulating. Colonoscopy is difficult when bleeding has slowed or stopped, since the view will be very poor. Such patient can be managed expectantly. It is always a difficult clinical decision whether to start preparing the bowels in anticipation of the need to intervene. Most gastroenterologists would opt to "let things cool," for fear of dislodging the clot, and to pursue the watchful policy. Such a regimen is appropriate, provided emergency therapeutic colonoscopy is on standby if and when the patient starts to bleed, when the self-cleansing action of hematochezia makes emergency colonoscopy possible. If the bleeding stump is distal to the splenic flexure, especially in the sigmoid, the bowel is easy to clean and therapeutic colonoscopy should be attempted before the next bleed. The alternative is emergency surgery if rebleeding resumes while the patient is being watched.

Delayed hemorrhage may also occur, presenting as a major bleeding 10 to 14 days after polypectomy, presumably the secondary hemorrhage from sloughing of the eschar. Many of these patients may have taken aspirin or anticoagulants. Shinya[45] recorded 24 instances out of 5,500 patients. Diagnosis is less straightforward, especially when diverticulosis has been documented in the colonoscopy, or when multiple polyps have been removed. The diagnostic routine, including angiography (described in Chapter 7), should be followed. Treatment is no different from immediate bleeding, but surgical operation is more likely to be required. Unlike bleeding from a stalk, bleeding from a slough is less likely to be amenable to therapeutic endoscopy.

PERFORATION

The incidence of this complication is between 3 to 4 per 1,000 procedures of polypectomy,[2,32,43] about twice as high as for diagnostic colonoscopy, and all patients must be informed of this risk. The mechanism of perforation is varied. Most commonly, inclusion of colonic wall in the snare has resulted in resection of a disc of the wall. There should have been clues to alert the endoscopist that all is not well during the procedure, such as excessive current requirement, excessive thickness of the stalk, excessive mechanical force needed for strangulation, and sometimes excessive bleeding. The maneuver of moving the ensnared stalk to and fro before passing current prevents most accidental inclusion of the colonic wall, but it is not foolproof, especially in a thin-walled redundant segment. The endoscopist should pause and review the situation whenever doubt exists and to resnare the polyp as necessary.

Mechanical perforation from avulsion with the snare can occur but is accompanied by so much bleeding that it would have been recognized at once. Perforation of a diverticulum, away from the site of polypectomy, as a result of excessive air distention, can be prevented if excessive insufflation is habitually avoided. Delayed perforation, taking many days to manifest, is usually the progression of transmural injury from electrocoagulation (see Full-Thickness Burn).

The predominant symptom of perforation is pain, persisting even after the procedure, becoming generalized and radiating to the shoulders. Tachycardia, tympanitic abdomen, guarding, fever, and leukocytosis renders the diagnosis clear without any need for radiographs to demonstrate pneumoperitoneum. In the absence of symptoms, pneumoperitoneum sometimes occurs, particularly in association with pneumophylloides intestinalis, the condition being distinguished by the term *benign pneumoperitoneum* and requires no treatment.

Emergent operation is mandatory. With the bowels well prepared and the process of peritonitis only beginning, the tissue is still fresh and the rent can be repaired by direct suturing. Most will heal without incident, although a few may leak and develop an abscess in the postoperative period. For perforation discovered late (after 24 hours), the process of peritonitis is usually well advanced, with abscesses and edematous and friable intestines, then exteriorization of the injured segment as a diversion colostomy after draining the abscesses is the safest procedure. Commonly the area of injury cannot be mobilized due to edema; a proximal diversion colostomy should then be performed in addition to repair (if possible) or drainage of the area of injury to form a controlled fistula, similar to treatment of diverticulitis with perforation. Whenever there is a question of malignancy at the time of endoscopy, urgent examination of the resected tissue prior to laparotomy is vital as a different operation may be needed when malignancy is present at the resection margin (see Malignant Polyp). When peritonitis is not severe and contamination minimal, colectomy can be performed as for any cancer with primary anastomosis. When peritonitis is advanced rendering it unsafe for anastomosis, a cancer operation can still be done, except that a temporary colostomy should be established, to be closed 6 weeks later.

FULL-THICKNESS BURN (CLOSED PERFORATION)

The main difficulty is to differentiate this complication from perforation since the pathogenesis is the same, differing only in degrees. Clinically the patient has localized or mild pain, and GI function is undisturbed. Leukocytosis, fever, and tachycardia may develop. If pain is persistent or worsening with loss of bowel function, operation is indicated. If pain improves with conservative treatment with bowel rest (NPO, nasogastric tube suction) and intravenous antibiotics, the presumptive diagnosis of full-thickness burn is supported. Such a lesion is expected to recover without need for operation.

EXPLOSION

The bacterial production of the explosive gases, hydrogen and methane, depends on glycoproteins as a substrate.[41] Mannitol has also been shown to be a potent substrate and must not be used for colonic preparation.[47] When the bowel is not well prepared, the endoscopist should take the necessary precaution before using electrocautery. On the other hand, routine use of CO_2 for insufflation has been found to be unnecessary by most endoscopists, since in the well-prepared colon this risk is practically nonexistent.

IMPACTION OF THE SNARE

This can be an embarrassing occurrence. The snare sometimes gets stuck in thick eschar and cannot be removed without causing pain. Experienced endoscopists frequently recommend using the homemade snare (consisting of a loop made with one continuous long wire) on the basis that if such entrapment occurs, the wire loop can be removed easily by pulling on one end. Unfortunately most of the time the regular snare has been used, when it must be cut at the handle, and the sheath and endoscope removed. The wire element is cut short so that only a few centimeters are exposed from the anus, and it is then secured to the skin with tape. Within a day or so softening of the eschar occurs and the wire element of the snare can be removed. The polyp should be retrieved by enema, but autolysis may have rendered histology unreadable.

Results

The results of large series of colonoscopic polypectomy fully demonstrated the superiority of this procedure to surgical polypectomy via colotomy. Especially in the hands of the experts, the complication rate can be very low. Thus in Shinya's series of more than 5,500 patients, the total complication rate was 0.5 percent with no mortality. In the American Society of Gastrointestinal Endoscopy survey of a series of more than 6,000 patients the total complication rate was under 4 percent, and the mortality was 0.03 percent.[43] A similar figure was reported from the survey of the American Society of Colorectal Surgeons in 1978,[32] the complication

rate was under 2 percent (including 1 percent for hemorrhage and 0.5 percent for perforation), and the mortality was 0.03 percent. This figure is far lower than any surgical operation, let alone colonic operation, for which wound infection alone is many times higher. The mortality for open colotomy was under 1 percent,[21] but if intraoperative endoscopy via the open bowel was performed to localize polyps, wound infection and other complication rate could be as high as 20 percent.[26] Without a doubt colonoscopic polypectomy has revolutionized the management of colonic polyps.

On the basis of the current knowledge of the natural history of adenomatous polyps and other conditions predisposing to carcinoma in the colon, a well organized regimen is desirable in the follow-up management of the patient who has had colonic polypectomy.[45] For those who had a hyperplastic polyp removed, nothing further need be done. For those who had a simple adenoma removed, a repeat examination every 1 to 3 years will suffice. Those who had multiple adenomas, a family history of polyps, or colonic carcinoma should be examined annually if they are over the age of 40. For patients who had carcinoma in situ or widebased polyps with marked villous components, or those with pronounced dysplasia in the polyps, the first repeat examination should be scheduled at 3 months and 6 months (to look for signs of recurrence), and if normal they should then be colonoscoped once every 1 to 3 years. For those who have had surgical resection for carcinoma, a colonoscopy should be performed every 6 months for the first 2 years (for early signs of suture line recurrence), and every 1 to 2 years thereafter, supplemented by testing of the stool for occult blood every 6 months and possibly determination of carcinoembryonic antigen (CEA). For patients with long-standing inflammatory bowel disease or who are members of a family with any of the inherited polyposes but without overt manifestation, a barium enema or colonoscopy or both should be performed at least once a year. When strictures appear in the radiographs of patients with inflammatory bowel disease, these should be biopsied and repeat colonoscopic biopsy and cytology performed every 6 months. All the above patients should have colonoscopy if at any time they develop occult or overt colonic bleeding that cannot be explained on the basis of anal disease.

GASTRIC POLYPS

The natural history of gastric polyps is dependent on their histological classification, and has been considerably clarified in recent years as a result of detailed pathological studies.[33,48] Since the endoscopist can only recognize polypoid lesions, the pathologic diagnosis and further management can only be determined after polypectomy or biopsy and cytology. Gastric polypectomy therefore is primarily a diagnostic procedure. When early cancer is found in the colonic polyp, polypectomy frequently is curative; however, this is not the case in the stomach. Polypectomy or excisional biopsy is indicated for all gastric polyps when discovered unless it is not technically feasible. Polypectomy is contraindicated when the lesion is grossly suspicious of carcinoma. Therapeutic endoscopic ablation of early cancer is discussed in the last section of this chapter.

Table 8-2 lists the different entities a gastric polypoid lesion can be. The only benign lesion with true malignant potential is the adenomatous polyp. However, since gastric cancer can be found in no fewer than 10 percent of stomachs that harbor hyperplastic polyps (although independent and unrelated to them), the presence of polyps should heighten the awareness of early gastric cancer and intensify the search for it.

Table 8-2. Polypoid Lesions of the Stomach

Neoplastic
   Adenomatous polyps
   Adenocarcinoma
   Mesenchymal tumors (leiomyoma, fibroma, lipoma, lymphoma)
Harmartomatous
   Peutz-Jeghers polyp
   Hemangioma
Others
   Hyperplastic
   Ectopic pancreas
   Inflammatory polyp or pseudotumor

The most common gastric polypoid lesion is the hyperplastic polyp, which occurs about 8 to 10 times more frequently than the adenomatous polyp.[33] Because adenomatous polyps tend to be larger when discovered, the chances of a polyp larger than 2 cm being adenomatous are higher. Hyperplastic polyps are usually smooth and may be slightly lobulated; while adenomatous polyps are usually covered with fine, velvety papillary projections and sometimes deeper fissures. Hyperplastic polyps can be anywhere in the stomach and tend to be multiple (30 percent of cases), but the adenomatous polyps occur predominantly in the antrum.

Mesenchymal tumors and hematomatous lesions occur much less frequently. Most of these are covered with more or less normal gastric mucosa, and many of them do not have a recognizable stalk when they are small. Some Japanese endoscopists use the term *protuberant* or *elevated* lesions rather than *polypoid* for this reason. Any of these lesions, when large enough, can acquire a stalk made up of normal gastric mucosa and submucosa. The author has seen a large antral leiomyoma prolapse into the duodenum at endoscopy. A larger leiomyoma often has an ulcerated crater that may be the source of massive hemorrhage. A large gastric varix may be mistaken for a polyp and cause massive bleeding if snared by mistake.

Technique

The technique of polypectomy described for colonic polyp can be totally applied to the stomach; maneuvering, however, is much easier in the stomach, as it is much more spacious. The duodenal scope can be used with advantage for some cardiac and fundic locations, eliminating the need for reverse gastroscopy. The right-angled snare is also helpful in many instances. Because the gastric mucosa is considerably more vascular and thicker than the colonic mucosa, there is a higher risk of bleeding than with colonic polypectomy. The bipolar snare technique (both double or single snare) is even more useful in the stomach due its vascularity.

For some broad-based lesions, this author has injected saline submucosally in order to facilitate the use of the snare. Saline is injected submucosally around the lesion using the sclerotherapy injector, resulting in diffuse swelling. The snare is reduced to form a loop just larger than the base, and is applied flat against the hillock to cause a circumferential cut surrounding the lesion. The saline will ooze, but the snare can now be tightened to form a pseudostalk and polypectomy can be completed in the usual manner. The purpose of the saline injection is to increase the thickness of the submucosa artificially, from which a pseudostalk can be fashioned. This technique is not as applicable to the colon where the submucosa is not as easily separable.

The technique attributed to Shinya for removal of submucosal lipoma in the colon can be readily applied to the stomach (Fig. 8-13). This is a technique for the experts; however, the risk of perforation is probably less in the stomach than in the colon. With a fine-pointed monopolar electrode, a cut is made in the mucosa over the mass. The snare loop is applied flat against the mass and tightened gradually, exerting a squeezing action which in effect enucleates the submucosal tumor. The pedicle is finally transected by closure of the snare. Not all submucosal tumor can be removed as some are very adherent. Lipomas are the only easy ones. Shinya described the cushion sign to test for lipomas: pushing with the tip of the snare on a submucosal lipoma regularly produces a dimple. It should be noted that a varix may be nodular in shape and that it will give the same sign.

Polyps 0.5 cm or smaller are suitable for

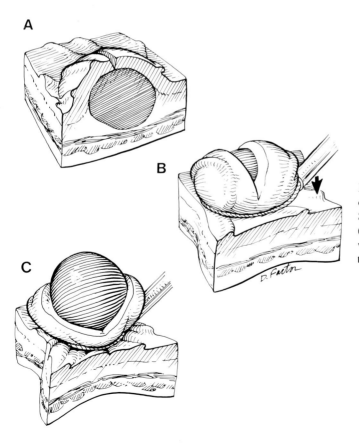

A

B

C

Fig. 8-13 Technique for excision of submucosal tumors (after Shinya). (A) Incision over tumor. (B) Downward pressure combined with closure of snare. (C) Enucleation of tumor.

removal with the hot biopsy technique described under colonoscopic polypectomy. For sessile lesions or broad-based lesions not suitable for snare removal and yet too large for the hot biopsy technique, laser photocoagulation is an increasingly recognized method of treatment, especially in Japan.

Postoperative care consists of empirical administration of antacids and H_2-receptor blockers to assist healing of the ulcer created by electrosurgery. In asymptomatic patients routine repeat endoscopy to monitor healing is probably not necessary, although endoscopy should be repeated if epigastric discomfort persists or if there is doubt as to the completeness of resection.

Complications

All complications of polypectomy described under colonic polyps may occur, although hemorrhage is more often in the stomach because of increased vascularity. Perforation is less likely on account of a thicker wall. Persistent ulceration at the site of electrosurgery (for polypectomy as well as for electrocoagulation of bleeding ulcers) has been observed by the author, who considers it justified to use antacids and H_2-receptor blocker routinely in the postoperative management.

Results

Gastric polypectomy can be safely performed with a complication rate of 1 to 2 percent.[9,17,23,24] The major contribution, however, is its diagnostic value in the management of early gastric cancer.

The results of treatment of gastric cancer remain disappointing unless early gastric cancer (EGC) is discovered through polypectomy. A 5-year survival of 80 percent can be expected from surgical treatment in these patients.[18,36] This is in contrast to advanced gastric cancer

(AGC) where a 5-year survival after curative resection is 20 percent at best. [25,28]

SCHEME OF MANAGEMENT OF GASTRIC POLYPOID LESIONS

In the patient presenting with a radiographic diagnosis of polypoid lesion in the stomach, gastroscopy is the first logical study (see Fig. 8-14). The entire stomach is carefully surveyed for associated lesions, and then the polypoid lesion itself is examined for its gross morphologic characteristics. Further action depends on the morphology of the lesion: The pragmatic classification suggested by Yamada and Ichikawa[52] is quite useful. Figure 8-15 shows how the lesion is graded as Type I through IV depending on the degree of protrusion into the lumen; this is not to be confused with the morphological classification of gastric carcinoma espoused by the Japanese Endoscopic Society. Type I lesions barely cause an elevation and is regarded as submucosal; type IV is a polyp complete with a well-defined stalk, while types II and III are grades in between. Snare removal is probably possible for most type III, but not type II, lesions. When the lesions are smaller than 0.5 cm, the hot biopsy technique will remove them satisfactorily at the same time providing good material for histologic study. For those lesions (type II, and an occasional type III) not removable by endoscopic means for histologic examination, open surgical wedge biopsy, performed by excision of the entire thickness of the wall bearing the lesion with a clear margin, is indicated. For type I, biopsy and brush cytology must be obtained. It is possible to obtain submucosal biopsies with the ordinary forceps by repeated biopsies through the same site, but a normal mucosa histology also helps to establish its submucosal nature. The vast majority of these are benign lesions, which may only require periodic observation. Occasionally a submucosal lipoma may be enucleated endoscopically (see Technique). Type IV lesions can be removed by polypectomy and

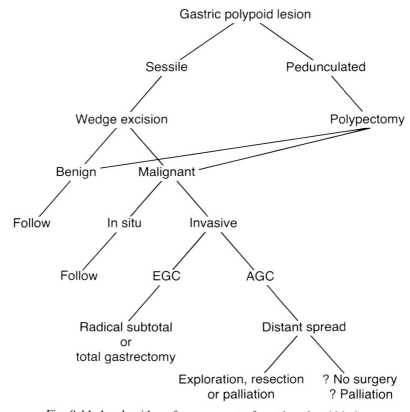

Fig. 8-14 An algorithm of management of gastric polypoid lesion.

the entire specimen examined for its nature and the presence of carcinoma. If the lesion is a hyperplastic polyp or some other benign mesenchymal curiosity and there are no other associated lesions, no further treatment is required. When the lesion is an adenomatous polyp without carcinoma foci, the patient should be entered in a surveillance program to be gastroscoped annually or biannually, since these tend to recur, and since carcinoma is found in 30 percent of these stomachs. When foci of cancer are found,

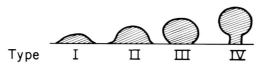

Fig. 8-15 Classification of polypoid lesions of the stomach. (Yamada T, Ichikawa H: X-ray diagnosis of elevated lesions of the stomach. Radiology 110:79, 1976.)

the lesion should be classified as early or advanced. Early cancer is defined as invasion up to the submucosa but not the muscularis (Fig. 8-16), and so if the specimen shows invasion up to the polypectomy resection margin the lesion must be read tentatively as advanced, pending further excisional biopsy of the stomach. The terms early gastric cancer (EGC) and advanced gastric cancer (AGC) do not necessarily denote time of onset or curability. It is likely that EGC progresses eventually to AGC, but in a proportion of cases, including many of those reported in Japan, the two lesions have different biologic behavior, with some EGCs having a good prognosis, even though some are known to have lymph node involvement. Surgery is indicated for all patients with carcinoma diagnosed by polypectomy, irrespective of resection margin. For all resectable cases, including those with free resection margin in

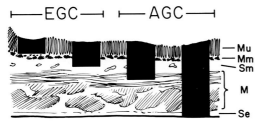

Fig. 8-16 The definition of early gastric cancer (EGC) and advanced gastric cancer (AGC) depends on depth of invasion. Advanced cancer is defined as invasion of the muscularis and beyond. Mu, mucosa; Mm, muscularis mucosae; Sm, submucosa; M, muscularis; Se, serosa.

the polypectomy specimen, subtotal gastric resection to include the lymphatic drainage is indicated, since about one-quarter of EGCs will have lymph node metastasis. For AGC, the choice of operation depends on extent of the disease.

Surgical resection of the polypoid lesion with a rim of gastric wall is indicated when endoscopic removal is not feasible, such as in some large sessile polypoid lesions more than 2 cm, or when cancer is suspected on endoscopic appearance alone. Frozen section must be obtained. For hyperplastic polyps and other benign lesions, the incision can be closed. For adenomatous polyps without cancer, or for those with only carcinoma in situ, the wedge resection so performed can be considered adequate treatment, but the patient's condition must be diligently followed up with endoscopic examinations. If the final histology reveals an invasive cancer foci, even though preliminary frozen section has exonerated the lesion, the management then will be the same as for EGC. Multiple pedunculated lesions (fewer than 10) are resected endoscopically, but multiple sessile lesions are most expeditiously dealt with by open operation through one single gastrotomy, excising the lesions with a full-thickness wedge, and submitting to frozen section. When the lesions are too many to resect individually, as in Menetrier's disease, major gastric resection may be justified on the grounds of protein losing gastropathy, inability to sample and to rule out adenomatous polyps, and a certain risk of cancer complicating the disease in future. In other cases when many samples have consistently showed hyperplastic polyps, laser photoablation of the smaller ones is probably justified in patients who are poor surgical risks, provided they are followed in a well-structured surveillance program.

There is some argument as to what surgical resection should be undertaken for early gastric cancer demonstrated to be confined in the polyp and for EGC in general. Because of higher operative mortality and higher morbidity, most surgeons do not advocate total gastrectomy despite the theoretical multifocal nature of the carcinogenesis. One factor that governs the selection of operation is the location of the polyp. For polyps in the antrum and body, a subtotal resection removing as well the lesser and greater omentum (radical subtotal gastrectomy) appears to fulfill the criteria of a cancer operation, except that the lymphatics to pancreas are untouched. Clinical results of such an operation for early gastric cancer show an operative mortality of under 2 percent and a 5-year survival of about 80 percent.[18,20,36] For polyps in the fundus, proximal or total gastrectomy with removal of the spleen and associated lymphatics appears justified. Advocates of total gastrectomy in this group of patients feel that the procedure would obviate the low recurrence rate in the gastric remnant, which, by the time it is diagnosed, is usually nonresectable.

For AGC, an exploratory laparatomy to determine resectability is usually justified if no distant metastasis is demonstrable. Surgery is undertaken with the philosophy to cure if possible, and to palliate if not. Exploration must be thorough, and frozen section biopsy must be resorted to whenever the extent is in doubt. For lesions confined to the stomach, the type and extent of resection is dependent on location of the tumor. For distal gastric cancer, a radical subtotal gastrectomy is usually advocated. For a high gastrectomy, the spleen is removed with the specimen. Total gastrectomy is indicated only in those tumors not resectable with lesser procedure, but unfortunately most such procedures prove palliative only.

ENDOSCOPIC ABLATION OF SMALL TUMORS OF THE GASTROINTESTINAL TRACT

Rationale and Indications

Therapeutic endoscopy for palliation of advanced malignancy is discussed in Chapter 10. Historically it was found that, for some rectal cancers, aggressive electrocoagulation in patients who are unsuitable for surgery resulted in occasional long-term survival.[12,15,31] However, to date it has not been possible to predict who would respond, and therefore therapeutic endoscopy for rectal cancer can not be offered except when surgical treatment is impractical by virtue of poor health.

Electrofulguration of small polyps has been employed with notable success in controlling development of new rectal polyps in familial polyposis after subtotal colectomy with ileorectal anastomosis.[7]

Laser photoablation of polyps is eminently practical with the Nd:YAG laser; however, no tissue is available for histologic study and the clinician is always worried that early cancer is being treated in this manner. In the stomach, at least, EGCs may have lymphatic involvement and endoscopic ablation certainly does not cure them. The indication for this method of treatment is therefore limited to benign lesions or only potentially malignant lesions. An example is the early crop of polyps encountered in patients being followed for familial polyposis. A special use of laser photoablation is in conjunction with subtotal colectomy in such patients.

Technique

LASER PHOTOABLATION

Both the Argon and the Nd:YAG laser may be used for fiberoptic endoscopy; CO_2 laser (penetration 0.1 mm) is suitable for shallow carpet-like villous growths in the rectum, if it can be exposed through the operating proctoscope. In addition, a contact probe has been developed for use with Nd:YAG laser. (See Chapters 2 and 10.) The choice of modality is dependent on the size of the lesion and the thickness of the wall of the gut. In general, the Nd:YAG laser is preferred for larger tumors, for the rectum, esophagus, and stomach, while the Argon laser or the Nd:YAG delivered by contact laser probe are preferred for the colon and cecum.

If appropriate precaution is used, it is possible to remove larger benign lesions (over 0.5 cm), with or without a distinct stalk with a snare, using modified technique if necessary. If removal is incomplete, the residual tissue can be safely photocoagulated, since histologic examination of most of the tissue would have been available. By the same token, this author firmly believes in preliminary hot biopsy excision of all smaller sessile lesions (0.5 cm and smaller) to obtain tissue for histologic study. Photocoagulation is applied only to the residual tissue after hot biopsy. If special hot biopsy forceps with larger cups are used, even larger polyps can be dealt with by this technique, decreasing the need for photoablation.

For extensive villous growth carpeting much of the circumference of a segment of the gut, multiple random hot biopsies should be taken prior to photocoagulation.

Argon laser is used with a power setting in the range of 5 to 10 watts in the continuous wave mode. A gas flow of 1 to 2 L/min is suitable for stomach and rectum, and a treatment distance of 0.5 to 2 cm is usually recommended.[3,4] For colonic and cecal lesions, similar parameters except a lower gas flow may be used. Smaller tumors are ablated in several seconds.

Nd:YAG laser is best used for larger lesions. A power setting of 40 to 70 watts is generally required, with pulse duration limited to 2 seconds, applied at a treatment distance of 1 to 2 cm.[5] A basal coaxial gas flow is set at 1 to 2 L/min, which may be doubled shortly before shooting, with appropriate venting provisions.

For contact delivery of Nd:YAG laser using sapphire crystal-tipped probes, a power setting of 10 to 15 watts is recommended. Application time usually does not exceed 1 to 2 seconds, being guided by the visible coagulation as no delay effect occurs with this mode of delivery.

Multiple sessions, 2 to 3 days apart, are required to treat larger lesions when noncontact lasers are used due to delayed necrosis from the effect of scattering. Overtreatment with no allowance of this effect may result in perforation.

Bowers recommended treating a polypoid lesion at the center first and then going to the periphery in concentric circles until the entire lesion is destroyed. The zone of delayed necrosis for larger polyps is deeper at the center than at the periphery of the base, making it clear that the edge, rather than the base, requires subsequent treatment.

In all patients undergoing endoscopic ablation, follow-up endoscopic examination is mandatory at 6-month intervals or sooner to look for and manage recurrent tumors or residual tumor.

OTHER MODALITIES

Electrocoagulation/Electrofulguration

Electrofulguration for rectal cancer is described in Chapter 10. Careful palpation and aggressive repeat sessions are necessary to treat malignant lesions. Long-term survival is possible with such local treatment.[12,15,31] Hot-biopsy technique as applied to small polyps is a classical application of electrocoagulation for tumor ablation.

Ethanol Injection

Ethanol injection for bleeding ulcers is described in Chapter 2. Otani first utilized this modality, however, in the treatment of smaller polypoid lesions in the stomach, noting the predictable depth of necrosis (dose dependent) following injection of 98 percent ethanol.[40] No significant experience in this country has been published.

Complications

The complication of most concern to the endoscopist is missing an early cancer when photoablation has been used exclusively. This risk is diminished by combining other methods such as snare excision or hot biopsy to obtain tissue. Early reexamination (within 3 to 6 months) is nevertheless mandatory just to be certain residual growth can be treated in time. If recurrent growth is detected, an overlooked malignant lesion is likely. Perforation and hemorrhage are the other major risks which are no different from other situations. Delayed hemorrhage from separation of slough is more apt to occur when large areas has been photocoagulated, manifesting as bleeding after 7 to 10 days. When circumferential mucosal coagulation has been required, rectal stenosis resulted in some cases. The overall incidence of complications is said to be small, but the real incidence is not known as the technique is still young.

Results

Bowers[3] has reported careful follow-up data after argon laser photocoagulation of benign polyps. Only one recurrence (in a large villous adenoma) was noted after 14 months of observation, successfully treated with Nd:YAG laser without further recurrence in 12 months. Dixon[13] used argon laser to treat new and residual polyps in the rectal remnants in patients with familial polyposis after subtotal colectomy. In one patient opting for rectal resection after completing photocoagulation shortly before surgery, no residual polyp was demonstrable and photocoagulation depth was only to the submucosa. Good success was also reported by Japanese workers.[34,44] For villous adenoma particularly, where removal with the snare is difficult, the Nd:YAG laser performed admirably. Lambert[27] reported 35 cures out of 39 patients, including 12 patients with demonstrated malignant foci. Kiefhaber reported cures in all 14 patients in one series.[25] Brunetaud[4,5] used argon and Nd:YAG lasers (depending on the volume of tumor to be treated) and documented complete tumor ablation in 42 of 56 patients. Some of their patients with more than two-thirds of the circumference involved received 5 to 26 sessions. Complications were minor, including bloody rectal discharge, low-grade fever, and one incident of delayed rectal bleeding. Even so, data in the literature are still insufficient to define the role of this modality in the treatment of GI tumors.

REFERENCES

1. Asaki S, Nishimura T, Sato M, et al: Endoscopic polypectomy using high frequency current: Double-snare method of polypectomy for prevention of incidental bleeding and perforation. Tohoku J Exp Med 136:215, 1982
2. Berci G, Panish JF, Schapiro M, et al: Complications of colonoscopy and polypectomy. Gastroenterology 67:584, 1974
3. Bowers JH: Laser therapy of colonic neoplasms, p. 139. In Fleischer D. Jensen D, Bright-Asare P (eds): Therapeutic Laser Endoscopy in Gastrointestinal Disease. Martinus Nijhoff, Boston, 1983
4. Brunetaud JM, Mosquet L, Bourez J, et al: Laser applications in nonhemorrhagic digestive lesions, p. 455. In Atsumi K (ed): New Frontiers in Laser Medicine and Surgery. Excerpta Medica, Amsterdam, 1983
5. Brunetaud JM, Mosquet L, Houcke M, et al: Villous adenomas of the rectum. Results of endoscopic treatment with argon and ND:YAG lasers. Gastroenterology 89:832, 1985
6. Bussey HJR, Wallace MH, Morson BC: Metachronous carcinoma of the large intestine and intestinal polyps. Proc R Soc Med 60:208, 1967
7. Bussy HJR: Familial Polyposis Coli. Johns Hopkins University Press, Baltimore, 1975
8. Castleman B: Current approach to the polyp–cancer controversy. Gastroenterology 51:108, 1966
9. Classen M, Demling L: Operative gastroskopie: Fiberendoskopische polypenatrogung in magen. Dtsch Med Wochenschr 96:1466, 1971
10. Cotton PB, Williams CB: Practical Gastrointestinal Endoscopy. 2nd Ed. Blackwell Scientific Publications, Oxford, 1982
11. Coutsoftides T, Sivak MV Jr, Benjamin SP, et al: Colonoscopy and the management of polyps containing carcinoma. Ann Surg 188:638, 1978
12. Crile G, Turnbull RB: The role of electrocoagulation in the treatment of carcinoma of the rectum. Surg Gynecol Obstet 135:391, 1972
13. Dixon JA, Burt RW, Rotering RH, et al: Endoscopic argon laser photocoagulation of sessile colonic polyps. Gastrointest Endosc 28:162, 1982
14. Eide TJ, Stalsberg H: Polyps of the large intestine in northern Norway. Cancer 42:2839, 1978
15. Eisenstat TE, Deak ST, Rubin RJ, et al: Five year survival in patients with carcinoma of the rectum treated by electrocoagulation. Am J Surg 143:127, 1982
16. Fucini C, Wolff BG, Spencer RJ: An appraisal of endoscopic removal of malignant colonic polyps. Mayo Clin Proc 61:123, 1986
17. Gaisford W: Gastrointestinal polypectomy via the fiberendoscope. Arch Surg 106:458, 1973
18. Gentsch HH, Groitl H, Giedl J: Results of surgical treatment of early gastric cancer in 113 patients. World J Surg 5:103, 1981
19. Gilbertsen VA: Proctosigmoidoscopy and polypectomy in reducing the incidence of rectal cancer. Cancer 34:936, 1974
20. Green PHR, O'Toole KM, Weinberg LM, et al. Early gastric cancer. Gastroenterology 81:247, 1981
21. Grinnell RS, Lane N: Benign and malignant adenomatuous polyps and papillary adenomas of the colon and rectum. An analysis of 1856 tumors in 1335 patients. Surgery 106:519, 1958
22. Haggitt RC, Glotzbach RE, Soffer EE, et al: Prognostic factors in colorectal carcinomas arising in adenomas: Implications for lesions removed by endoscopic polypectomy. Gastroenterology 89:328, 1985
23. Hargrove RL, Overholt BF: Polypectomy via the fiberoptic gastroscope. JAMA 224:904, 1973
24. Jacobs WH: Endoscopic electrosurgical polypectomies of the upper gastrointestinal tract. Am J Gastroenterol 68:241, 1977
25. Kieffhaber P, Kiefhaber K: Present endoscopic laser therapy in the gastrointestinal tract, p. 439. In Atsumi K (ed): New Frontiers in Laser Medicine and Surgery. Excerpta Medica, Amsterdam, 1983
26. Kleinfeld G, Gump FE: Complications of colotomy and polypectomy. Surg Gynecol Obstet 111:726, 1960

27. Lambert R, Sabber G: Laser therapy in colorectal tumors, early results. Gastroenterology 84:1223, 1983

28. Langer JC, Cohen Z, Taylor BR, et al: Management of patient with polyps containing malignancy removed by colonoscopic polypectomy. Dis Colon Rectum 27:6, 1984

29. Lipper S, Kahn LB, Ackerman LV: The significance of microscopic invasive cancer is endoscopically removed polyps of large bowel: A clinicopathologic study of 51 cases. Cancer 52:1691, 1983

30. Lumpkin WM, Crow RL, Hernandez CM, et al: Carcinoma of the stomach: Review of 1035 cases. Ann Surg 159:919, 1964

31. Madden JL, Kandalaft S: Electrocoagulation in the treatment of cancer of the rectum: A continuing study. Ann Surg 174:530, 1971

32. Marino AWM Jr: Complications of colonoscopy. Dis Colon Rectum 21:1, 1978

33. Ming SG, Goldman H: Gastric polyps: A histogenetic classification and the relation to carcinoma. Cancer 18:721, 1965

34. Mizushima K, Namiki M, Harada K, et al: Endoscopic laser therapy of gastric cancer and polyps, p. 470. In Atsumi K (ed): New Frontiers in Laser Medicine and Surgery. Excerpta Medica, Amsterdam, 1983.

35. Morson BC, Bussey HJR, Samoorian S: Policy of local excision for early cancer of the colorectum. Gut 18:1045, 1977

36. Morson BC: The Pathogenesis of Colorectal Cancer. WB Saunders, Philadelphia, 1978

37. Morson BC, Whiteway JE, Jones EA, et al: Histopathology and prognosis of colorectal polyps treated by endoscopic polypectomy. Gut 25:437, 1984

38. Murakami T: Early cancer of the stomach. World J Surg 3:685, 1979

39. Nivatongs S, Goldberg SM: Management of patients who have polyps containing invasive carcinoma removed via colonoscope. Dis Colon Rectum 21:8, 1978

40. Otani T, Tatsuker T, Kanamaru K, et al: Intramural injection of ethanol under direct vision for the treatment of protuberant lesions of the stomach. Gastroenterology 69:123, 1975

41. Perman JA, Modler S: Glycoproteins as substrates for production of hydrogen and methane by colonic bacterial flora. Gastroenterology 83:338, 1982

42. Rickert RR, Auerbach O, Garfinkel L, et al: Adenomatous lesions of the large bowel. An autopsy study. Cancer 43:1847 1979

43. Rogers BHG, Silvis SE, Nebel OT, et al: Complications of flexible fiberoptic colonoscopy and polypectomy. Gastrointest Endosc 22:2, 1975

44. Sasako M, Iwasaki M, Konishi T, et al: Clinical application of the Nd:YAG laser endoscopy. Lasers Surg Med 2:137 1982

45. Shinya H: Colonoscopy: Diagnosis and Treatment of Colonic Diseases. Igaku-Shoin, New York, 1982

46. Spratt JS, Ackerman LV, Moyer C: Relationship of polyps of the colon to colonic cancer. Ann Surg 148:682, 1958

47. Taylor EW, Bentley S, Youngs D, et al: Bowel preparation and the safety of colonoscopic polypectomy. Gastroenterology 81:1, 1981

48. Tomasulo J: Gastric polyp. Histologic types and their relationship to gastric carcinoma. Cancer 27:1346, 1971

49. Treat M, Forde K: Bipolar electrocautery snare for safer endoscopic polypectomy, Gastrointest Endosc. 28:147, 1982

50. Wolff WI, Shinya H: Definitive treatment of malignant polyps of the colon. Ann Surg 182:516, 1975

51. Yamada E, Miyashi S, Nakazato H, et al: The surgical treatment of cancer of the stomach. Int Surg 65:387, 1980

52. Yamada T, Ichikawa H: X-ray diagnosis of elevated lesions of the stomach. Radiology 110:79, 1976

9

Dilation of Strictures

Strictures of the GI tract within reach of the endoscope may be treated successfully with dilation. The basic principle of dilation is to stretch a fibrous scar gradually by means of a series of dilators inserted into the lumen. The art is ancient, and the procedure has long been known as an effective and safe treatment for strictures if performed correctly. The only significant advance introduced recently is visual monitoring of the process of dilation. The best means of monitoring is by endoscopy, but fluoroscopy is very useful as well; there are also situations in which both are simultaneously used with advantage. Although direct bouginage is possible for many esophageal and rectal strictures, without endoscopic visual control more complicated maneuvers cannot be performed. The techniques of dilation are described in detail for the esophagus because these are the strictures that provide most endoscopists with their first learning experience in using dilators. Very similar techniques can be applied to dilating obstructive lesions elsewhere in the GI tract; and these are discussed in order in this chapter.

BENIGN ESOPHAGEAL STRICTURES

Pathologic Anatomy

Strictures arise as a result of cicatrization reducing the luminal passage. Most commonly the process of scarring involves the mucosa, submucosa, and a varying amount of the muscle coat, but a thin diaphragm or web of mucosal stenosis without deeper components may be seen on occasion, as in Vinson-Plummer syndrome. The response to dilation is clearly dependent on the depth of scarring. In the extensive and deep injuries of corrosive ingestion, for example, where the entire muscle coat may have been replaced with fibrous tissue, repeated stretching will be necessary over time first to attain and then to maintain an adequate lumen. In less severe injuries in which most of the muscle coat remains intact, the lumen is much more readily restored and may not require repeated dilation if no further inflammation perpetuates the process of cicatrization. The intact peristaltic function is important in facilitating dilation and above all in maintaining the lumen by ingestion of solid food.

The mechanism of action of dilation is to enlarge the lumen with a tapered device, converting the axially directed force to a radial force counteracting the stenosis (Fig. 9-1A). New dilators operating on this principle are being introduced as frequently as new models of automobiles, a higher price being the most notable feature. In treating a long stricture with this type of dilator, as dilation progresses, the stricture is first shortened progressively before the last of the narrow segment is assessible to the action of the dilator (Fig. 9-1A). In 1979 the balloon catheter, also called the Gruntzig cath-

181

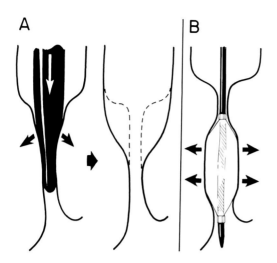

Fig. 9-1 Mechanisms of action of dilation of benign strictures. (A) The axially directed force is converted to a radial force by the conical shape of the dilator tip. As a long stricture is dilated, it is progressively shortened. (B) Direct radial force to widen the stricture is imparted by the balloon dilators.

eter, was introduced for transluminal dilation of stenotic arteries, and the same principles were utilized for dilation of esophageal strictures.[12,32] This new type of dilator uses a preshaped balloon which maintains its limiting diameter over a wide range of intraballoon pressure. Direct radial force is applied at the stricture instead of at the shelf at the beginning of the stricture (Fig. 9-1B). The principle appears sound, but there are practical disadvantages in its execution (see technique); consequently, this dilator has not replaced the time-proven devices.

What size lumen is considered adequate depends as much on the condition of the patient as on the underlying disease process. The main variable often overlooked is the intrinsic motility of the esophagus. For the otherwise healthy patient with good motility of the esophagus, a 36 Fr. lumen (or 1.1-cm diameter) enables the patient to swallow most masticated food except red meat or bread; even these foods may produce only mild "sticking," although regurgitation is the rule. A 44 Fr. lumen in these patients may completely abolish symptoms. By the same token, esophageal cancer gives rise to few symp-

toms in stronger patients until the lumen is markedly encroached upon. On the other hand, in the frail and the elderly, and in those strictures with long segments of muscle destruction (e.g., lye burns), a 36 Fr. lumen bestows mostly liquid swallowing. A lumen of 50 Fr. or more is required to abolish symptoms, a goal that is often impossible to attain.

Clinical Types of Benign Strictures

The etiology of esophageal stricture is listed in order of frequency in Table 9-1. By far the most common stricture is secondary to peptic esophagitis, the result of uncontrolled gastroesophageal reflux. The diagnosis is suggested by the clinical history of chronic reflux esophagitis prior to the onset of dysphagia and the radiologic appearance of the stricture, confirmed by the endoscopic examination and biopsy. Departures from the typical presentation should raise the possibility of a carcinoma, and biopsy and cytology must be obtained. In this regard it should be stressed that biopsy alone has a surprisingly high rate of false-negative results (20 percent or more[41]). It is not unusual to have to rebiopsy, since the endoscopic appearance is so characteristic of carcinoma. To overcome the errors of sampling, a large number of biopsies[6-10] should be obtained. However, if biopsy is combined with cytology, the accuracy is greatly improved.[28]

While most peptic strictures are located at the lower third of the esophagus with or without an associated hiatal hernia, the presence of a mid-esophageal stricture is likely to be associated with columnar epithelium lining the esopha-

Table 9-1. Etiology of Benign Strictures

Reflux esophagitis
  Columnar-lined (Barrett's) esophagus

Chemical esophagitis
  Corrosive ingestion
  Sclerotherapy for varices

Achalasia

Anastomotic

Webs and rings

gus below the stricture, the Barrett's esophagus. The diagnosis is made endoscopically by exclusion of malignancy with cytology and biopsy and by the demonstration of columnar epithelium distal to the stricture. The condition has been shown to have malignant potential and thus requires close follow-up evaluation.

A form of benign stricture, seen only recently since the reintroduction of sclerotherapy for esophageal varices, is the stricture resulting from sclerotherapy. Unlike peptic strictures, which are lined with granulation tissue resting on top of mature fibrous tissue, these strictures have only minimal or no mucosal inflammation. The pathology appears to be mainly fibrosis of the mucosa and submucosa extending into the muscular coats due to deep injection of the sclerosant. A deep ulcer may mark the site of injection, but otherwise the mucosa appears pale and atrophic, but free of inflammation. A striking finding is that varices are either very small or absent above the stricture. These strictures respond well to dilation and are further discussed under complications in Chapter 3.

A short stricture, weblike in some cases, may mark the site of an anastomosis, particularly when the anastomosis has been constructed with the stapler. Many of the staples will have been passed or hidden by epithelialization, but radiologic identification remains possible indefinitely, since the fine staples are not easily missed. These strictures are readily dilatable, although it should not be done too soon after the operation (e.g., 4 to 6 weeks).

Strictures due to corrosive injury vary widely in extent and severity. Suicidal ingestion of lye, in the worst cases, results in mediastinitis from virtual dissolution of the esophagus, for which the clinical manifestations are obvious. Those presenting with strictures may have one long and dense stricture affecting most of the esophagus or two or more short segments interposed with normal esophagus. Furthermore, stricture of the gastric antrum and pylorus from the same ingestion is not uncommon. The history and distribution of the chronic injury are thus diagnostic.

In achalasia the radiologic appearance is often striking. Esophageal manometry shows repetitive simultaneous contractions of swallowing and a high resting tone of the lower esophageal sphincter with incomplete or no relaxation induced by swallowing. Endoscopy is unnecessary to make a diagnosis, although malignancy is best ruled out endoscopically. In the capacious esophagus with a complete lack of peristalsis, chronic changes in the epithelium secondary to stasis provide a dramatic endoscopic sight. The endoscope enters the stomach surprisingly easily despite the degree of functional obstruction.

Indications and Contraindications

Dilation with bougies is the first treatment considered for benign strictures. Mild strictures calibrating 34 Fr. or larger may be readily dilated with blind dilation, using the Hurst or Maloney dilator (Fig. 9-2). For tighter strictures, or when blind bouginage has failed, endoscopic dilation

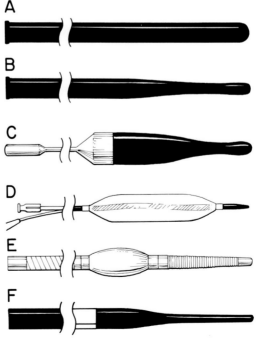

Fig. 9-2 The commonly used dilators, all about 60 cm long. (A) Hurst. (B) Maloney. (C) Jackson. (D) Balloon. (E) Eder-Puestow. (F) Savary.

is indicated. Before commencing dilation, however, the first priority is to make sure that the stricture is indeed benign. It is a tragic error, usually on the basis of radiologic appearance, to engage in a course of dilation for carcinoma with the mistaken assumption that a benign stricture is being treated. By the time the error is realized, it is often too late for any worthwhile surgical treatment.

It is the credo of the esophagologist that no matter how severe the disease, a dilatable esophagus serves the patient infinitely better than any surgical substitute or reconstruction. Considering the operative mortality and the side effects of resection of the gastroesophageal junction, open surgical treatment is generally reserved only for extremely complicated cases not amenable to endoscopic dilation. Such complicated strictures include those with fistulas from chronic perforation, long and tortuous ones from multiple false passages, and those in patients who recovered from an acute perforation due to instrumentation. Dilation may also be considered a failure when the effect is too transient or when dilation cannot be performed at the required frequency for any reason.

Performing dilation in dehydrated and nutritionally depleted patients is unwise, as the risk of complication is very high. These patients must be replenished first, either with parenteral or enteral alimentation by jejunostomy or gastrostomy, before the stricture can be treated endoscopically. The mere presence of a large thoracic aortic aneurysm is not necessarily a contraindication, although dysphagia may be the symptom from pressure of a large aneurysm on the esophagus; in such cases, dilation would not improve the symptoms.

While resection of strictures should be reserved as a last resort, the same is not true for antireflux operations. These operations carry much lower morbidity and mortality, and the functional results of the modern operations are excellent.[3,23,29,35,39,44,46] Most strictures (about 80 percent) do not require maintenance dilations following a successful antireflux operation.[23,24,29,39,46] Without surgery, many but not all peptic strictures tend to persist as long as

reflux continues and require repeated maintenance dilations. There is no reliable indicator to predict which patient will do well requiring only infrequent dilation and which will remain symptomatic requiring an antireflux operation.[36] However, in the patient considered a poor surgical risk, regular maintenance dilation works surprisingly well for many years. A perspective of relative risks in surgical and nonsurgical treatment is further discussed under Results.

Technique

DIRECT BOUGINAGE

Direct bouginage is usually done without local anesthetics or sedation in the adult. Some clinicians argue that such patients need to be taught that there is nothing to fear in the manipulation and that the sooner they learn to help themselves with a problem they will have to live with for many years the better off they will be. This is true for those requiring self-dilation and for those motivated to help themselves; but for the nervous patient who does not require many dilations, intravenous meperidine works wonders; in my experience it has never interfered with the clinical end point of knowing when to stop. Children should be spared the emotional trauma of dilation and all esophageal manipulation can be done under general anesthesia.

Endoscopists have long been concerned about the possibility of vagovagal reflexes on the heart induced by pharyngeal stimulation, but there is no satisfactory prevention. Routine use of atropine constitutes overkill; the side effects are especially dangerous in the elderly, in whom dysrhythmia is of prime concern. My practice is to monitor the occasional patient who has a known history of coronary disease and cardiac dysrhythmia during a manipulative procedure of the pharynx and esophagus, rather than routine atropinization. All dilations must be done after overnight fasting to reduce the risk of regurgitation and aspiration of collected food debris above the stricture.

The old standbys are the mercury-filled bougies, which have been used extensively for many decades. The Hurst and the Maloney dilators are both made of a heavy rubber shell filled with mercury; the Hurst is blunt tipped, while the Maloney has a short-rat-tailed tip of more gradual taper. These bougies are suitable for use by patients who have been taught how to self-dilate. The procedure should be done with the patient seated, holding an emesis dish and draped with an apron. The thinly lubricated bougie is swallowed by the patient but is actually guided to the cricopharyngeus by the physician. To prevent the heavy dilator from dangling, the physician holds it coiled in the right hand. The tip is guided by the left hand to the hypopharynx and comes to rest just behind the epiglottis, without pressure on the tongue and keeping strictly in the midline. The patient is then asked to swallow. Gentle pressure is maintained during the act of swallowing, and entry into the esophagus is sensed as an automatic advance of the dilator. Once in the esophagus, the physician reaches deep behind the tongue with the index finger and thumb to push the dilator along, uncoiling the dilator in the other hand. When the stricture is encountered, insertion pressure is increased gently. It is the give when it enters the stricture that guides the physician as to the adequacy of the treatment. To confirm that the stricture has been engaged, the dilator is pulled back slightly, when a little tug will be felt as the dilator is being gripped by the stricture. At times the feel and the tug may be vague, and it is uncertain whether the dilator is merely coiling up above the stricture or has passed it. If the dilator can be passed until it almost disappears, it is unlikely to be coiled. A good rule of safety is to dilate no more than three sizes larger than the calibration of the stricture in one session. If difficulty occurs such as undue pain, repeated coiling, and failure to pass the obstruction, dilation guided by endoscopy is indicated.

Dilators with more body have been in fashion off and on over the past five decades. A very popular dilator used 20 years ago is the Plummer dilator, consisting of a set of metal olives mounted on whalebone, to be used with a guidewire or preswallowed string. The modern equivalent is the Savary dilator (Fig. 9-2), which is made of a softer solid plastic with a central lumen to accept a guidewire; it is not wobbly like the mercury-filled rubber shells and is therefore better suited for transmitting the pushing effort to the stricture. The more gradual taper and very flexible tip distinguish the Savary from the Maloney dilator. A series of 10 bougies cover the sizes of 16 Fr. through 47 Fr. (5 to 15 mm). To pass the Savary dilator without the guidewire the tip is guided to behind the epiglottis as it is for the mercury-filled dilators. (For use with the guidewire, which is the recommended method, see the section on the guidewire method.) The patient then swallows the tip, the physician synchronizing a gentle push with the swallowing. After the esophagus is entered, the patient is asked to extend the neck. The dilator enables the operator to have a good feel for the stricture, its tightness, and the degree of yield. The patient is allowed to take over advancing it and thus to self-dilate at his or her own pace. Withdrawal should be done by the physician, who should note the tightness and whether any blood streaks are present on the bougie. The Savary dilators are unsuitable for dilating any stricture that lacks room beyond to accommodate the relatively long tip, such as a strictured gastrojejunostomy.

Direct bouginage is the method of choice for low-grade strictures, with a lumen larger than 36 Fr. This is the only method for dilating to 50 to 60 Fr. In the author's own practice, it is employed in almost every case. Even in high-grade stenosis, after dilating to 36 Fr. with other methods, direct bouginage is used to bring the lumen to the desired size, 46 to 50 Fr.

DILATION THROUGH RIGID ESOPHAGOSCOPY

The rigid esophagoscope itself may be used to dilate a mild stricture, (e.g., 38 Fr. or so), taking advantage of the beveled end. Such a stricture appears to the endoscopist as a rim, almost ready to admit the endoscope. Parthetically it should be stressed that with a fiberoptic endoscope, when a stricture appears as a thin rim framing the lumen, the lumen is somewhat larger than the objective (depending on the angle of view and the distance from the objective), 3 to 4 mm in diameter, and by no means ready to accept the endoscope, which is usually 9 to 12 mm in diameter. (Fig. 9-3). The cross section of the Jackson esophagoscope is oblong but will be accommodated by a lumen the equivalent of 42 Fr. For somewhat tighter strictures, a rigid bronchoscope may be used in the same manner. High-grade strictures can be dilated by Jackson dilators inserted into the lumen of the rigid scope, much like using the lumen finders to aid passing the rigid endoscope into the cricophayngeus. The disadvantages of this method are many. For example, the largest dilator admitted into the adult esophagoscope is only 26 Fr., and insertion of the dilator renders the already inferior view unacceptable. The view

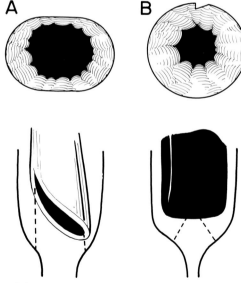

Fig. 9-3 (A) When the stricture appears as a rim in the view through the rigid endoscope, it is just narrower than the endoscope, which may be used to dilate it. (B) When it appears as a thin rim through a fiberoptic endoscope, however, the stricture is just smaller than the objective, depending on the distance away from it, and far too small for dilation with the endoscope.

can be improved by means of a telescope attachment, but the lumen will then be too narrow to be used for dilation. The use of general anesthesia required for rigid endoscopy eliminates the patient's reaction, generally considered a safeguard in preventing overenthusiastic dilation. Nevertheless, rigid endoscopic dilation is direct and simple and is probably the best method for dilating a high stricture where only a short instrument (e.g., pharyngoscope) is needed.

The safe performance of rigid esophagoscopy requires considerable training and skill. The author prefers the supine position under general anesthesia with endotracheal intubation. The left lateral position, without general anesthesia or controlled ventilation, is commonly used by gastroenterologists. The patient may also be seated on a bronchoscopy chair (a low back stool with arms) with the endoscopist standing behind; the procedure is done under sedation and topical anesthesia. In whatever position, control of the position of the head is crucial; the best assistant is the expert headholder, particularly for the supine position.

To begin the procedure with the patient in the supine position, the patient's eyes are covered for protection, and gauze pads are used to protect the upper lip, teeth, and gum. The ocular end of the rigid esophagoscope is held by the right hand, handle pointing up, or suction channel dependent, while the left hand controls the patient's jaw. To begin the insertion, the patient's head must be flexed. The thinly lubricated endoscope is introduced almost vertically into the mouth onto the base of the tongue, which is lifted forward by the tip of the instrument. The left hand controls the distal shaft like a billiard cue; the left index finger at the same time separates the lip from being crushed by the shaft. First the base of the tongue and then the epiglottis or the endotracheal tube, which hides it partially, are seen. The endotracheal tube is followed until it disappears into the laryngeal aditus, bounded posteriorly by the aryepiglottic folds. At this stage it is most important to mentally visualize the axis of the hypopharynx and the esophagus and to align the endoscope accordingly. The headholder flexes and lifts the head, while the left thumb of the endoscopist presses the shaft of the esophago-scope anteriorly to lift the cricoid cartilage for-ward, both to prevent crushing the delicate pos-terior pharyngeal wall against the cervical spine and to align the endoscope for visualization of the cricopharygeus. Some advocate passing the tip of the endoscope over the right aryepiglottic fold into the right pyriform fossa, and then, at the bottom of the fossa, move into the midline, the level of the cricopharyngeus. The author prefers to keep strictly to the midline and to recognize the transverse slitlike cricopharyngeus (with the round openings of the pyriform fossae on either end of the slit, although they would not be visible if the slit were in full view) and insinuate into the slitlike lumen while the left thumb continues to press forward on the shaft. When in doubt, the lumen finder (a small-caliber Jackson dilator, 6 to 8 Fr.) is most helpful at this stage. If it falls into the transverse slit with-out encountering resistance, the endoscope is in correct alignment and can be advanced over the finder.

A rigid endoscope must never be advanced without the lumen in full view. The most com-mon site of injury is the posterior pharyngeal wall, both as a result of crushing by the tip against the cervical vertebrae and perforation by the tip when advanced without seeing the lumen at this point. Once inside the esophagus, the lumen is easy to see. Little force is needed to advance if the headholder now extends the head. To survey the entire circumference, how-ever, the endoscope should not be rotated; rather, the head should be moved from side to side. Bear in mind that the esophagus gradually courses to the left, the head is rotated gently to the right as the lower esophagus is reached, and the lower esophageal sphincter can then be entered. Shifting the axis of the endoscope to attempt straightening out the esophagus and advancing without seeing the lumen is the cause of perforation just above the gastroesophageal junction, the next most common site of instru-mental injury.

In a strictured esophagus, the advance must stop as soon as the stricture comes into view. If the perimeter of the stricture is almost to the rim of the endoscopic view, gentle insinua-tion of the endoscope into it is permissible, but experience in recognizing appropriate resis-tance is essential, as no amount of didactic in-struction can be an adequate substitute. The endoscope must not come too close to a tight stricture, to avoid undue stretching above an unyielding scar. Transendoscopic dilation may be done with the Jackson dilator. After guilding the top of the dilator into the stricture, the rest of the dilation goes largely by feel, since the dilator blocks most of the endoscopic lumen. A good view, however, is possible with a tele-scopic attachment. Strong suction and lavage are the strong points of the rigid endoscope, but that hardly makes up for the poor view. Dilation cannot progress beyond 26 Fr. using the adult Jackson esophagoscope, or 30 Fr. with the Negus model.

Despite the apparent technical difficulty, the rigid endoscopic method is the method of choice for dilating a high-grade stenosis in the upper third of the esophagus, especially at the cricopharyngeus. A rigid pharyngoscope (a short esophagoscope) can be used, and many of the disadvantages of the long esophagoscope, such as examination of the lower esophagus as it deviates to the left, do not apply. The main reason is that the short rigid endoscope is stable and affords a direct route to the anatomi-cal region. This is the ideal method for the rare case in which a Zenker's diverticulum coex-ists with a high-grade upper esophageal stric-ture.

Over a decade ago Hirschowitz[25] stated that rigid esophagoscopy should no longer be per-formed except for dilation of esophageal stric-tures. He argued that rigid esophagoscopy is difficult and hazardous in the hands of the nonex-pert; in these days of increasing specialization, esophagoscopy is done by the gastroenterologist and by general, thoracic, and ENT surgeons. As a result, the concentration of experience nec-essary to train an expert is no longer available. It is thus surprising that 20 years after the intro-duction of the flexible endoscope few specialty surgeons are conversant with its use. It takes some exposure to fiberoptic endoscopy to appreciate the limitation of the rigid endoscope. The following endoscopic methods are superior to dilation via rigid esophagoscopy.

PARAENDOSCOPIC METHOD USING JACKSON DILATORS

This method is ideally suited for the simple peptic strictures encountered in the lower third of the esophagus.[10] The instruments required are a set of Jackson dilators and a small-caliber fiberoptic endoscope. The Jackson dilators (Fr. 6 to 40 in even sizes) (Fig. 9-2) are made of silk-woven olives impregnated with lacquer and mounted on thin steel spring handles. At endoscopy the area is lavaged, suctioned, and carefully inspected. The degree of previous trauma (from self-dilation or otherwise), the presence of pseudodiverticula and false passages, the estimated size, and the eccentricity of the lumen are carefully noted. It is unwise to undertake dilation immediately following biopsy, as the weakened area may become the site of a serious tear; in any case, the pathology of the stricture should have been established beforehand by a previous diagnostic endoscopy.

With the endoscope positioned 5 to 8 cm above the stricture, the lubricated Jackson dilator of appropriate size is passed alongside the endoscope. The tip is guided to the posterior pharyngeal wall and behind the epiglottis. By following the shaft of the fiberscope, the cricopharyngeus, felt as a short band of slight resistance, is passed. The dilator is advanced until it comes within view, and the endoscope is withdrawn a few centimeters, if necessary, to make room. Under visual control, advancing the endoscope if necessary for a closer view, the tip of the dilator is manipulated into the opening of the stricture (Fig. 9-4). A rotary motion helps negotiate an eccentric opening. If the dilator does not seem to move freely, it is because the endoscope is too close and interferes with the movement of the olive portion of the Jackson dilator. Withdrawing the endoscope to make

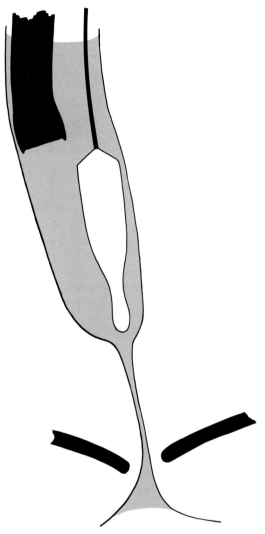

Fig. 9-4 The Jackson dilator in use in the paraendoscopic method. (Chung RS: Therapeutic endoscopy. p. 63. In Fromm D (ed) Gastrointestinal Surgery. Churchill Livingstone, New York. 1985.)

room will correct the situation. The actual dilation is performed by gentle forward pressure combined with rotation. One must resist the temptation to dilate too rapidly at one session. A commonly observed rule of safety is not to go up more than three sizes (e.g., from 22 Fr. to 28 Fr.) after the stricture has been calibrated. The patient should not be anesthetized or so narcotized as to be unable to report pain. A short sharp catch without lasting pain need not elicit alarm; it is normal for the patient to experience this every time the dilator passes the tightest spot. After withdrawal of the last Jackson dilator, the stricture is irrigated and inspected for major hemorrhage, mucosal tears, and the size of the final opening. Multiple passage of the dilator is uncomfortable to the patient; therefore, the topical anesthetization of the throat must be especially thorough.

DILATION WITH THE GRUNTZIG BALLOON DILATOR

In this method the balloon dilator modified from the Gruntzig balloon catheter for angioplasty, is used. Smaller balloon dilators can be inserted via the instrument channel into the strictures under vision and be inflated with water for visually monitored dilation. This is the technique generally used for dilation of strictures distal to the esophagus. For esophageal work, the larger balloons cannot be used endoscopically; they are mounted on shorter catheters, to be passed deflated over a guidewire until the balloon is positioned inside the stricture as monitored fluoroscopically. They are then inflated with dilute contrast agents. The balloons (Fig. 9-2) come in various diameters and are preshaped with tapered ends; the shape and diameter are maintained over a range of pressure and will burst when pressure is grossly exceeded, rather than expand in volume. In contrast to the conventional dilators, balloon dilators exert a radial force, which is much more efficient (indeed, at times too efficient) than the conventional dilating force, which acts axially, directed initially at the shelf of the stricture (Fig. 1-1C). For this reason, the technique is especially suited for long strictures. The 180-cm-long dilator with a balloon smaller than 8 mm can be inserted via the usual 2.5-mm instrument channel; however, dilators with larger balloons (e.g., 1-cm balloon and larger) require a 3.6 or larger channel and are mostly used with the guidewires.

Balloon dilators require some preparation be-fore use (see also Chapter 6). This involves priming the system with water or dilute contrast, such as 15 to 30 percent diatrizoate, to remove all air from the system in an effort to obtain even transmission of hydrostatic pressure. To facilitate removal of the collapsed balloon. When used in the instrument channel of the endoscope, it should be made to fold when collapsed. The primed balloon is aspirated to empty and folded as two wings in a clockwise or counterclockwise direction, using the supplied balloon folder. It is then immersed in a water bath of 65°C for 1 minute to impart to it a memory, so that it will collapse in the same manner in which it has been folded. The balloon is next cooled in a cold water bath for 10 seconds.

Under direct vision, the appropriate sized dilator with collapsed balloon is inserted into the stricture. Using a 20-ml glass syringe, contrast medium is slowly instilled to inflate the balloon to acquire a feel for the stricture, to experience how rigid the wall is and how much it will give. This is only possible if the dilator is larger than the stricture. Guided by endoscopic appearance as well as the patient's reaction to discomfort, the pressure is held at a level without producing pain and the volume instilled is read off. The pressure is maintained for 1 minute and released. After resting for a moment, the balloon is inflated first to the same volume, then a little more, and the cycle repeated. Soon it is found that a slightly larger volume can be accommodated without generating discomfort. If a pressure gauge is used, this becomes very obvious: a larger volume of water is accommodated by the balloon without raising the pressure, or a much lower pressure is registered when the same volume is instilled, provided that the balloon has not been fully inflated. Once the maximum volume has been attained, further pressure from the plunger only causes a sharp rise in the internal pressure of the balloon, causing it to become almost rigid. A pressure of 4 to 6 atm (58.4 to 87.6 psi) is accommodated without deformation of the balloon. It is also important to realize that the smaller the syringe, the greater the pressure that can be generated by hand and that to use a syringe smaller than

10 ml is hazardous. With a 50-ml syringe, it is difficult to generate more than 70 to 80 psi of pressure manually, so is quite safe to use even without the pressure gauge. The balloon dilator may not be used like the conventional Jackson dilator after it has been inflated with water, since the catheter is too flexible to transmit pressure to the stricture.

Multiple balloon dilators can be used sequentially when the dilation is done with fluoroscopic rather than endoscopic monitoring. The deformation of that balloon appears as a "waist" under fluoroscopy if the stricture is short, but in strictures longer than the balloon, deformation cannot be relied on to indicate correct position. To ensure correct positioning, the technique for the pneumatic dilators used for achalasia (see Achalasia) can be modified for this purpose. This is the basis of the recently described retrograde technique[19] for the balloon dilators. In this method, correct positioning of the balloon into the stricture can be accomplished without the need for either endoscopy or fluoroscopy. The deflated dilator is first inserted well past the stricture. It is then inflated and withdrawn until resistance to withdrawal is met. At this point the length is read, which indicates the lower limit of the stricture. The balloon is then deflated and the catheter withdrawn 2 cm or so, depending on the estimated length of the stricture. In this position, inflating the balloon will accomplish dilation by means of a radial force.

The true retrograde action, comparable to the Tucker's dilator (see Retrograde Dilation), is realized when the deflated dilator, after first being inserted past the stricture well into the stomach, is inflated to the predetermined diameter and pulled back (Fig. 9-5). The advantage of retrograde dilation is that it starts to work on the side of the stricture that has been protected from repeated trauma; the tissue is usually pliable and easy to stretch. By the time the worst scarred segment is reached, the funnel already formed confers a mechanical advantage for dilating this segment. This technique has the combined advantages of retrograde dilation and prograde insertion. A major advantage over the

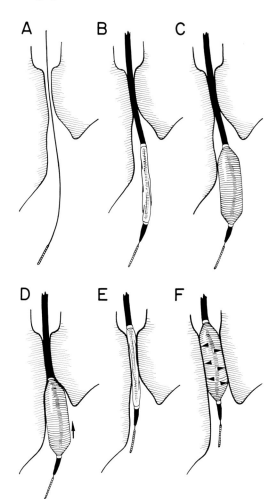

Fig. 9-5 Balloon dilators being used for retrograde dilation. First, guidewire is passed (A). Deflated dilator is next passed into the stomach over the guidewire (B), and then inflated (C). The dilator is withdrawn until the balloon catches at the stricture (D), then deflated until it passes into the stricture (E). Dilation is effected by reinflation (F). (After Graham DY, Smith JL: Balloon dilatation of benign and malignant esophageal strictures. Gastrointest Endosc 31:171, 1985.)

classic retrograde dilation is that the per oral insertion of a balloon dilator makes it unnecessary to establish a preliminary gastrostomy.

The balloon dilator is best used for high-grade strictures longer than 2 cm. It is the most useful technique for strictures occurring beyond the esophagus, such as a stenotic gastrojejunostomy, or pyloric stenosis, wherein the dilator is most conveniently and accurately positioned via the instrument channel at endoscopy.

GUIDEWIRE METHOD

The guidewire method is suitable for the high-grade stricture treated in the past with string-guided dilation using a hollow metal olive mounted on a flexible shaft made of whale bone (the Plummer sound).[30,42] The patient is given a string to swallow, some hours beforehand. The oral end of the string is threaded through a central lumen in the olive (Fig. 9-2). Dilation is effected by holding the string taut and sliding the olive down to the stricture. The major disadvantage is that the string may take a long time to pass. When it is finally anchored, traction on the string may rarely cut into the mesenteric side of the intestines. These disadvantages have been eliminated by the endoscopic guidewire method, using the Eder-Puestow and balloon dilators.

This technique is made more difficult now that the shorter flexible esophagoscope has been replaced by the longer panendoscope. The guidewire has to be very long, at least 300 cm, creating problems in handling. The guidewire must be held taut at all stages, since coiling is hazardous of perforation. The modern esophagologist may do well to invest in a modern fiberoptic sigmoidoscope (60 cm) dedicated to esophageal work. Most of these are slim (1-cm diameter or less), have a large channel, and have optics quite suitable for inspection of the esophageal lumen. Such an endoscope is ideal for dilators used through the instrument channel because the shorter length of these channels offers much less friction for the balloon catheters, and the guidewires do not have to be as long.

The guidewire is first passed through the stricture at endoscopy. The flexible spring tip of this wire facilitates negotiation of the stricture and reduces the chance of false passage. Since the tip of the wire is invisible once inserted into the stricture, however, the feel becomes the only guide unless fluoroscopy is used at the same time. When in good position, the wire can be withdrawn and advanced equally easily, without a sensation of coiling (increased resistance on advance and decreased resistance on withdrawal). Between 10 to 15 cm of the wire should be placed beyond the stricture, too much slack would invite coiling and increase the hazards of injury. When in doubt, fluoroscopy should be used. Three types of dilators may be passed over the guide, but the actual dilation should still be monitored with either fluoroscopy or endoscopy. The first is the balloon dilator described under Endoscopic Method. This dilator has a central lumen to accept the guidewire and radiopaque markers marking the balloon-bearing segment. When monitored by fluoroscopy, the uninflated balloon is first positioned to span the entire stricture, as judged by previously obtained distance from the incisors; dilute contrast is then instilled to distend the balloon, exerting a radial force to enlarge the lumen.

The second type of dilator that can be used with the guidewire is the Eder-Puestow dilator, probably the most common dilator used today. This dilator comes in the form of a set with interchangeable metal olives to be mounted on a hollow semiflexible metal handle (Fig. 9-6). The assembled dilator is threaded over the guidewire and guided past the cricopharyngeus into the esophagus. The stricture is dilated in the conventional manner by steady but gentle forward pressure combined with rotation, guided by feel and the patient's reaction.

The third type is the currently popular Savary dilator, described under the section of direct bouginage. This is a gradual tapering dilator resembling the Maloney in shape, but it is made of solid plastic, marked with radiopaque marker so that dilation can be monitored under fluoroscopy. A central lumen accepts the guidewire. Both the Eder-Puestow and the Savary are less efficient in operating principle than the Gruntzig balloon. Restrospective comparison of the results using the Eder-Puestow and the Savary at two centers has been published;[13] no signifi-

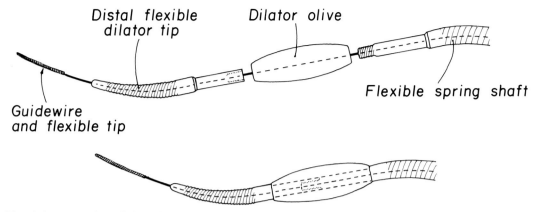

Fig. 9-6 Assembling of the Eder-Puestow dilators. (Chung RS: Therapeutic endoscopy. p. 64. In Fromm D (ed) Gastrointestinal surgery, Chruchill Livingstone, New York, 1985.)

cant difference was reported in a total experience of 300 patients.

No matter what dilator is used, the guidewire must be prevented from being pushed farther into the gut as the dilator is advanced. Such action invites perforation by the soldered junction of the wire and the spring (see under Mechanisms of Perforation) (Fig. 9-9D). Also, there must be no coiling of the wire anywhere, and excess wire must not be inserted. The coil acts like a blade wherever it is formed (see Fig. 9-9E); movement transmitted to the coil may cut into many structures, commonly the esophagus. To prevent this from happening, the guidewire must be kept straight and taut at all times by the assistant.

When fluoroscopy is not available, monitoring of the actual dilation can be accomplished very simply by endoscopy, except in the case of the Savary dilator. A clear view is readily obtained by reinserting the endoscope alongside either the balloon catheter, or the Eder-Puestow dilator. A small caliber endoscope is helpful; but even with the regular-sized endoscope the movement of the dilator is not impeded. The position of the balloon is verifiable at endoscopy, as are early signs of injury, such as hemorrhage and mucosal tears. The injury due to metal olives usually starts at the entrance of the stricture in the form of a longitudinal split in the mucosa. When fluoroscopy is used as a monitor,

the first sign of trouble is perforation, since mucosal tears are not detectable by this means.

The Eder-Puestow dilators are a good choice for a high-grade lower esophageal strictures; in fact, they are the workhorse of most gastroenterologists. These dilators may be used interchangeably with the paraendoscopic method; both are indicated in the same situations. However, in order to monitor visually, the endoscope has to be reinserted, a minor inconvenience. The guidewire makes negotiation of a narrow opening more certain than the finer Jackson's, but some endoscopists have reservations about the invisible portion of the guidewire beyond the strictures, especially in the process of dilating (see mechanisms of perforation).

RETROGRADE DILATION VIA A PREESTABLISHED GASTROSTOMY

Retrograde dilation, using a previously established gastrostomy, has been considered the safest method of dilation of long strictures, such as those resulting from ingestion of corrosives. This method was popularized by Tucker and co-workers,[47,49] whose results are still unsurpassed. A gastrostomy is fashioned just below the gastroesophageal junction near the lesser curvature, using a large tube, and immediately put to good use in correcting nutritional depletion while the track is allowed to mature. The natural funnel of the gastroesophageal junction is said to help "shoehorn" the dilator into the correct axis, but a better reason may be that the soft tissue is always free from the repeated trauma of previous attempts at restoring the lumen. The traditional technique requires that a thread be first swallowed and retrieved from the gastrostomy. A series of Tucker's dilators (short spindles with ties on both ends) are tied in series with the two ends of the swallowed thread to form a continuous loop (Fig. 9-7).

Dilation is carried out by pulling the thread from the mouth, moving the dilators into the gastrostomy and up through the stricture. This method is easily modified for the endoscope. Through the gastrostomy, reverse esophagoscopy is performed, inserting the endoscope past the lower esophageal sphincter. The lower end of the stricture is visualized. A balloon dilator is inserted into the stricture and dilation is accomplished as described for balloon dilators. Other dilators can also be used. Endoscopic retrograde dilation has the advantage of obviating the need to pass a string as a preliminary step, a time-consuming procedure of uncertain result; in addition, there is no unsightly loop of string hanging from the patient's mouth for the duration of treatment. The new method of per-oral retrograde dilation using the balloon dilator has not been used for very long strictures, but if the results are promising it may well eliminate the gastrostomy method.

This method should be reserved as a final resort for the most difficult stricture, after other methods have failed or complications have developed. It should be tried before deciding on the esophageal replacement with colon for chronic lye burn, according to Tucker. Although it involves a preliminary gastrostomy, the operation is needed for correction of nutritional depletion, which is always serious in such difficult strictures. It is the surest method of dilation in my experience, but it may be underutilized these days because of the inhibition to do a preliminary gastrostomy.

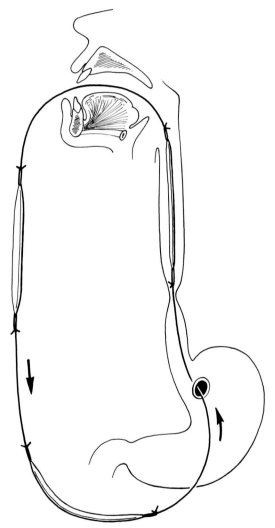

Fig. 9-7 Tucker's retrograde dilators in action. The string tying the series of dilators has been knotted as a continuous loop during dilation. When not in use, the string only is taped to the abdomen and nose until next session. (Chung RS: Therapeutic endoscopy. p. 65. In Fromm D (ed) Gastrointestinal Surgery, Churchill Livingstone, New York, 1985.)

OPERATIVE DILATION

Hayward[22] first showed that good results can be obtained with dilation of dense strictures at laparotomy followed by repair of the hiatal hernia, a simple method yielding far more superior results than resection or bypass, the surgical operations advocated before the 1960s. Considerable clinical experience has since substantiated the claim that, if reflux has been corrected, maintenance dilation is needed in only 10 to 20 percent of cases.[3,23,46] The only controversy appears to be one of technical detail: When the esophagus is shortened, it has not been conclusively shown whether intrathoracic fundoplication suffices[45] or whether the esophagus has to be lengthened with some form of plastic procedure (e.g., Collis gastroplasy) (Fig. 9-8) before performing the Nissen fundoplication.[35,38] In any case, the stricture itself is dilated both shortly before and at operation. At laparotomy or thoracotomy, depending on the location of the stricture, the esophagus is dissected and the stricture identified. With the stricture supported on the outside by both hands of the surgeon, the assistant (or the anesthesiologist) passes a Maloney dilator of appropriate size into the stricture, using steady, gentle pressure coordinated with the supporting effort of the surgeon. Dilation to 50 Fr. is recommended. The plication is then performed with the dilator in the esophagus.

This method is only feasible for the low-grade stricture. In the opinion of this author, it is almost always possible to dilate at a leisurely pace to the desired size before the patient comes to operation. The expediency of operative dilation must be balanced with the risk of rupturing the esophagus by a procedure carried out by a person other than the operating surgeon, and often with too much haste.

Although many different methods are described, a combination of techniques often works best, particularly for the most difficult strictures. For example, for the long and narrow corrosive strictures, retrograde balloon dilation over a guidewire under fluoroscopy should be initiated. Once the lumen has been fully dilated by the 1-cm balloon (31 Fr.), the dilation may be continued with the Savary or Jackson dilators until 40 Fr. is reached. Thereafter, the Maloney or Hurst mercury bougies may be used to attain a size of 50 Fr. or more. The patient should be taught how to self-dilate with the mercury bougie and sent home with one for maintenance dilation.

Complications

HEMORRHAGE

A small amount of oozing from the granulation lining of the stricture is inevitable and requires no more action than rinsing and watching. Spontaneous clearing is the rule. Rarely, brisk hemorrhage is encountered, usually associated with more serious injury, such as extension of a tear to the submucosa, where the larger vessels are located. Where accurate electrocautery is feasible, it is the most effective measure. Often

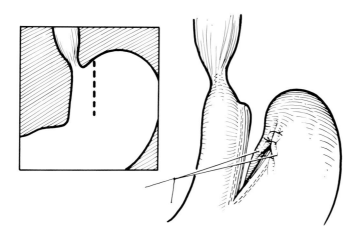

Fig. 9-8 Collis gastroplasty. The esophagus is lengthened by utilizing the fundus of the stomach to form a tube.

Fig. 9-9 Mechanisms of perforation. (A) The Maloney dilator perforating a pseudodiverticulum. (B) The tip of the rigid endoscope perforating the esophagus above the stricture. (C) Coiling of the Maloney dilator, misdirecting the force. (D) When the guidewire spring tip is bent at the soldered wire–spring junction, the flexibility is lost. (E) A kinked guidewire perforating the esophageal wall. (F) The metal olives are unsuitable for dilating anastomses such as the gastrojejunostomy as the rigid dilators do not conform to the shape of the intestinal lumen. (G) Splitting of the stricture by too much stretching force. (H) Air is trapped in the stomach when stricture is blocked by dilator. Perforation of acute duodenal ulcer may occur if the patient retches while being dilated.

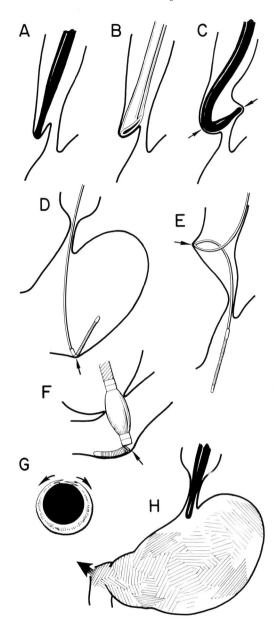

bleeding is seen coming from the bottom of a tear, so hidden that accurate electrocautery is out of the question. Tamponade with thrombin soaked gelfoam may be tried, but one must be wary of converting the tear into a full-thickness perforation by too enthusiastic applications. Anecdotal success has been reported with a single subcutaneous injection of bethanechol, as well as with intravenous injection of vasopressin.

FALSE PASSAGE

False passage is a chronic state—a common cause of failure of self-dilation after initial success. A pseudodiverticulum is formed next to the mouth of the stricture, forming a trap for the tip of dilators. It can only be surmised that self- or blind dilation initiated a small injury, and subsequent dilations only served to aggravate this lesion (Fig. 9-9A). The clinical significance of this finding is that (1) the stricture is symptomatic and is not being managed well by self-dilation, and (2) endoscopic dilation and surgical correction of the condition causing the stricture (if applicable) are indicated.

PERFORATION

Perforation is the most frequent serious complication, a possibility that is never lightly dismissed by the experienced endoscopist. The usual location of perforation from endoscopy alone is at the cricopharyngeus, but when dilation is added to the procedure, the location is often just proximal to or at the stricture.

Figure 9-9A–H illustrates the many possible mechanisms of perforation. Although it covers most of the commoner situations, it is by no means exhaustive. The tip of a dilator may perforate the esophagus at the shelf or a pseudodiverticulum during direct bouginage (blind); likewise the tip of the rigid endoscope can cause similar injury. Too rapid stretching caused by too large a dilator produces a splitting of the granulation lining, which may extend to become a full-thickness rupture. Splitting at the weakened area occasioned by deep biopsy (e.g., suctional biopsy) performed at the same session has been documented.[27] Coiling of the tip of a Maloney dilator misdirects the shaft, resulting in a rupture just above the stricture. Coiling or acute kinking of a guidewire cuts into the wall of the esophagus like a knife blade and can occur at any level. Perforation distal to the stricture can occur as well. A deformed guidewire tip, bent at the soldered junction between the wire and the spring, is a frequent culprit, as that spring becomes ineffective and the inflexible soldered junction can perforate the normal gastric wall. Even a new guidewire may perforate the small intestine by catching at a fold. Perforation of a duodenal ulcer has been reported[11] due to retching while air was trapped in the stomach as the stricture is blocked by the dilator. The rigid metal olive section of the Eder-Puestow does a good deal of damage if used for dilating the gastrojejunostomy: Each time it springs past the stricture, it imparts a jab to the jejunal wall.

Most series report a high mortality for esophageal perforation, in excess of 20 percent.[42] This is understandable if one appreciates how the odds are stacked against the patient. Impaired nutrition may have been long standing from dysphagia; the tissue surrounding the perforation has been traumatized by repeated dilation, resulting in chronic scarring and decreased blood supply, and above all there is the unrelieved obstruction distal to the perforation. Mortality increases steeply with delay in diagnosis; hours can make a substantial difference. The perforation can be large, such as that inflicted with the tip of a rigid endoscope. When it is caused by the dilator, it can range in size from a gross rent to a fine hairline split; the latter may account for subacute onset of symptoms. A routine chest radiograph in search of pneumomediastinum after the first dilation is prudent; in any case, it should be obtained after a difficult session. The most prominent symptom is pain on swallowing,

especially when perforation occurs at the cricopharyngeus. Perforation in the chest may also be associated with substernal chest pain, radiating to the back or chin. Crepitus may be palpable at the root of the neck or even higher in the face. Tachycardia and fever soon develop. Emergency gastrografin swallow must be obtained. If no extravasation is demonstrable, it may be assumed that the perforation is small, and the patient may be managed on a trial basis with a regimen of NPO broad-spectrum antibiotics, parenteral fluids, and nutrition, with close monitoring of symptoms and vital signs. Operative treatment is indicated if there is no response within 12 hours or sooner if the patient's condition deteriorates while so managed. When a leak has been demonstrated by contrast study, emergency operative treatment is mandatory. Primary repairs only occasionally heal, for not only is the tissue friable from local sepsis, trauma, and ischemia, but it is also proximal to an unrelieved obstruction. When conditions are not favorable for resection or plastic reconstruction in the emergency setting, consideration should be given to a multistaged treatment plan with an exclusion-diversion-drainage procedure as the emergency stage. Accurate intercostal drainage or, in the case of perforation in the neck, drainage of the cervical prevertebral fascial plane (cervical mediastinotomy) must be instituted. One simple and effective diversion is T-tube drainage of the perforation with gastrostomy drainage, originally described by Abbott et al.[1] If possible, the short limb of the T-tube should be intubating the stricture while the long limb drains to the exterior. Formal resection and reconstruction are undertaken electively after recovery. If the diagnosis has been early and the conditions favorable, immediate resection and reconstruction may be feasible. For resectable cancer complicated by instrumental perforation, resection is often the only choice.

Perforation distal to the esophagus is suspected by acute onset of symptoms and signs suggestive of acute abdominal catastrophy; it is confirmed by radiologic demonstration of free air in the peritoneal cavity. The treatment is laparotomy; it does not appear to carry the excessively high mortality as that for esophageal perforation resulting in mediastinitis.

Results

The main difficulties in assessing the published results of dilation are the severity of the lesion and the variability of subsequent progress. In general, the surgical series tend to be weighted with better-risk patients with more severe stenosis, while the medical series tend to show more spontaneous improvement after the initial dilation and prolonged follow-up. In one such series, the natural history of benign strictures was described by Patterson et al.,[36] who clearly showed the variability of the course. Over a period of 4 years, one-third of their patients required no dilations. About one-half of the patients required repeated dilations, but the median frequency was less than once per year for the total series. In this series, as in others,[31,51] the overall success rate in endoscopic treatment without surgical correction of reflux was said to be more than 80 percent.

It would be a reasonable estimate that approximately some 20 percent of all patients with benign stricture would require surgical treatment. Surgical treatment of strictures is basically dilation followed by correction of gastroesophageal reflux, although plastic procedures such as lengthening or widening have also been used as an adjunct in selected circumstances.[35] Resection is reserved for the most complicated cases. The surgical mortality for dilation and antireflux procedure is in the region of 3 percent, with 67 to 76 percent excellent results sustained over 5 to 10 years and a 12 to 15 percent failure rate.[3,23] The mortality for resection and replacement with colon or jejunum for benign disease is higher, as it is technically more demanding, although in expert hands it is still under 5 percent.[4]

In a personal series of 64 patients (all peptic strictures except two) treated between 1974 to 1981, 139 sessions of endoscopic dilations were performed. In about 60 percent of sessions, the paraendoscopic technique was employed, although for most patients a mixture of techniques had been used in different stages. There was

one perforation, occurring in the thoracic esophagus above a dense stricture. The Eder-Puestow dilator had been used. The perforation was treated by a diversion–exclusion procedure with delayed reconstruction by colonic replacement. Pursuing an aggressive policy of surgical correction for reflux in all patients deemed reasonable surgical risks, 49 patients underwent Nissen fundoplication after dilation, and only five of these required postoperative dilations (up to three sessions) during a minimum of 4 years follow-up. Symptomatic relief was maintained in 42 patients. There was no operative mortality, but six patients unsuitable for surgery later died of unrelated causes. Four of these patients survived long enough to require maintenance dilations (nine sessions total) over a 3-year period. Six other patients were treated with dilations alone without surgery, as they either did not have reflux or refused surgery: Two of these were long strictures from lye ingestion, for which retrograde dilations via a gastrostomy was the primary initial therapy. All six had good symptomatic relief. Five patients in the entire series were lost to follow-up.

The Mayo clinic's experience with balloon dilation monitored by fluoroscopy was recently published.[31] Of 69 patients with benign esophageal strictures, initial symptomatic improvement was 90 percent after dilation; 35 percent of these required further dilations after a median duration of improvement of 12 months. Of 36 postoperative (14 gastric and 22 esophageal) strictures, 76 percent had initial improvement, with a median duration of reponse of 8 months; 43 percent of these patients required repeated dilations. In the case of esophageal strictures, the complication rate appears to be superior to other methods. The rate of success for gastric and pyloric strictures is the same as for esophageal strictures.

ACHALASIA

In achalasia, where loss of peristalsis and failure of the lower esophageal sphincter to relax occur concurrently, the treatment principle is directed toward weakening the lower esophageal sphincter. The results of nonsurgical treatment are variable, and the comparison of different methods of dilation can be very difficult. The experienced clinician will not hesitate to switch treatment modalities when optimal results have not been attained. Very transient relief is occasionally obtainable by dilation to a very large diameter (e.g., 56 Fr.) with one of the methods described for peptic strictures, but prolonged relief requires forceful stretching (called brusque dilation) using special dilators. Unlike dilation for strictures, for which mature fibrous tissue is being stretched gradually to avoid disruption, the opposite is aimed for in achalasia. It is the relatively normal lower esophageal sphincter in the aperistaltic esophagus that has to be disrupted, effectively performing a blunt myotomy, as it were. It is next to impossible to divulse normal muscle fibers if they are relaxed: The surgeon knows it only too well when trying in vain to palpate for the internal anal sphincter under caudal anesthesia in performing sphincterotomy for anal fissures. Sudden forcible stretching without warning, eliciting muscular spasm, yields the desired results by tearing some muscle fibers, a difficult process to control. Understretching is ineffective, while overstretching may end up in perforation. The margin of safety is fine and difficult to appreciate. Perhaps the variability of the results is a measure of the uncertainty of achieving a complete myotomy.

Surgical myotomy is indicated after brusque dilation has failed to give a good result or when dilated esophagus is so tortuous as to render dilation hazardous. Some surgeons who consistently achieve good results would offer surgical treatment to every patient with this condition.[16] As in brusque dilation, the importance of technique cannot be overemphasized. If performed correctly, surgical myotomy is precise and controllable, and the results are more predictable and reliable. Nevertheless, the occasional failure of surgical myotomy may still benefit from brusque dilation, possibly by improving on an inadequate myotomy. There is some controversy as to whether an adequate myotomy may be followed by reflux; some advocate performing a Nissen fundoplication over a very large bougie at the completion of the myotomy.[40] Many experienced surgeons claim that reflux is not a problem if myotomy does not extend downward onto the stomach for more than a few millimeters[14] and that a significant incidence of dysphagia may result if a fundoplication is added to the myotomy. Reflux infrequently occurs following successful brusque dilation, estimated in one series to be about 17 percent, but no patients suffered disabling symptoms from it.[6]

Forcible stretching is effected through skillful use of pneumatic or expandable metal dilators. Each technique has its proponents.

Technique

PNEUMATIC DILATORS

The inflatable cuff mounted on the shaft of a Hurst dilator (Hurst–Tucker dilator) or, as preferred by most endoscopists, on the shaft of an endoscope, is both simple and effective. A fine catheter connects the cuff with the air pump and pressure gauge. The cuff is a cylindrical silk and rubber bag that, when fully inflated, has a maximum diameter of 3 cm. A pediatric fiberscope may be used. The cuff is mounted with the "waist" positioned over the 30-cm mark on the endoscope; the cuff itself measuring 15 cm long. If the esophagus is tortuous and contains much retained food, it should first be extensively lavaged by preliminary intubation or endoscopy. Malignancy must also be ruled out in the preliminary examination. Premedication with some analgesic, such as meperidine, is indicated. The specially prepared endoscope, with the pneumatic cuff correctly mounted, is passed into the stomach. By retroflexion, the inflatable cuff can be seen clearly to straddle the lower esophageal sphincter (Fig. 9-10). The cuff is inflated rapidly with the sphygmomanometer to 200 mmHg and held for 60 seconds. If the patient is forewarned of pain, an excessive anxiety reaction can be avoided. At the end of 1 minute, the pressure is raised to 300 mmHg and held for 2 minutes, if possible. Besides pain, minor bleeding and submucosal bruising may be seen endoscopically. One advantage of

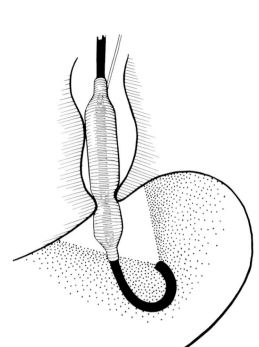

Fig. 9-10 Pneumatic dilator mounted on the endoscope for dilating achalasia. The dilation is monitored by retroflexion.

this method of dilation is that the extent of damage may be surveyed immediately, eliminating guesswork.

If the endoscopic method is not used, the position of the cuff must be monitored with fluoroscopy. One such dilator is the Browne-McHardy dilator, which is a balloon mounted on the Hurst dilator equipped with a nylon limiting sac to prevent overexpansion. The Rider-Moeller pneumatic dilator is similar, except that it has a metal tip and a central lumen in a flexible shaft similar to the Eder-Puestow dilator to accept a guidewire, a possible advantage for the tortuous esophagus. When a satisfactory position has been attained, as verified on fluoroscopy, the balloon is quickly inflated with the sphygmomanometer to the pressure specified for the instrument, usually 200 to 300 mmHg, and maintained for the specified duration, from 30 seconds to 2 minutes, depending on tolerance. As most endoscopists prefer monitoring with endoscopy, these instruments are not their favorite.

The pain elicited is visceral in character, dull, crushing, and substernal to interscapular, almost like angina, causing as much anxiety in the physician as in the patient. Occasionally this is accompanied by orthostatic hypotension or syncope, so the patient should be observed at bed rest and kept NPO. Vital signs are monitored closely, looking for persistent tachycardia and fever. The neck is periodically palpated for crepitus. A chest radiograph is obtained in all patients after brusque dilation for the first time. A contrast study is obtained whenever there are signs or symptoms suggestive of perforation, and the management is then along the lines described for the complication following dilation for strictures.

THE EXPANDABLE METAL DILATOR

A method utilizing a different principle is the Starck or Henning expandable metal dilator (Fig. 9-11). Despite its formidable appearance, its proponents favor it because of the unsurpassed control the operator can have owing to sensitive feel. Rigid esophagoscopy is sometimes used to pass the dilator under direct vision until the expandable portion is over the narrowing. The dilator is manually opened by squeezing the handle, and the resistance felt by the endoscopist provides good feedback. As general anesthesia is usually employed with rigid esophagoscopy, the muscle is relaxed and divulsion is not as effective; it is also easy to overstretch and produce mediastinitis. The original method circumvents such a disadvantage: It is used alone without endoscopy or anesthesia. The instrument is passed much like any other dilator but is first inserted all the way to ensure that it is in the stomach. As it is withdrawn, the handle is given a series of quick squeezes until resistance is felt. This indicates that the expandable portion is now in the region of the stricture. A 5-second firm squeeze at this time will produce effective stretching, at the same time inducing pain. A most unpleasant crunching sensation is felt, indicating breaking of the muscle fibers. Symptomatic relief may not last

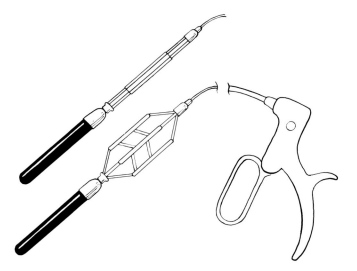

Fig. 9-11   The Henning dilator.

if this is not felt. The quick squeezes continue up the esophagus until mid-esophagus is reached; it is then withdrawn in the closed position. A worthwhile modification of this technique is to cover the metal cage with a rubber sheath (e.g., the esophageal balloon taken from a Sengstaken-Blakemore tube) to prevent catching of the mucosa. The dilator is opened after it has been inserted all the way (intragastric). It is then withdrawn slowly in the open position. As soon as resistance to withdrawal is met, the dilator is closed and withdrawn for 3 to 4 more centimeters. Following a quick, light squeeze of the handle to confirm that it is in position at the gastroesophageal junction, as 5-second hard squeeze is given immediately.

The position of the expandable portion can also be confirmed by fluoroscopy. The process can be monitored endoscopically by introducing the endoscope to verify the position of the dilator as well as to watch the stretching action. Some form of monitoring is recommended to clinicians using the dilators for the first time.

RESULTS

Although lasting relief from brusque dilation is variable in incidence and duration, short-term results are good. The pain disappears in hours, and the dysphagia is immediately improved. Between 60 and 70 percent of patients obtained lasting relief for 4 to 16 years. A 2.5 percent incidence of esophageal rupture has been reported in the Mayo Clinic series[37] of more than 400 patients in whom the pneumatic dilator was mainly used. Experience with the Starck or Henning dilator is similar. Treatment of this complication is similar to perforation following dilation of esophageal strictures. Some bleeding is to be expected, but rarely it may continue and require transfusion, causing concern for possible rupture or mucosal tear. Transient bacteremia, manifested as fever, is an occasional complication that may be difficult to differentiate from pulmonary causes.

Surgical myotomy, in the same Mayo experience, is superior to brusque dilation, both mortality and complications are lower, and more patients obtained lasting relief than with pneumatic dilation.[14] Presumably some element of selection must have biased the results for surgery, since only the better-risks patients were operated on. Early failure after the operation may mean an inadequate myotomy; late failure may indicate healing or scarring across the divided muscle fibers. For this group of patients, either further brusque dilation or reoperation may still improve the symptoms.

DIFFUSE ESOPHAGEAL SPASM

For reasons not entirely clear, dilation often provides transient alleviation of the symptoms of pain and dysphagia in patients in whom investigations, including manometry, have established the diagnosis of diffuse esophageal spasm. Often this is attributed to muscles stretching, but it is doubtful how significant a stretch is obtainable with even the largest dilators. In any case, since there is no stricture, the largest mercury-filled dilators (e.g., 50 to 56 Fr.) are used. For a motivated patient, this simple treatment is quite practical: the patient is taught how to use the dilator for regular self-dilation at home, as the relief obtainable from such treatment is quite short lived. After a varying amount of experience, depending on the aptitude of the individual, very little supervision is needed. Many such patients are known to be quite skilled at self-dilation and have lived comfortably for many years with a once-a-week ritual.

More effective stretching is obtainable with pneumatic dilators used exactly as for achalasia. However, symptomatic relief does not last as long as for achalasia, and dilations may have to be repeated more often.

Ellis[16] reported good results with long myotomy, carried from the lower esophageal sphincter as for achalasia to just above the aortic arch. The operation may be offered to patients with disabling symptoms not responding to dilations.

CORROSIVE INJURY OF THE ESOPHAGUS

The unpredictability of both the extent and course of corrosive injuries of the upper GI tract makes it a challenging condition to treat. Certain guiding principles may help the inexperienced in formulating a treatment plan.

Burns of the mouth and pharynx afford no guide as to the presence or absence of distal lesions. The patient may have vomited or regurgitated the material, causing more contact with the mouth and tongue. Yet in other patients in whom no oral or pharyngeal burns are found, the esophagus, or often the gastric antrum, may have sustained a full-thickness injury due to prolonged contact with more dilute corrosives. Immediate flexible endoscopic examination does not pose an overwhelming threat of perforation or aggravation of the injury, provided it is done with care. Except for the most severe injury in which dissolution of the organ may have already occurred with early signs of mediastinitis and sepsis or even shock, the vast majority of cases have either erythema, edema, contact bleeding, or spasm, where a flexible endoscope does little harm when used skillfully. The utter lack of predictability in the distribution is thus the major reason for a thorough examination.

Broad-spectrum antibiotic therapy has been shown to reduce the speed of bacterial colonization of the necrotic tissue[21,26] and is used prophylactically in most centers, but it is certainly indicated when early sepsis is present. Anaerobic oral bacteria must be included in the consideration. The effects of steroids are still controversial, although there is some good laboratory evidence to support the claim that stricture formation is reduced in alkali burns.[50] Antidotes and lavage are too late to do any good and may actually do harm.

A thorough endoscopic evaluation is the basis of planning for therapy. Even though it may not be clearcut because of changes due to healing or superinfection, the patient's injury can usually be placed among one of the following groups and managed accordingly.

Full-thickness Necrosis, Liquefaction, and Impending Perforation

History of a large amount of corrosive ingested, evidence of shock, mediastinal involvement such as persistent tachycardia, midline chest pain (front or back), pleural effusion, fever, epigastric pain, nausea, peritoneal irritation, ileus, and distention are all ominous signs.

Many of these patients may have dyspnea from laryngeal injury, for which tracheotomy may be necessary. Dehydration and mental confusion are late signs. Radiologic signs such as intramural gas, pneumoperitoneum, or extravasation of contrast are also late. The most helpful early sign is the endoscopic detection of a large area of black, necrotic mucosa; when it is extensive, full-thickness necrosis is almost certain.[2,9]

Early operation offers the best chance of survival in this group of patients. In full-blown cases, the diagnosis is seldom in doubt, and the course of action is clear. After the fluid volume status has been restored and antibiotic therapy started, the patient is explored for resection of necrotic esophagus and stomach and for establishing a diversion cervical esophagostomy. A feeding jejunostomy is an essential step. Reconstruction utilizing the ileum or colon is left for a later stage. The major difficulty is in doubtful cases, in which it is impossible to predict whether the patient, now stable, will go on to perforation. Such a patient must be observed in the intensive care unit for any evidence of deterioration and radiologic or endoscopic evaluation repeated whenever necessary. Antibiotics and steroids are used. Severe mucosal injury without full-thickness necrosis may not progress to perforation; such patients are managed as in the next group.

Extensive Mucosal–submucosal Injury

Endoscopically, this appears as fiery red areas with contact bleeding, edema, and spasm. Superficial ulcerations may range from extensive confluent denudation to small isolated patches. Blisters may form. Black areas are minimal or absent. Granulation lining may be seen when the lesions are a few days old. Serial endoscopic examinations show that the hyperemic areas decrease in size,[9] although with the ingrowth of granulation tissue contact bleeding may be more troublesome a few days later. Some attempt has been made to grade the severity, but this is not widely used, as it is artificial and offers little help in either management or prognosis. A more practical index of severity is the mucosal surface area burned.

The priority is to prevent dense cicatrization in this group of patients, yet the means of achieving this is controversial. There is consensus that the patient must be allowed to eat and drink as tolerated. Most of the controversy, however, resolves around the advisability of early bouginage at this stage, whether it is risky and whether it is necessary. On the basis of experimental pathology, the injured area would be at its weakest at 10 to 14 days or at 4 weeks when steroids have been administered; therefore, the theoretical hazard of perforation is the greatest at those times. There have been no clinical data to support this fear, and in any case the proponents of early dilation argue that it is not true dilation but rather prevention of early stricture. If patients with minimal injury are excluded after careful esophagoscopic examination, the incidence of stricture formation in the untreated patients is high; stricture being invariable in severe injury. Also, Silastic stents (50 Fr.) placed at operation successfully prevented stricture formation in very severe injuries.[18,34] For these reasons, it appears justified to begin soft bouginage early, as soon as endoscopic evaluation has been accomplished, using the Hurst dilators. The dilation routine is established as a drill: It is performed daily by the same physician, as the feel and changes experienced in performing the procedure give important clues to the progress of the lesion. For adults a 40 Fr. and for children a 24 to 26 Fr. Hurst dilator may be used in the beginning. At first the dilator passes easily; some minor blood staining is not unusual. Days later, the passage begins to be resistant, causing gagging and discomfort, and a smaller size may have to be used. After 2 weeks, it should be possible to dilate progressively again as in a chronic peptic stricture without causing much discomfort, using any of the methods of dilation. The adult patient should be discharged after settling to a diligent habit of daily self-dilation, using a 46 Fr. Hurst bougie. At follow-up visits, the frequency of dilation may be decreased from daily to every other day, but any failure to self-dilate should be followed by dilation performed by the physician with endoscopic evaluation if necessary.

The patient must be educated as to the life-long need to be watchful for recurrent dysphagia and a return to dilation periodically for months to years. Periodic reevaluation with endoscopy is necessary indefinitely. The late development of carcinoma manifests as progressive worsening of dysphagia years after apparent cure of the corrosive burn and is only detected by the alert physician or patient.

It is the patient who has not been managed with early bouginage, through either fear of early endoscopic assessment or instrumental injury, who presents with long or multiple tight strictures with malnutrition or dehydration. Tucker has successfully managed this condition with retrograde dilations via a preliminary gastrostomy and has shown that resection was avoidable for all but the most severe cases (1 of 111). Many of the methods of dilation, especially endoscopic methods, described under peptic strictures, may be used as well. A favorite alternative to Tucker's retrograde dilation for this lesion is the guidewire Eder-Puestow method. The objective is to dilate gradually until a wide enough lumen is reached (e.g., 36 to 38 Fr.) to permit the effective use of the mercury-filled bougies, so the patient can take over with self-dilation. Over a period of months, the frequency of self-dilation is regulated, and the patient's attitude as well as the difficulty of the stricture.

The indication for esophageal replacement is generally clear, although the timing is not. For really difficult strictures with multiple pocketing, fistulae, and chronic abscess, surgical replacement is clearly indicated. Indeed, surgery should have been undertaken at an earlier stage. These patients usually have a history of dysphagia despite skilled dilation and supportive treatment. For borderline cases, the cumulative risks of repeated dilations, the duration of disability, as well as the chance of restoration of the esophagus to reasonable function must be weighed against the risks and benefits of surgical resection. A patient may get on well with daily bouginage if no complication arises, but should the patient perforate or cause false passage even once, the subsequent dilations are much more risky and surgical reconstruction should be considered.

Colonic replacement of the esophagus is indicated when almost the entire esophagus has to be resected. The colon is selected because of adequate length; the abdominal anastomosis can be performed at the gastric antrum, while the upper anastomosis can be performed in the neck. For replacement of the lower third or half of the esophagus, jejunal interposition between the upper esophagus and the stomach can be used as an alternative to colon. The stomach can also be brought up into the chest for a esophagogastrostomy. Alternatively a reverse gastric tube, fashioned out of the greater curvature of the stomach, may be brought up to anastomose to the esophagus. Instead of resection, some investigators champion simple bypass of the nonfunctional esophagus with a colon conduit,[17] claiming a decrease of operative morbidity by eliminating difficult and hazardous dissection. However, some risk of malignant degeneration of the diseased esophagus is a remote possibility.

Even successful prevention of strictures of the esophagus by early dilation has not totally eliminated the need for surgery. Some patients may later present with stenosis of the pylorus and antrum from corrosive injury is not amenable to daily dilation. These are most expeditiously treated with surgical resection.

Transient Hyperemia of the Pharynx, Esophagus, and Gastric Antrum

These are the mildest lesions and can be treated by early bouginage. However, if reevaluation in 2 weeks shows no trace of injury whatsoever, dilation may be stopped and the patient instructed to return for periodic endoscopic examination. Fortunately, the majority of cases in most series fall into this category. There is some risk of late-occurring stenosis, although it is difficult to assess how real such a risk is.

Results

The overall mortality varies from 0 to 37 percent[8] but is generally 3 to 4 percent in larger recent series.[20] The operative mortality for resection and reconstruction is between 5 and 14 percent,[4] somewhat higher when the stomach is used and somewhat lower when the esophagus was not resected.[17] Fatal complications include leakage of anastomosis, ischemic necrosis of the transposed loop, in addition to the usual major surgical complications. A 15 percent incidence of stenosis of the esophagogastrostomy can be expected; the incidence of stenosis is lower for other anastomoses.

ANASTOMOTIC STRICTURES OF THE ESOPHAGUS AND STOMACH

Some anastomotic strictures following esophageal or gastric operations are amenable to dilation. These include esophageal anastomoses, especially those constructed with the stapler, and those following reconstruction for lye burns; the gastrojejunostomy of the Billroth II and the gastroduodenostomy of Billroth I gastrectomy; and the increasingly common complication following gastric-limiting procedures for morbid obesity, such as the gastric bypass, the gastrogastrostomy, and the vertical-banded gastroplasty. Endoscopic dilation is indicated when the anatomic configuration of the lesion is such that would lend itself well to dilation, such as a thin diaphragm-like stricture.

The secret of success is in careful planning. The radiologic study must first be examined carefully to determine the length as well as the diameter of the stricture, the axis of the gut above and below the anastomosis, and any evidence of adjacent abscess or displacement. For angulated anastomosis, such as the side-to-side

gastrojejunostomies, inflexible metal olives (e.g., Eder-Puestow) may not be used due to the lack of room beyond the stricture, running a risk of perforation of the jejunum. For diaphragmlike strictures, electrocautery incisions may enhance the effect of dilation. A sharply angulated axis may require preshaping of the balloon dilator (when a guidewire is not used), much as the angiographers preshape their catheters. Sometimes at endoscopy additional findings may alter the plan. For example, an unsuspected Marlex band erosion was discovered in a patient thought to be suffering from simple stenosis of the gastroplasty stoma based on radiologic study. The band had to be divided completely with endoscopic scissors before the stoma could be dilated.

Technique

At endoscopy the size and the apparent axis of the anastomosis are estimated. If the anastomosis is more or less in the same axis as the esophagus, such as the gastrojejunostomy of the gastric bypass operation or the stomas of various types of gastroplasties, any one of the methods of dilation can be used. The author prefers the balloon dilator, which is particularly suitable when the anastomosis is some distance away from the gastroesophageal junction. The balloon is only inflated after it has been inserted beyond the stricture, and dilation is effected by withdrawal of the balloon. The guidewire method also works well, but the metal olives are unsuitable for dilating a gastrojejunostomy. Visible foreign bodies such as polypropylene sutures or strands of mesh used for reinforcement of stomas in gastric-limiting procedures, having eroded into the lumen, should be cut with scissors and removed as much as possible by forceps. Marlex band erosion into the lumen months or years following vertical banded gastroplasty performed for weight reduction is more common than the literature suggests, and the band must be first divided before the stenotic stoma can be dilated. Such a band most commonly erodes at the lesser curvature. When the radiograph shows that the stenosis is in the form of a weblike membrane, a sphincterotome may be used to make cuts prior to dilation, usually requiring two cuts 180 degrees apart. This author has treated a patient who, following vertical banded gastroplasty and weight loss, presented with almost complete obstruction of the marlex reinforced stoma from scarring. Fortunately she also developed a tiny separation (2 mm) of the staple line, which appeared on radiographs as a diaphragm across the fundus. By means of the sphincterotome, the separation was enlarged by incising the direction of the staple line until the gastrogastrostomy so created admitted a 32 Fr. dilator. This was done over several sessions to lessen the risk of incising into the free peritoneal cavity.

Experience shows that it is unwise to overdilate in gastric-limiting procedures. The usual size of these stomas created at the original operation is 28 to 30 Fr. If the stoma is enlarged enough to admit a regular endoscope (36 Fr.), it may already be too large, and subsequent spontaneous enlargement and weight gain become inevitable. Dumping and bile gastritis have also appeared following overdilation of strictured anastomosis in gastric bypass patients.

PYLORIC STENOSIS

The role of endoscopic dilation in pyloric stenosis is unclear. While it is technically possible to dilate a stenotic pylorus secondary to peptic ulcer disease, it is not clear how often lasting results can be obtained. A reasonable indication to dilate pyloric stenosis is when a patient who is considered a poor surgical risk is receiving successful medical treatment for the ulcer diasthesis. The result of surgical treatment for this condition is so predictably good that the endoscopic treatment, uncertain at best, is not usually recommended without extenuating circumstances. A better example of application of this technique is in dilating the pylorus in a thoracic stomach after esophagectomy. Some surgeons do not perform pyloroplasty after esophagectomy with esophagogastrostomy recon-struction (with the mandatory vagotomy), claiming that the resulting bile reflux creates more problems than an occasional case of delayed gastric emptying, which can be treated by endoscopic dilation. Since the nonemptying is transient, the true efficacy of dilation can not be easily assessed in this condition.

Technique

The only dilators suitable for this application are the balloon dilators. Suitable sizes are the 1- and 1.5-cm balloons. A therapeutic endoscope with a large instrument channel (3.7 mm or larger) for passing the balloon dilators is essential if endoscopic dilation is desired. Otherwise at endoscopy a 300-cm guidewire is first passed into the stenosis, making sure that it can be easily advanced and withdrawn. The endoscope is withdrawn without dislodging the guidewire. The balloon dilator (9 Fr.), well lubricated with silicone spray, is threaded over the guidewire into the stomach. The endoscope is reinserted and directed to the antrum for a clear view of the pylorus. The dilator is advanced over the guidewire into the stenosis. Actual dilation is done by inflation of the balloon with diluted Gastrografin and is monitored by both fluoroscopy and endoscopy, since it is possible for the duodenum to be perforated at the superior duodenal angle by the tapered tip of the balloon dilator. Because the retroperitoneal duodenum is relatively immobile, and because the tip may catch at the plica semicurcularis, flouroscopy is an added safety.

ANTRAL WEBS AND DIAPHRAGMS

An antral diaphragm is diagnosed radiologically as a thin membranous partition just proximal to the pylorus. When the opening is small, the true pylorus may not be delineated well because of inadequate filling, and the diaphragm may then be mistaken for the pylorus. The endoscopic appearance is almost indistinguishable from pyloric stenosis that the antral side of the pylorus is remarkably smooth. A radiologically well-demonstrated diaphragm may be incised with the sphincterotome and then dilated with the balloon dilator, as for pyloric stenosis. Because of the propensity for the incision to remain as a chronic ulcer, this author prefers one clean cut to two diametrically opposite cuts, and certainly not a cut in each quadrant. The chronic ulcers may take weeks to heal.

ANAL STENOSIS AND STRICTURE

In children the cause of anal stenosis and stricture is congenital, but in adults it is often secondary to operative treatment of hemorrhoids and anal warts, as well as from veneral disease. Chronic inhibition of defecation results in poor bowel habits, and even the adult patient may present with a massively dilated rectum and sigmoid loaded with stool. The first dilation should be done under general anesthesia using Hegar dilators until digital examination is possible and then followed by sigmoidoscopic examination. If the bowel movements are assisted with stool softener, the daily movements tend to diminish the number of maintenance dilations required.

ANASTOMOTIC STRICTURE OF THE RECTUM AND SIGMOID COLON

Anastomotic complications for low anterior resection of the rectosigmoid colon are frequent; of these, leakage and stricture are the most common. Routine digital or radiographic examination of the low rectal anastomosis frequently reveals narrowing, but symptoms may not occur. Many of these strictures disappear with time. However, those who are symptomatic with constipation, narrowed or ribbon stool, and lower abdominal cramps shortly after the operation are likely to continue to experience symptoms and are candidates for therapeutic endoscopy.

The radiologic study is all important in planning. For strictures below the peritoneal reflexion, dilation is quite straightforward, since the rectum is well supported, within easy reach, and safe. Blunt-tipped dilators such as the Hegar dilators work well. For strictures above the reflexion, the axis of the bowel above and below the stenosis must be examined with great care, using double contrast if necessary, for clear differentiation of a membranous obstruction at the anastomosis from bowel folded upon itself. Balloon dilators may be helpful in some cases of membranous obstruction, while in others electrocautery incision with a sphincterotome may be necessary. If the bowel is simply folded on itself at the site of anastomosis, it is unsuitable for therapeutic endoscopy, and formal revisional surgery is indicated.

REFERENCES

1. Abbott OA, Mansour KA, Logan WD Jr, et al: Atraumatic so-called ''spontaneous'' rupture of the esophagus—A review of 47 personal cases with comments on a new method of surgical therapy. J Thorac Cardiovasc Surg 59:67, 1970
2. Ashbaugh DG, Jenkins DW, Gainey MD: Gastroscopy in corrosive burn of the stomach. JAMA 216:1638, 1971
3. Belsey RHR, Skinner DB: Management of esophageal strictures. p. 173. In Skinner DB, Belsey RHR, Hendrix TR, Zuidema GD (eds): Gastroesophageal Reflux and Hiatal Hernia. Little, Brown, Boston, 1972
4. Belsey RHR: Reconstruction of the esophagus with left colon. J Thorac Cardiovasc Surg 49:33, 1965
5. Benedict EG: Peptic stenosis of the esophagus. Am J Dig Dis 11:761, 1966
6. Bennett JR, Hendrix TR: Treatment of achalasia with pneumatic dilatation. Mod Treatm 7:1217, 1970
7. Bill AH Jr, Mebust WK, Sauvage LR: Evaluation of techniques of esophageal dilatation in relation to the danger of perforation: A study of 441 dilatations of benign strictures in children. J Thorac Cardiovasc Surg 45:510, 1963
8. Cardona JC, Daly JF: Current management of corrosive esophagitis—An evaluation of results in 239 cases. Ann Otol 80:521, 1971
9. Chung RS, DenBesten L: Fiberoptic endoscopy in treatment of corrosive injury of the stomach. Arch Surg 110:725, 1975

10. Chung RS, Shirazi SS, DenBesten L: Dilation of esophageal strictures. Arch Surg 111:795, 1976

11. Chung RS, Gurll NJ, Shirazi SS: Perforation of peptic ulcers related to fiberoptic endoscopy. Dig Dis Sci 24:926, 1979

12. Cohen R, Gray S, Hersh T: Balloon dilation of benign and malignant esophageal strictures—A new technique. Gastrointest Endosc 29:181, 1983

13. Dumon JF, Meric B, Sivak MV, Fleischer D: A new method of esophageal dilation using Savary-Gilliard bougies. Gastrointestinal Endos 31:379, 1985

14. Ellis FH Jr, Gibb SP, Corzier RF: Esophagomyotomy for achalasia of the esophagus. Ann Surg 192:157, 1980

15. Ellis FH Jr, Olsen AM, Schlegel JF: Surgical treatment of esophageal hypermotility disturbances. JAMA 188:862, 1964

16. Ellis HF: Disorder of the esophagus in the adult. p. 765. In Sabiston DC Jr, Spencer FC (ed): Gibbon's Surgery of the Chest. 4th Ed. WB Saunders, Philadelphia, 1983

17. Fati L, Marchand D, Crawshaw GR: The treatment of caustic strictures of the esophagus. Surg Gynecol Obstet 102:195, 1956

18. Fell SC, Denize A, Becker NH, Hurwitt E: The effect of intraluminal splinting in the prevention of caustic stricture of the esophagus. J Thorac Cardiovasc Surg 52:675, 1966

19. Graham DY, Smith JL: Balloon dilatation of benign and malignant esophageal strictures. Gastrointest Endosc: 31:171, 1985

20. Haller JA Jr, Andrews HG, White JJ, et al: Pathology and management of acute corrosive burns of the esophagus: Results of treatment in 285 children. J Pediatr Surg 6:578, 1971

21. Haller AJ Jr, Bachman K: The comparative effect of current therapy on experimental caustic burns on the esophagus. Pediatrics 34:236, 1964

22. Hayward J: The treatment of fibrous stricture of the esophagus associated with hiatal hernia. Thorax 16:45, 1961

23. Hill LD, Gelfand M, Bauermeister D: Simplified management of reflux esophagitis with stricture. Ann Surg 172:638, 1970

24. Hill LD, Velasco N: p. 797. In Sabiston DC, Spencer FC (eds): Gibbon's Surgery of the Chest. 4th Ed. WB Saunders, Philadelphia, 1983

25. Hirschowitz BI: Progress in esophagoscopy. Endoscopy 2:75, 1970

26. Johnson EE: A study of corrosive esophagitis. Laryngoscope 73:1651, 1963

27. Jones JD, Bozymski EM: Instrumental esophageal perforation. Dig Dis Sci 24:319, 1979

28. Kobayashi P. Prolla JC, Winan CS, et al: Improved endoscopic diagnosis of gastroesophageal malignancy with combined use of direct vision brushing, and cytology and biopsy. JAMA 212:2086, 1970

29. Larrain A, Csendes A, Pope CE II: Surgical correction of reflux—An effective therapy for esophageal strictures. Gastroenterology 69:578, 1975

30. Lilly JO, McCaffery TD: Esophageal stricture dilatation: A new method adapted to the fiberoptic esophagoscope. Am J Dig Dis 16:1137, 1971

31. Lindor KE, Ott BJ, Huges RW Jr: Balloon dilatation of upper digestive tract strictures. Gastroenterology 89:545, 1985

32. London RL, Trotman BW, DiMarino AF Jr, et al: Dilatation of severe esophageal strictures by an inflatable balloon catheter. Gastroenterology 80:173, 1981

33. Mansour KA, Symbas PH, Jones EL: A combined surgical approach in the management of achalasia of the esophagus. Ann Surg 42:192, 1976

34. Mills LJ, Estrera AS, Platt MR: Avoidance of esophageal stricture following severe caustic burns by the use of intraluminal stent. Ann Thorac Surg 28:60, 1979

35. Orringer MB: Short esophagus with peptic stricture. p. 809. In Sabiston DC Jr, Spencer FC (eds): Gibbon's Surgery of the Chest. WB Saunders, Philadelphia, 1983

36. Patterson DJ, Graham DY, Lacey Smith J, et al: Natural history of benign stricture treated by dilatation. Gastroenterology 85:346, 1983

37. Payne WS, Donoghue FE: Surgical treatment of achalasia. Mod Treatm 7:1229, 1970

38. Pearson FG, Langer B, Henderson RD: Gastroplasty and Belsey hiatus hernia repair. J Thorac Cardiovasc Surg 61:50, 1971

39. Pearson FG, Henderson RD: Long-term follow-up of peptic stricture managed by dilatation, modified Collis gastroplasty and Belsey hiatus hernia repair. Surgery 80:396, 1976

40. Peyton MD, Greenfield LJ, Elkins RC: Combined myotomy and hiatal herniorrhaphy: A new approach to achalasia. Am J Surg 128:786, 1974

41. Pope CE II: Tumors of the esophagus. p. 579. In Sleisenger MH and Fordtran JS (eds): Gas-

trointestinal Disease. 2nd Ed. WB Saunders, Philadelphia, 1976

42. Postlethwait RW: Perforation and rupture. p. 152. In Postlethwait RW (ed): Surgery of the Esophagus. Appelton-Century-Crofts, New York, 1979

43. Rockman S, Morrissey JF: A simple approach to narrow esophageal strictures. Gastrointest Endosc 16:212, 1970

44. Rosetti M, Allgower M: Fundoplication for treatment of hiatal hernia. Prog Surg 12:1, 1973

45. Safai-Shirazi S, Zike WL, Anuras S, et al: Nissen fundoplication without crural repair. Arch Surg 108:424, 1974

46. Safai-Shirazi S, Zike WL, Mason EE: Esophageal strictures secondary to reflux esophagitis. Arch Surg 110:629, 1975

47. Tucker GF Jr: Cicatricial stenosis of the esophagus, with particular reference to treatment by continuous string, retrograde bougienage with the author's bougie. Ann Otol Rhinol Laryngol 33:1180, 1924

48. Tucker G, Hawthorne HR: Follow-up observations on the treatment of benign stenosis of the esophagus. Ann Otol Rhinol Laryngol 60:731, 1951

49. Tucker JA, Turtz ML, Silberman HD, Tucker GF Jr: Tucker retrograde esophageal dilatation 1924–1974. A historical review. Ann Otol Rhinol Laryngol 83 (suppl 16):1, 1974

50. Weiskoff A: Effects of cortisone on experimental lye burns of the esophagus. Ann Otol 61:681, 1952

51. Wesdrop ICE, Bartelsman JFWM, Den Hartog Jager FCA, et al: Results of conservative treatment of benign esophageal strictures: A follow up study in 100 patients. Gastroenterology 82:487, 1982

10

Endoscopic Palliation of Advanced Carcinoma

CARCINOMA OF THE ESOPHAGUS AND THE GASTRIC CARDIA

The choice of treatment for carcinoma of the esophagus is influenced by the stage and location of the lesion. Curative treatment is possible with only surgery and radiotherapy, alone or combined, although the high operative mortality, typically 20 to 30 percent, and the low survival rate, typically no better than a 15 percent 5-year survival, make this a discouraging condition to cure.[22] The symptoms of esophageal carcinoma are so disabling that major resection, with its mortality and morbidity, has been considered worthwhile even when performed as a palliative treatment.[8,21,22] Survival after palliation is 10 to 12 months as compared with 3 months for the untreated condition.[8,21] It is alleged that the patient runs a much lower risk of dying from aspiration, the major cause of death in esophageal obstruction, if palliation has been successful. The optimal modality of palliation has not yet been found, the argument still rages among proponents of endoscopic, surgical, and radiotherapeutic measures. Neither radiotherapy nor chemotherapy reliably restores

a useful lumen, and certainly not immediately. A spit fistula and a feeding gastrostomy or jejunostomy are considered poor palliation as they do not relieve the symptoms of obstruction; in addition, the patient has to put up with the indignity imposed by the artificial stomas. Most patients with advanced disease are malnourished and do not tolerate major operations well. Bypass procedures using the colon, or the stomach (e.g., the Kirschner operation) carry a significant mortality.[21] Endoscopic palliation is therefore appealing not so much on its own merits but because of the disadvantages of all other methods. Even if its success is temporary, it may be repeated when obstruction recurs. Best of all, the patient does not have to sacrifice a substantial portion of his remaining days for convalescing in the hospital. Among the current endoscopic options are: dilation followed by irradiation, dilation with prosthesis insertion, and endoscopic ablation by laser or electrocautery. Except for its resistance to radiotherapy, inoperable carcinoma of the gastric cardia can be palliated by similar endoscopic techniques when obstruction at the gastroesophageal junction is the main symptom.

Dilation and Intubation with Endoprosthesis for Advanced Esophageal Carcinoma

INDICATIONS

All patients suffering from advanced esophageal carcinoma should be considered for any of the available modalities of endoscopic palliation. However, not all tumors are dilatable or intubatable. For the terminally ill patient with aspiration, inanition, mediastinal sepsis, or other serious complications, therapeutic endoscopy is contraindicated, as it is too late to do any good and it is meddlesome not to let nature take its course.

It must be conceded that the concept involved in this method of treatment is not entirely sound. *Dilation of a malignant stricture,* a term of ancient lineage, is unfortunately inaccurate and misleading. The procedure is easily misconstrued as being similar to dilation of the benign stricture, the confusion is further compounded by the usage of the term *malignant stricture*

for carcinoma. Most carcinomas are exophytic lesions causing obstruction by virtue of their bulk. Invasion into the surrounding tissue is almost the rule. Thus where the lumen is narrowest the tumor is also at its broadest (Fig. 10-1). Not only is cancerous tissue less yielding, but it is often much more bulky than the normal esophageal wall. It is therefore misleading to talk of dilating a cancerous segment of the esophagus as though it is a fibrous stricture, which does not have bulk. For truly advanced lesions with tortuous lumens, dilation is technically impossible or extremely hazardous (Fig. 10-2A). While the neoplastic tissue can be compressed somewhat by pressure with the dilators, any real opening up of the lumen is more likely to be due to removal of the superficial necrotic layer by mechanical curettage through the pushing action of the dilators. If the esophagus has not been circumferentially involved (not uncommon even in advanced cases), the apparent dilation is actually the yielding of the uninvolved esophagus to stretching (Fig. 10-2B). Unless the lumen is kept open by wedging a tube in

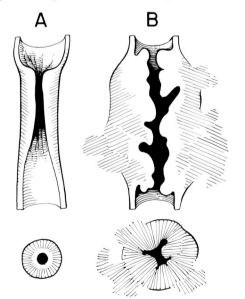

Fig. 10-1 Schematic diagrams comparing the cross sections of a fibrous stricture (A) with carcinoma of the esophagus (B). Even without infiltration into surrounding organs, a carcinoma is bulky and hard, completely different from a fibrous stricture.

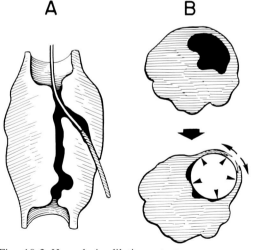

Fig. 10-2 Hazards in dilating a tortuous cancerous lumen. (A) The guidewire has entered a branch of the cancerous lumen; perforation readily results if the tip is pushed through the necrotic tissue. (B) The more pliable sector takes up most of the stretching force, leading to a splitting type of perforation.

place, the enlargement of the lumen is extremely short lived. Endoprosthesis, a tube designed to be wedged into the lumen, is placed after maximal dilation; the correct position of the prosthesis can only be maintained by pressure or friction. Too much pressure generates necrosis; this is followed by loss of friction and migration of the prosthesis. If pressure is continued, such as with excessively tight wedging, the endoprosthesis may erode through the tumor or even through the normal structure. The placement technique is thus very critical. In the opinion of this author it is almost impossible to ride the fine line, if there is one, between migration of the tube on the one hand and erosion of the tumor on the other. What friction would suffice to hold the prosthesis in place for 6 months, and what friction would be considered too great, ending up in perforation? This is a question that defies scientific answer. It is therefore not surprising that despite quantum advances in technique and equipment, the modern result has not perceptibly improved compared to the results of the original Souttar tube introduced more than 60 years ago.[21] The most common complications are still migration and erosion; the latter is almost impossible to treat and is usually lethal, although in some centers the reported mortality is not as great as one may expect.

Despite an unsound theory, the palliation is surprisingly good quality, and the clinical result is at times nothing short of spectacular, especially considering the relative simplicity of the procedure. The saliva no longer has to be expectorated, the incessant coughs and laryngeal irritation from small aspirations are gone, and, most importantly, the patient is happy to be able to swallow again, all of which is accomplished without an external wound. The endoscopist cannot help but be impressed by this first successful intubation. It may well be that the observed complication rate is low as the patients have a short time to live, which actually further emphasizes the virtue of endoscopic palliation.

Placement of various tubes through the tumor by open operation has been performed for many decades. The operative technique of intubation across an esophageal tumor is often called the pull method, as distinguished from the endoscopic technique, the push method. The tapered tube (e.g., the Celestin tube), with a funnel at the upper end is inserted by mouth, and the tapered end is pulled at laparotomy via a gastrostomy, to cause it to become wedged firmly in the tumor. The tube is then sutured to the stomach, and the gastrostomy is either closed or separately intubated. The position of the tube can only be surmised by a chest radiograph taken before the abdomen is closed. When compared with the operative intubation, the endoscopic technique really appears superior. Wound infection alone in such debilitated patients is 26 percent, and hospital mortality is averaging three times higher than endoscopic insertion (see Results). Everything that operative placement can do can be done endoscopically. This author believes that operative intubation for inoperable esophageal carcinoma is about as outdated a procedure as the operation of polypectomy through laparotomy and colotomy. If endoscopic intubation is impossible, so is operative placement.

A special role for placement of endoprosthesis is in the treatment of malignant fistula of the trachea or bronchus, when the disabling symptoms cannot be palliated effectively by any other means. If the prosthesis is placed accurately, symptomatic relief is almost always striking.

In addition to the obviously terminal patient, there are a few contraindications for placement of endoprosthesis. When the tumor is located just below the cricopharyngeus, intubation does not palliate well, since the constant presence of the endoprosthesis felt by the patient is by itself an intolerable symptom, and the prosthesis is likely to be regurgitated. If the tube spans both upper and lower esophageal sphincters, death from aspiration can be expected. Intubating across the lower esophageal sphincter alone is not an absolute contraindication, although the physician must be prepared to treat the resulting reflux medically. When the tumor is not dilatable, where the lumen is extremely narrow and the tumor is more sclerotic than necrotic, or when there had been some form of chronic perforation, curettage with the metal dilators is extremely hazardous and other endoscopic methods should be considered.

TECHNIQUE

Intubation aided by the endoscope[14] is an appealing technique because of its simplicity and safety and because it is inexpensive. The malignant stricture is dilated gradually and patiently to 46 to 50 Fr., taking multiple sessions over many days (see Fig. 10-3). Some endoscopists use only sedation and topical anesthesia, but others advocate general anesthesia for difficult lesions, because of the discomfort of the large bouginage and the aggressive dilation, accepting the increase in hazards. In bulky tumors, partial

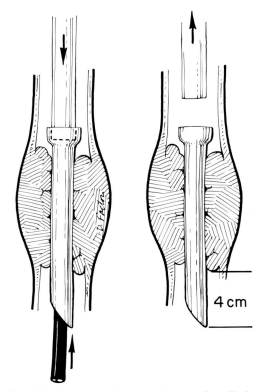

Fig. 10-3 Insertion of endoprosthesis. After dilation to 50 Fr., the endoprosthesis is inserted with pusher tube, both mounted over an endoscope. The position must be checked with fluoroscopy. The endoscope is first removed, followed by removal of the pusher tube, leaving endoprosthesis in place.

resection with the polypectomy snare hastens the process of dilation, but it is risky of perforation if dilation is performed either simultaneously or soon afterward (see Photoablation). The Eder-Puestow dilator over the guidewire technique is preferable because the sliding and pushing action of the metal olives probably remove more of the necrotic layers than do other dilators. Monitoring with fluoroscopy is essential if dilation is not monitored endoscopically. After dilating to an adequate diameter, the lesion is thoroughly irrigated and examined; both the proximal and distal levels of the tumor are measured as distances from the incisor. Based on this measurement, an endoprosthesis is custom made from stock polyvinyl tubing (Tygon R3693). This tubing has an internal diameter of 12.5 mm and a wall thickness of 1.6 mm. The external diameter is therefore 15.7 mm (49 Fr.). The tube should be 4 cm longer than the tumor for construction of the flare end. Particularly for tumors arising from the gastric cardia, a tube longer than the tumor and extending into the stomach for a short distance is less likely to be dislodged by respiratory movements.

To custom-make the endoprosthesis (Fig. 10-4A–E), the required length is cut with a distal end beveled at 45 degrees, while a funnel shaped upper end is created by first immersing the tubing in hot mineral oil (110°C) for 3 minutes and immediately pushing it over the rounded end of a test tube of appropriate size until the flare is about twice as wide (25 mm).[4] The sharp edges are sanded round. An optional distal-retaining flange may be glued on; the flared end cut off from a softer tubing serves well. Alternatively, a spiral groove can be etched into the outside of the Tygon tubing by winding a steel spring tightly around it and heating it in the mineral oil bath. When the spring is removed, the grooved impression remains. Radiopaque marker strips, cut from a Salem sump suction nasogastric tube, can also be glued on; a ring marks the beginning of the upper flare and another for the lower end.

Expensive commercially available endoprosthesis may also be used. They are made with inert plastics and come in various sizes.

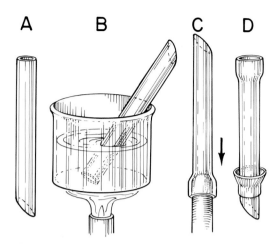

Fig. 10-4 Method of fashioning an endoprosthesis from polyvinyl tubing. (A) Tygon tubing cut 4 cm longer than the tumor. (B) Square end heated in mineral oil bath. (C) Heat-softened end wedged on the round end of the test tube to shape it into a funnel. (D) Endoprosthesis with optional retaining flange glued on.

They all have a flared upper end and a retaining flange at the lower end that tends to prevent upward or downward migration. The material may be silicone rubber, nylon-reinforced Latex, or a steel spring coil embedded in silicone. The internal diameter is 11 to 12 mm, while the external diameter is about 16 mm (50 Fr.). The endoprosthesis typically costs $150 apiece. Most come with introducers or specially modified bougies, and the set can cost $600 to $2,000. Despite the cost, there have been no real design innovations and no special advantages are offered other than convenience.

Insertion is done immediately after the final dilation. A pusher tubing is mounted onto a smaller-caliber endoscope (e.g., Olympus GIF Q), followed by the endoprosthesis (Fig. 10-4). Under topical or general anesthesia, the assembly is passed. The endoscope is advanced into the stomach. The prosthesis is first pushed over the endoscope with the pusher tube until it is wedged in place into the tumor-bearing stricture. Advancement of the prosthesis is much easier than withdrawal, which requires moving the endoscope to the upper rim of the prosthesis and grasping it with a pair of rat-toothed forceps

inserted via the instrument channel. The correct position is best adjusted under fluoroscopy. While maintaining pressure on the pusher tube, the endoscope is withdrawn. The endoscopist should get a good look at the lower and the upper margins (since the tube is transparent) before removal. The pusher tube is first disengaged from the prosthesis by twisting and is then removed.

Insertion may be monitored by fluoroscopy alone. To take the place of the endoscope, a special introducer (e.g., the Nottingham introducer), essentially a Eder-Puestow shaft with a device for holding the prosthesis through internal friction, is used. Other introducers hold the prosthesis by internal friction provided by an inflated balloon (e.g., Celestin introducer). Both the prosthesis and the rammer (a pusher tube) are assembled over the introducer, and the entire assembly is passed over the preplaced guidewire (Fig. 10-5). The ideal position is attained when the prosthesis spans the entire tumor, with the anchoring parts (the funnel and the retaining flange) wedged above and below the tumor. The introducer is first loosened from the endoprosthesis once fluoroscopy shows that correct positioning has been attained and is removed while pressure is maintained on the rammer. Finally the rammer is removed.

Postprocedure care is important to ensure continued function. The patient must be instructed

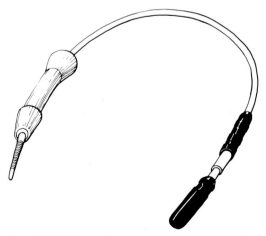

Fig. 10-5 Endoprosthesis mounted on the Nottingham introducer, ready for insertion.

to avoid chunky and stringy foods, which will plug the lumen. If the patient does not have proper dentition or dentures, a food processor must be used until the dental problem is corrected. Some gastroenterologists advise the routine use of papaine, 1 teaspoonful stirred into 60 ml of water, to be taken after each meal as an effective preventive measure against clogging by food debris.

The major cause of failure of intubation is the undilatable tumor. Dilating to 50 Fr. is no mean feat, and one often has to be content with dilating to a smaller diameter and inserting a smaller prosthesis. However, a prosthesis smaller than 42 Fr. is unlikely to function well, and food blockage tends to be troublesome.

COMPLICATIONS

Food Blockage

Despite good judgment on the patient's part, 10 to 20 percent of them still experience food blockage, usually shortly after discharge from the hospital, requiring disimpaction. This represents early blockage as distinct from the late blockage, which is usually due to overgrowth of tumor. A sudden return of dysphagia with or without aspiration symptoms is the typical complaint, and the diagnosis is usually made by the patient. First a nasogastric tube may be passed. If obstruction is encountered, the reservoir of retained secretions is suctioned and a solution of papaine is then instilled. The nasogastric tube is passed again after waiting for an hour or so. If it still does not dislodge, endoscopy is undertaken. Meat and vegetable fibers may be removed by snares, forceps, or polyp retrievers; often the initial picking loose of a hard impaction permits passage of the biopsy forceps into the prosthesis lumen. The rest of the disimpaction is then accomplished by combined stirring with the forceps and irrigation. For extreme cases, the prosthesis must be removed and replaced. The blocked prosthesis may be extracted by simply snaring the flared end with the polypectomy snare. If the retaining flange has been glued on and should come off

during extraction, it may be retrieved by a second insertion of the endoscope or be pushed into the stomach to be passed per anum. A new prosthesis should be inserted before restenosis, which can occur with surprising rapidity.

Migration

A prosthesis may migrate upward or downward, even when placed properly. A 22 percent incidence was observed in the Amsterdam series.[14] Shrinkage of tumor may be expected when radiotherapy is used after insertion of the endoprosthesis, but mostly pressure necrosis of the tumor is the cause of dislodgement. If the patient brings in the regurgitated prosthesis, a new copy is made and inserted as soon as the patient is ready. For distal migration, endoscopic retrieval is undertaken if possible; the simple method of tugging with a rat-toothed forceps is often successful although the softer tubes may disintegrate at the site of purchase. The prosthesis can be left in the stomach, where it may remain for the rest of the patient's life, if it does not pass by itself. A new prosthesis is then reinserted.

Reflux Esophagitis

When the lower esophageal sphincter has been stented by the prosthesis, gastroesophageal reflux occurs regularly. To prevent emergence of new symptoms after palliating dysphagia, the patient with the prosthesis spanning the lower esophageal sphincter must be instructed to sleep with the head of bed up on blocks, to avoid bending and straining, and to take antacids.

Bleeding

Bleeding episodes may herald the erosion into an adjacent organ, but often it simply occurs and then stops spontaneously. It appears to be more often following placement by open operation. Severe reflux esophagitis is another cause.

Obstruction by Tumor

Late obstruction is more likely from tumor growth than from food although this is not substantiated by studies.[14] The recurrence of dysphagia is more gradual. The preferred diagnostic modality is endoscopy, since restoration of function may still be possible by excising the overgrowth by either photoablation or electrosurgery, if it is obstructing the upper end. If a lower end obstruction is found after the upper end has been cleared, the prosthesis has to be removed, the tumor curetted with dilators, and a new prosthesis inserted. Sometimes the endoprosthesis may be firmly embedded in tumor growth and cannot be removed. Recannalization of the lumen with photocoagulation may be the only option.

Perforation

Instrumental perforation from endoscopy (usually the rigid endoscope) and from dilation account for most of the immediate perforations, while erosion by the prosthesis presents more insidiously. Instrumental perforation, an incidence of 8 to 10 percent in large series, is managed conservatively with antibiotics, intravenous fluids and nasogastric decompression. A 50 percent mortality is expected. Chronic perforation is the result of erosion of the prosthesis, which may find its way into the pleural cavities, or the mediastinum, and may fistualize into the respiratory tract, the pericardium, and other or-gans. Since spontaneous fistula develops frequently in the late stages of the disease, the real incidence of perforation from the foreign body cannot be determined with great certainty.

Airway Obstruction

When intubating a tumor with extensive extraesophageal spread, encroaching on the trachea or main-stem bronchi, airway obstruction can result.[26] The mechanism appears to be compression of the airway encased in the tumor. Since the airway is more compressible than the tumor mass, the endoprosthesis creates the space at the expense of the airway (Fig. 10-6). The diagnosis is made only when the endoscopist is aware of this possibility: When there is abrupt onset of severe respiratory distress after the endoprosthesis has been inserted, the diagnosis must be entertained. There is no time to await confirmation with CT scan; once tension pneumothorax has been ruled out clinically, the endoprosthesis must be removed forthwith.

RESULTS

Of 175 patients with obstruction by advanced esophagogastric carcinoma in the Amsterdam series,[14] the procedure-related mortality was 2 percent; 53 percent lived more than 2 months and 17 percent more than 6 months, all with good symptomatic palliation. There were 16 perforations, with only one death resulting di-

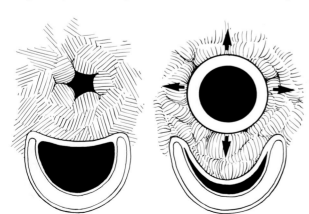

Fig. 10-6 Compression of trachea or bronchi by endoprosthesis when extra-esophageal spread is extensive.

rectly from it. Thirty instances of obstruction occurred, food or tumor obstruction being almost equal in frequency. Forty-four instances of tube migration were reported.

Of 65 patients in Atkinson's series,[1] 40 survived more than 1 month, most of whom tolerated solid or soft food. There was a 10 percent rate of acute perforation, most of these the result of dilation. When obstruction could be circumvented by successful intubation, conservative treatment of the perforation may have a 50 percent salvage rate.

In a collective review by Giradet et al. covering 2128 patients,[12] the rate of acute perforation was 4 percent. Rigid esophagoscopy was used in almost all of these patients. Dislodgement was 9.9 percent and tube obstruction 8.6 percent. Postlethwait[21] compared the collected results of over 1,300 patients having the pull type of operative placement, to another 1,300 patients with the push type (endoscopic) of intubations. While complications of the two methods were similar (27 percent versus 30 percent respectively), the pull type was associated with a hospital mortality of 21 percent, when the push type was only 7 percent. Wound infection following operative intubation was 25.8 percent. The superiority of endoscopic intubation is thus well supported.

Nd:YAG Laser Photoablation

Endoscopic fulguration to reduce the bulk of tumor has been employed for decades to palliate advanced rectal cancer, but the same principle can be applied to esophageal tumors. In the case of the rectum, tenesmus is not completely relieved by fulguration, as local infection and discharge cannot be totally eliminated; but since this is not the main cause of symptoms in the esophagus, this modality seems to work better. The theoretical objections to dilation and intubation, discussed in the previous section, do not apply to endoscopic ablation. Endoscopic piecemeal removal of the tumor bulk provides a better lumen than dilation, yet without the risk of late erosion due to a chronic indwelling endoprosthesis. There is no tube to dislodge

or plug up, although repeat procedures are probably also needed in the long term, for which there are no data. Forcible dilations and intubations involve the use of large-diameter instruments, and the procedures carry much more discomfort for the patient. Photoablation requires a large initial investment in equipment. The current experience, concentrated in a few individuals, is insufficient to allow a general statement to be made, but the soundness of principles is supported at least by initial good results. Within a few years, with widespread use of this modality, we should be able to make more conclusive statements.

INDICATIONS AND CONTRAINDICATIONS

The indications are similar to insertion of endoprosthesis although there are some specific situations particularly suited to photoablation. For upper esophageal carcinomas, in the vicinity of the cricopharyngeus, intubation is contraindicated, as the constant presence of the endoprosthesis will be felt by the patient. Photoablation is superior in this region although it may call for some special techniques. Similarly, in the presence of a large thoracic aneurysm, forcible dilation and intubation are best avoided, but photoablation does not carry additional risks.

Symptoms due to tracheoesophageal fistulas are not helped by photoablation, and is best treated by endoprosthesis. Photoablation is only used to enlarge the lumen prior to intubation. Extrinsic compression, such as from bronchogenic carcinoma, is not suitable for photoablation, as the tumor is separated by normal esophageal wall. Dysphagia from cancerous infiltration causing disordered motility is not relieved by photoablation, since luminal obstruction is not the problem. Extensive submucosal tumor has been cited as an unfavorable prognostic factor for laser photoablation.[11]

In carcinoma of the gastric cardia, the fundic extension of the tumor may not be easily reached by the conventional end-viewing endoscope.[11] However, removal of the obstructive component, which is the portion presenting into the eosphageal lumen, affords significant palliation of dysphagia.

TECHNIQUE

Preparation

The conventional barium swallow provides limited but important information. In addition to location, length of tumor, and size of lumen, the axis of the stricture can be determined. A lumen in the axis of the endoscope is easier to enlarge with the laser than a horizontal axis, sometimes found near the gastroesophageal junction. A CT scan of the chest or abdomen is usually performed to evaluate resectability, but the cross sections of the tumor in the esophagus bear close scrutiny. The thinnest quadrant at any level must be noted, since the lumen is not always concentric. If it is anticipated that a large tumor may take many sessions to debulk (calling for more than 1 week of hospitalization), parenteral nutrition may be started, since the patient's nutrition may markedly deteriorate with the additional fasting imposed prior to each session. Premedication should include atropine to diminish the amount of secretions, and the likelihood of aspiration. Intravenous meperidine in small doses and topical anesthetic spray are sufficient for most cases, but general anesthesia may be considered if the patient has experienced significant pain in a previous session.

Equipment

The physics of medical lasers and the commonly used Nd:YAG laser generator and waveguide is discussed in Chapter 2. In brief, the laser is conducted in a closed system by a quartz fiber inserted down the instrument channel and directed at the tissue to be ablated. Lower energy delivery effected by longer treatment distance, larger beam spot, and lower power setting, induces coagulative necrosis, appearing as a whitish spot. Higher energy delivery (shorter treatment distance, longer burst, and higher power setting) results in tissue ablation in the form of explosive cavitation from evaporation of water. Both forms of tissue destruction are involved in clinical use: The bottom of the cavitation produced may undergo further necrosis due to tissue "scatter" of the laser energy, evident some 48 hours later. The endoscope must be modified for use with laser. The tip must be made heat resistant, usually coated white to reflect light and heat. A built-in filter should be installed behind the eyepiece to safeguard retinal damage from reflected laser traveling up the image bundle; otherwise, the cumbersome goggles will have to be worn. Other safety regulations must also be heeded, including prominent posting of laser biohazard signs in the area of use and an enclosed area with an outside warning light while the machine is activated.

A double-channel endoscope has certain advantages. It allows for simultaneous suction of smoke or venting of gas from the coaxial jet of the waveguide (see Chapter 2, under Equipment for Laser Photocoagulation for Gastric Hemorrhage). A small-caliber single-channel endoscope is also useful, since at times one has to enter the stricture to get to the narrowest portion of the lumen. An efficient irrigating system, such as the pulsating water jet, is helpful in dislodging debris. Polypectomy snares, polyp retrievers, and dilators are essential accessories on standby.

ENDOSCOPIC TECHNIQUE

In the preliminary assessment, the tumor is surveyed for eccentricity of the lumen, exophytic bulk, and submucosal extensions. If there are polypoid protrusions into the lumen, excision of some of these with the polypectomy snare (see next section) greatly shortens the procedure. If only a tiny lumen is seen, a guidewire may be passed and dilated with Eder-Puestow dilator as described in Chapter 1, monitored endoscopically, to 22 Fr. or so prior to using the laser. If no lumen can be discerned, the secretion is suctioned and the area is vigorously lavaged with the water jet attachment. Any semblance of a lumen is explored gently with the guidewire, being careful not to produce a false passage. In most instances, a true lumen can be found, signified by free entry and withdrawal of the guidewire, and so dilation to a small caliber can be done. The purpose of this manipulation is to define the lumen clearly, without which tumor ablation cannot be achieved safely. A transparent plastic cannula may be inserted into the lumen to aid further orientation during the sessions.

The laser power and energy required for palliative treatment of both esophageal[9] and gastric cardia cancers[10] have been published by Fleischer and are summarized in Table 10-1. For both cancers, identical setting for gas flow and pulse duration are used, although the power setting varied over a wider range for gastric cancers, depending on the estimated thickness of the lesion at the point of application. After endoscopic assessment, in which the center of the tumor is determined, the beam is aimed at the upper margin of the tumor just next to the lumen (Fig. 10-7) covering a disk of between 1 and 1.5 cm diameter. Initially a white spot is seen, but cavitation is produced by firing with the tip at about 0.5 to 1 cm away from the target, or when the burst is long enough (about 2 seconds). A charred area remains on the treated surface, due to coagulated blood. Steadiness of the hand is important and treatment distance is critical, as injury may arise if the tip is inadvertently moved too close to the target,

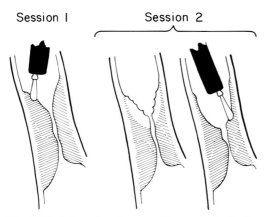

Fig. 10-7 Schematic diagram of laser photoablation of esophageal carcinoma (after Fleischer). Two days after the first session, more tumor necrosis can be found (white area), to be removed by forceps, lavage, or aspiration before more photoablation is performed.

since very high energy can be delivered to a small area in this way. It is safe to do a complete circumferential burn of the upper margin as long as exophytic tumor is being evaporated; when part of a wall is uninvolved or shows only submucosal involvement, that portion is left intact.

After irrigation the lumen is reevaluated. If it admits the endoscope, the next level of uncharred area is treated; if it does not, the session is ended for that day. A second session is scheduled 48 hours later, when the previously charred area will be seen to be necrotic and can be separated with cleaning brushes or irrigation jets, and removed with polyp retrievers, stone baskets or suction; or simply pushed distally if the lumen allows. A helpful device described by Fleischer is a suction tube modified from a 34 Fr. gastric lavage tube made by cutting off the tip and sanding smooth the sharp edges. It is passed to be wedged at the previously treated area. Strong suction is applied, and any separated necrotic tissue is thus debrided by withdrawing the tube while suction is engaged. A channel of irrigation can be added to the tube, and more dislodgement of necrotic debris is facilitated. Laser treatment can then be applied to the newly exposed cancerous tissue. The longer the vertical extent of the tumor, the more sessions it would take to restore the lumen; three to five sessions are required on the average for the nonexpert, but fewer sessions are needed by those with substantial experience.

For high esophageal carcinoma invading the cricopharyngeus, the short rigid endoscope, such as the pharyngoscope, may be the instrument of choice. Under general anesthesia with good muscle relaxation and complete control of the respiration and airway, the rigid endoscope requires only one hand to maintain exposure. A short waveguide, inserted into a narrow metal tubing to give it rigidity, is used exactly as for the fiberoptic endoscope. Venting through the open endoscope is generous, and gas flow parameters need not be changed. The regular suction tip used in rigid endoscopy is left in the lumen of the instrument to remove smoke.

For carcinoma of the gastric cardia, the objective of palliation is also lumen restoration; although Nd:YAG photocoagulation may have some as yet unproven value in reducing blood loss. For relief of obstruction, only the portion presenting into the esophageal lumen need be treated, and the technique is almost identical to that described above. It is important to avoid inadvertent damage to the opposite gastric wall as the lumen is being enlarged (Fig. 10-8A), even though the greater curvature is quite a distance away with the usual gas flow, this still has to be borne in mind. The fundic portion of the gastric cancer is difficult to get at with an end-viewing endoscope, retroflexion runs the risk of damaging the endoscope by the laser (Fig. 10-8B). To palliate diffuse oozing, the entire surface area of the tumor must be treated with coagulation. While it may be coated white or brown at completion of the session, its lasting efficacy in preventing further bleeding is entirely unknown.

It is quite practical to approach the gastric cardia via a preliminary gastrostomy, inserting the endoscope through the matured opening. A large gastric lavage tube may be inserted via the mouth as a guide, and the tumor surrounding the tube may be ablated sector by sector.

As shown by results published to date, the major difficulty in this technique is posed by

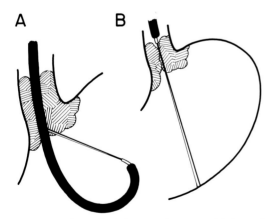

Fig. 10-8 Theoretical hazards in photoablation of the carcinoma of the gastric cardia. (A) Accidental injury of the opposite gastric wall. (B) Accidental damage of the endoscope by laser when working in the retroflexed position.

anatomical location (e.g., cervical esophageal tumor, fundic carcinoma);[11] the tumor histologic type did not influence the results. Such difficulties are likely to be solvable by future mechanical improvements.

COMPLICATIONS

Transient low-grade fever and leukocytosis are observed in a few patients but have little clinical significance. Pain during the procedure occurred in 5 percent of patients.[9]

Perforation related to the procedure occurred in 2 patients out of about 40 in Fleischer's experience;[9,10] in both cases, dilation had been used concomitantly. It appears to be unwise to dilate shortly after laser ablation since the weakened area tends to yield more and thus more susceptible to rupture, even though the photoirradiated area may take 48 hours to be frankly necrotic.

RESULTS

The quality of palliation is often very good. Relief from dysphagia is impressive; almost all patients can take all food at completion of therapy.[9] Odynophagia and chest pain, when present, are also markedly improved. Even early in the experience the complication rate, including perforation, compares very favorably with dilation and intubation. Thus Fleischer and Kessler[9] reported a series of 14 patients so treated without a mortality. The treatment time required was under 2 weeks, taking a mean of 5.3 sessions. In a subsequent report on palliation of carcinoma of the gastric cardia,[10] 15 patients were successfully treated without complications or mortality, taking a mean of 2.8 sessions over an average of 5.7 days. Several patients in this series lived to develop recurrent obstructions, which were again successfully treated by laser ablation. Encouraging experience has also been reported by Bown[3] and others.

There are as yet few published data on prolongation of survival, although historical controls have been used to show that treated patients seem to live longer. The data from the Washington D.C. VA series[20] indicate that, compared to patients of the same institution treated before the initiation of the laser protocol, median survival after laser photoablation was 36 weeks, significantly longer than that after radiotherapy alone (17 weeks, $P = 0.02$). However, the controls were historical and the numbers were small. Confirmation of the data is eagerly awaited.

Nd:YAG Contact Laser

A significant recent development in the technology of delivery of the laser photoablation is the introduction of artificial sapphire crystals as probes for delivering the laser by tissue contact[6,15] (see Chapter 2, under Physics for the Clinician). By virtue of different geometric shapes, such crystals allow contact irradiation to be delivered much like electrocautery, and yet without many of the disadvantages of electrocoagulation. Since the power density at the point of delivery is dependent on the surface area of the tip, a very high power density, appropriate for cutting, can be achieved using a probe with a fine tip. (See Fig. 2-5). A larger flat tip is appropriate for coagulation, especially when used in conjunction with pressure for coaptive coagulation, much like the heater probe. The crystals are interchangeably coupled to the tip of the conventional quartz fiber and can be used much like monopolar electrocautery electrodes. The outstanding advantages are improved ease of use and safety. The contact probe has no backscatter; and it has a predictable depth of penetration, doing away with the variables such as treatment distance, treatment angle, angle of divergence of the beam, and spot size. It does not burn up from staining by blood and debris. When used appropriately it is free from sticking, unlike electrocautery probes.

When applied to ablation of tumors at a power setting of about 10 watts, the exact spot coming in contact with the probe is seen to melt away, accompanied by little or no smoke. A large chunk of tumor may be removed by cutting away the base. Hemostasis is good. The treated area is coated with only a thin layer of charring. For more surface coagulation to stop oozing the larger tip probe may be inserted. Tissue damage is limited to 0.5 mm deep. There is no delayed necrosis, and good restoration of the lumen is possible in one session. Early experience by users of both conventional and contact laser seem to indicate a strong potential of the new system of delivery. Meaningful clinical data will soon be available.

Palliative Electrocautery Excision

Based on the same rationale as laser photoablation, electrocautery has been used to palliate obstructing esophagogastric carcinomas. In the opinion of this author, everything the laser can do in the gut lumen can be duplicated by electrocautery, given the necessary skill and ingenuity. Thus electrocoagulation in skilled hands gives the same results as laser photocoagulation for control of acute gastrointestinal bleeding (see Chapter 2), and also for control of potential bleeding lesions. Benign lesions can be removed by electrocautery as well as photoablation. The technologic sophistication of the laser confers only ease of use, but not necessarily increased capability or increased safety. Future technologic advance may yet make the laser the preferred modality and truly advance the therapeutic capability of the endoscopist, but while waiting for its development and for the cost to come down, let us not forget electrocautery that serves the surgeons so well for so long. It is fairly certain that, with development of better electrodes and the necessary technique to use them, the lowly electrosurgical generator may thrive for a long time to come.

TECHNIQUE

A simple polypectomy snare has been used to excise exophytic lesions as a debulking procedure prior to other methods of palliation, such as photoablation. As shown in figure 10-9A, the exophytic tumor is treated like a large sessile polyp; the irregularly protuberant portions may be excised in piecemeal fashion. When the tumor is friable, separation may occur before current is passed and bleeding results. This author uses medium-power electrocoagulation current even before the snare is closed, to cut down on the oozing. Sometimes a polypoid tumor may be dealt with by multiple cuts with the polypectomy snare, in the manner described for large colonic polyps by Shinya.[24] A sphincterotome may also be used to make cuts into the tumor parallel with the axis of the esophagus, followed by rotating cuts, effected by twisting the sphincterotome, to complete the excision (Fig. 10-9B). The author has devised a small right-angled snare (Fig. 10-9C) to reclaim the lumen much as the resectoscope of the urologist is used to enlarge the lumen of the prostatic urethra. This device is moved upward and downward axially, parallel with the lumen, while a blended electrocautery current is passed. Adjacent quadrants are treated in succession. Johnston et al.[16] recently described a prototype bipolar electrode in the form of a dilator that may be used to debulk esophageal cancers. The clinical data are too scanty to draw conclusions other than to suggest that the future holds much promise. The techniques described in this section are therefore for information purposes only and not for general adoption, as neither efficacy nor safety has been demonstrated.

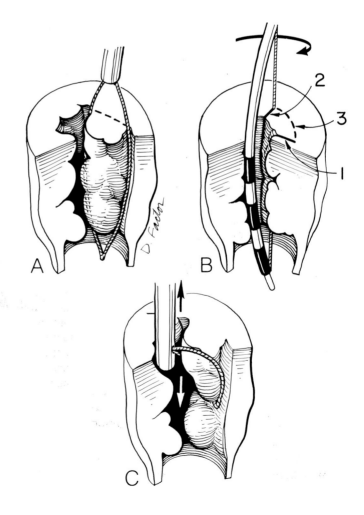

Fig. 10-9 (A) A polypectomy snare is used to remove necrotic tumor by piecemeal resection. (B) A sphincterotome is used to make two cuts parallel with the esophageal wall. A third cut, effected by rotating the sphincterotome, completes the resection of a portion of the tumor. (C) A small right-angled electrocautery snare is used to remove tumor. The wire is stiffer than the ordinary snare, and opens to form a loop 1 cm in diameter.

Results of Surgical Treatment

Postlethwait[21] reviewed the major series in the world literature and has summarized his series of 708 patients in his monograph. Resection procedures, curative and palliative taken together, yielded a 5-year survival of 8 percent, but when resection was deemed curative, the 5-year survival was 14 percent. There were no long-term survivors in nonresection treatment. With such a dismal prospect for cure, restoration of function of swallowing has become the principal goal of surgical treatment. In this regard, surgery has been quite successful, as both resection and bypass operations restore swallowing well; most patients retain the function until death. Mortality of surgical treatment varies with location of tumor and the patient's risk factors, an overall figure of 19 percent for resection operations was recorded in Postlethwait's series, quite representative of the literature. The simplest bypass procedures have a lower mortality, but not markedly so.

It would appear that surgical resection is still the treatment of choice for the fit patient even though it has a miserable cure rate. Granted the majority of them eventually die of the disease within months, the symptom of dysphagia is well treated by resection. When the patient is medically unfit, or when the disease is obviously advanced, nonsurgical palliation, aiming at restoration of swallowing, is a better choice because of the lower procedure-related mortality. The nonintubation endoscopic techniques appear to be the most promising.

CARCINOMA OF THE RECTUM

Treatment of carcinoma of the rectum is primarily surgical. When cure is an unattainable goal, palliative treatment should be considered. Unlike advanced carcinoma of the esophagus, for which the predominant symptom is dysphagia, symptoms other than those of obstruction are common and pronounced in advanced cancer of the rectum, including pain, tenesmus, malodorous discharge, and bleeding. Therefore, the efficacy of any palliative procedure should be evaluated in terms of relief of all or most of these symptoms. Reduction of the bulk of tumor tends to alleviate tenesmus, discharge, and bleeding, but pain may not be significantly reduced if it arises as a result of neural invasion. Despite such theoretical considerations, over the years considerable experience has accumulated supporting the efficacy of electrocoagulation and cryotherapy used locally to reduce the bulk of the tumor for palliation of advanced rectal cancer. Nd:YAG photoablation works similarly in principle, although clinical data are still scarce. Because of its adaptability to the fiberoptic endoscope, it has been used for higher lesions such as those in the sigmoid or the left colon.

Electrocoagulation

This modality was introduced in 1935 by Strauss et al.[25] and has since intermittently had strong advocates, including Crile and Turnbull[5] and Madden and Kandalaft[18,19] in more recent years.

The major indication for this modality is for patients with rectal cancer in poor general health considered a high surgical and anesthetic risk. The stage of the tumor is less of a selection factor: It may be an early lesion, such as a tumor on a stalk, or it may be frankly ulcerating and obstructive. For the carcinoma presenting as a polyp, diagnosed after pathological examination of the excised specimen, the decision to offer surgical resection is based on a number of considerations. This has been discussed lucidly by Goligher:[13] The degree of differentiation, the extent of involvement of the stalk, and the patient's reluctance to live with a colostomy are all factors to be considered in addition to the operative risks. Where pain is the predominant symptom, supplemental measures may be required for more certain pain relief.

TECHNIQUE

The procedure is best performed in the operating room under caudal anesthesia, which is ideal for relaxation of the anal sphincter. The patient may be in the left lateral, lithotomy, or jackknife position, depending on the preference of the operator as well as the quadrant in which the bulk of the tumor is located. Exposure is maintained by insertion of the self-retaining bivalve speculum, if the tumor is within reach of the finger, or by the operating sigmoidoscope, if it is just beyond. The fiberoptic sigmoidoscope is used for lesions above 12 or 13 cm from the anal verge. Electrocautery excision of the more discrete components by a snare should first be considered, as it would cut down on the bulk and the time required to electrocauterize the entire area. A fine ball-tipped hand-held operating electrode is suitable for use via the speculum and rigid sigmoidoscope, but the flexible coagulating electrode has to be used with higher lesions. The technique this author employs is more appropriately termed electrofulguration (see Chapter 2). Using medium coagulating current, the electrode is activated before it touches the tissue to induce a spark-gap action at close range. This prevents sticking, which fouls the electrode and causes bleeding when the electrode is removed. Electrofulguration delivers deeper tissue destruction and would thus be appropriate when much bulk has to be dealt with. Upon approaching a thin area, electrocoagulation may be used instead. In this mode, current is applied only after the electrode is in contact with the tumor. This technique requires frequent cleaning of the electrode, which has a tendency to stick to the eschar and cause bleeding when tearing lose. The entire surface of the visible tumor is treated until it is covered with a charred coagulum. The smoke should be cleared with a constant suction vent inserted next to the endoscope. The coagulum is then scraped off with a uterine curette, exposing the underlying tumor with a raw bleeding surface. Electrofulguration is then systematically applied and the coagulum curetted again until the induration is minimal by palpation, or an adequate lumen has been restored if it is too high to be palpable. It may take five or six fulguration–scraping cycles to achieve this goal according to Madden, but most surgeons would stop sooner at any one session to prevent delayed perforation due to cumulative devitalization from overtreatment. It may be more prudent not to aim for eradication of all induration during the first session. The patient must be examined after 2 weeks to assess the degree of response, and further sessions may be undertaken at biweekly intervals. All patients should be seen every 6 months to catch recurrences at an early stage, when recautery is relatively simple.

Cryotherapy

The cryoprobe is a fine, hollow probe cooled with internal circulating liquid nitrogen. It has an insulated handle and shaft. The tip, which is not insulated, is capable of delivering a temperature of $-180°C$.[23] The usual length of the instrument is such that lesions no higher than 10 to 12 cm from the anal verge can be dealt with. Cryotherapy is supposedly painless, but in order to obtain adequate exposure complete sphincteric relaxation must first be obtained through regional or general anesthesia. Exposure is maintained with the bivalved speculum or an operating sigmoidoscope. The thickest portion of the lesion is touched with the probe, and the coolant circulation is switched on. The probe turns white with frost and becomes adherent to the tumor. The tumor adjacent to the probe progressively turns white. After 1 to 2 minutes, a 5-mm disk of whitened tissue would be visible, with the probe at the center. The coolant circulation is turned off, and the frost over the probe disappears as it warms up, freeing it from the frozen tissue. It is important not to move the probe during treatment or tear it forcibly from the frozen tissue, which results in hemorrhage. The depth of tissue affected by the freezing approximates the diameter of the disk. A second spot may then be treated, and the procedure repeated until the area surrounding the lumen has been completely covered. Increased discharge, with the sloughing of treated area, would continue for the ensuing week. The patient should be re-examined in 2–3 weeks to ascertain the size of the lumen obtained and the need for further sessions.

Photoablation

A technique similar to that used to treat esophageal carcinoma may be used for palliation of advanced rectal cancer. For direct application with hand-held probes, three types of lasers are available—CO_2, argon, and Nd:YAG—in increasing order of depth of penetration. The CO_2 laser cannot be used via flexible waveguides. Below the peritoneal reflection, the Nd:YAG laser is an effective tool for tumor debulking. The settings should be lower than those used for esophageal tumors: Thus the power should be 30 to 60 watts, the maximum pulse duration 1 to 2 seconds, and the treatment distance 0.5 to 3.0 cm (Table 10-1). Between 1,000 to 5,000 joules/session have been used. The question of safety has not been systematically examined either here or elsewhere in the lower GI tract. Some authorities claim that the argon laser is more suitable for sigmoid lesions above the peritoneal reflection, as it is less penetrating, although it will take a longer time and more applications to get the task done. The operator should be on the lookout for technical difficulties not encountered in the esophagus. Thus a steady fecal stream may interfere with exposure once a small lumen has been reclaimed in the case of high-grade obstruction. The curvatures of the sigmoid make it harder to estimate the true axis of the lumen. The laser may also be more likely to damage the wall inadvertently at the bend beyond the lesion.

Contact laser probes made of artificial sapphire crystal (see under Esophageal Tumor) are easier to use in this location and may be the tool of choice for palliation of inoperable rectal tumor in the future. This claim has yet to be substantiated by wider clinical experience.

COMPLICATIONS

When electrocoagulation is used to irradicate all residual indurated areas, a higher rate of complications is expected. When used conservatively for larger tumors mainly for debulking, complications are few. A 29 percent complication rate was reported by Madden and Kandalaft.[18,19] Hemorrhage (17 of 77) was the most frequent complication, generally treatable with cautery, but perforation and rectal vaginal fistulae were also reported. An overall 10 percent complication rate was reported for cryotherapy, including stricture formation, bleeding, perforation (1.6 percent), and perirectal abscess.[23]

RESULTS

There is little question that electrocoagulation or fulguration of the smaller rectal tumors occasionally provides long-term survival, a truly surprising finding, considering the treatment is at variance with the generally accepted principles of cancer surgery. The first systematic clinical survey of this modality came from the Mayo Clinic,[27] reporting on 128 patients (out of 2,028 patients with rectal cancer) given electrocoagu-

Table 10-1. Nd:YAG Laser Photoablation of Gastrointestinal Cancers: Specifications[a,b]

	Esophagus[8]	Gastric[9]	Colorectal[2]
Power (watts)	50–70	40–90	30–70
Max pulse duration (seconds)	2	2	1–2
Treatment distance (cm)	0.5–3	0.5–3	0.5–3
Number of sessions	2–13	1–10	1–5
Total energy per session (joules)	1,200–6,500	1,000–12,000	1,000–5,000
Total energy per patient (joules)	2,500–70,000	1,500–30,000	1,000–20,000

[a] A basal gas flow at 20 to 30 ml/sec, with maximal flow rate at 40 to 60 ml/sec, may be set for all cases.

[b] Sources are cited as superscripts.

lation. Fifty-four (42 percent) of these patients survived more than 5 years, and 6 (5 percent) more than 10 years. Madden and Kandalaft[19] reported similarly surprising experience. Out of a total of 77 patients treated by electrocoagulation, 42 patients had been treated for 4 to 17 years, of whom 20 were alive and well. Crile and Turnbull[5] reported 62 patients so treated over a span of 13 years and found that 68 percent lived more than 5 years from the time of first treatment. The latest report, by Eisenstat et al.,[7] contained details of a group of 48 patients receiving electrocoagulation as the definitive initial treatment, aiming at cure. Nineteen were eventually operated on with abdominal perineal resection because of the finding of residual tumor at follow-up, while 29 continued to be observed. The 5-year survival in the resection group was 5 of 19 (26 percent), and that of the nonresected group was 20 of 29 (68 percent). All these studies stressed that this modality was only offered to patients not suitable for or having refused surgery. It is, however, completely unknown why occasional cures are obtained or which patients are likely to respond to this mode of therapy.

From the standpoint of palliation, the symptoms of obstruction, tenesmus, and discharge are relieved in this order of efficacy. Major bleeding episodes can be terminated effectively, but recurrence cannot be prevented. Pain relief is only fair since, when prominent, it is likely to be due to extraluminal spread. From the literature on laser, similar results have been reported,[2,17] but there are no long-term data comparable to those obtained with electrocoagulation.

REFERENCES

1. Atkinson M, Ferguson R, Parker GC: Tube introducer and modified Celestin tube for use in palliative intubation of esophago-gastric neoplasms at fiberoptic endoscopy. Gut 19:669, 1978
2. Bowers JH, Dixon JA: Laser palliation of gastrointestinal cancer. Lasers Surg Med 3:138, 1983 (abs.)
3. Bown S: p. 130. In Fleischer D, Jensen D, Bright-Asare P (eds): Therapeutic Laser Endoscopy in Gastrointestinal Disease. Martinus Nijhoff, Boston, 1983
4. Boyce HW Jr, Palmer ED: Techniques of Clinical Gastroenterology. Charles C Thomas, Springfield, Ill, 1975
5. Crile G Jr, Turnbull RB Jr: The role of electrocoagulation in the treatment of carcinoma of the rectum. Surg Gynecol Obstet 135:391, 1972
6. Daikuzono N, Joffe SN: Artificial sapphire probes for contact photocoagulation and tissue vaporization with Nd:YAG laser. Med Instrum 19:173, 1985
7. Eisenstat TE, Deak ST, Rugin RJ, et al: Five year survival in patients with carcinoma of the rectum treated by electrocoagulation. Am J Surg 143:127, 1982
8. Ellis FH: Disorders of the adult esophagus. p. 762. Sabiston DC Jr, Spencer FC (eds): In Surgery of the Chest. 4th Ed. WB Saunders, Philadelphia, 1983
9. Fleischer D, Kessler F: Endoscopic Nd:YAG laser therapy for carcinoma of the esophagus: A new form of palliative treatment. Gastroenterology 85:600, 1983
10. Fleischer D, Sivak MV: Endoscopic Nd:YAG laser therapy as palliative treatment for advanced adenocarcinoma of the gastric cardia. Gastroenterology 87:815, 1984
11. Fleischer D, Sivak MV: Endoscopic Nd:YAG laser therapy as palliation for esophagogastric cancer: Parameters affecting initial outcome. Gastroenterology 89:827, 1985
12. Girardet RE, Ransdell HT Jr, Wheat MW Jr: Palliative intubation in the management of esophageal carcinoma (collective review). Ann Thorac Surg 18:417, 1974
13. Goligher J: Surgery of the Anus, Rectum and Colon. 5th Ed. Bailliere Tindall, London, 1984
14. Hartog Jager DFCA, Bartelsman JR, Tytgat GNJ: Palliative treatment of obstructive esophago-gastric malignancy by endoscopic positioning of a plastic prosthesis. Gastroenterology 77:1008, 1979
15. Joffe SN: Contact Nd:YAG laser endoprobes. Endosc Rev 2:37, 1985
16. Johnston J, Quint R, Petruzzi C, Namihira Y: Development and testing of a large BICAP probe for palliative treatment of obstructing esophageal and rectal malignancies. Gastrointest Endosc 31:156, 1985
17. Kiefhaber P, Kiefhaber K, Huber F, et al: Tumor irradiation by Nd:YAG laser of stenosing carci-

nomas and neoplastic polyps in the upper and lower gastrointestinal tract. Lasers Surg Med 3:137, 1983 (abs.)

18. Madden JL, Kandalaft S: Electrocoagulation: a primary and preferred method of treatment for cancer of the rectum. Ann Surg 166:413, 1967
19. Madden JL, Kandalaft S: Electrocoagulation in the treatment of cancer of the rectum: a continuing study. Ann Surg 174:530, 1971
20. Mellow M, Pinkas H: Endoscopic therapy for esophageal carcinoma with Nd:YAG laser: Prospective evaluation of efficacy, complications, and survival. Gastrointest Endosc 30:334, 1984
21. Postlethwait RW: Carcinoma of the esophagus. p. 369. In Surgery of the Esophagus. Appleton-Century-Crofts, New York, 1979
22. Sanderson DR, Bernatz PE: Malignant tumors of the esophagus and cardia of the stomach. p. 245. In Payne WS, Olsen AM (eds): The Esophagus. Lea & Febiger, Philadelphia, 1974
23. Scholzell E, Langer S: Die Kryotherapie des mastdermkrebses. Helv Chir Acta 48:867, 1981
24. Shinya H: Colonoscopy. Diagnosis and Management of Colonic Diseases. Igaku-Shoin, New York, 1982
25. Strauss AA, Strauss SF, Crawford RA, Strauss HA: Surgical diathermy of carcinoma of rectum: Its clinical end results. JAMA 104:1480, 1935
26. Utts SJ, DiPalma JA, Wytock DH: Tracheobronchial obstruction complicating peroral prosthesis insertion. Gastrointest Endosc 31:383, 1985
27. Wittoesch JH, Jackman RT: Results of conservative management of cancer of the rectum in poor risk patients. Surg Gynecol Obstet 107:648, 1958

11

Removal of Foreign Bodies

RATIONALE

From the earliest days of endoscopy, removal of foreign bodies impacted in the GI or the respiratory tract has been an important use of the endoscope. Most biologically inert objects, once they passed the pylorus, are passed per rectum without mischief, but there are major exceptions. The important considerations are the size, shape, nature of the objects, and the anatomy of the alimentary canal of the individual patient. Occasionally the number of objects ingested may also have to be considered. For example, long needles or stiff wire may cause perforation in the intestines even though they may quickly pass the pylorus, and sharp and irregular objects (e.g., razor blades, open safety pins, and bone spicules) have a reputation for hazardous passage. Metallic and plastic objects change little when subjected to the chemical actions of the digestive tract, but other organic indigestible substances may swell or undergo chemical dissolution or hardening. Watch batteries are dangerous because of their potential for leaking corrosive and toxic chemicals rather than for their physical size.[13] After gastric operations in which the pylorus has either been bypassed or resected, foreign objects may leave the stomach quicker than anticipated and get beyond the reach of the endoscope much sooner. Previous abdominal operations may cause adhe-sions preventing the uneventful passage of the object, giving rise to intestinal obstruction days after the ingestion.

Indications for Endoscopic Extraction

The concept is to avoid unnecessary endoscopy on the one hand and forced surgical intervention on the other. Impaction or retention in the GI tract should be treated endoscopically first, whenever it is within the reach of the endoscope. All foreign bodies impacted in the esophagus should be removed upon diagnosis. This organ is designed for rapid transit of luminal contents; any object remaining in it indicates failure of normal function. For gastric foreign bodies, the vast majority will pass spontaneously even if the object appears two or three times larger than the size of the pylorus. However, if the size, shape, and nature indicate a hazardous journey ahead, endoscopic removal should be undertaken without delay. This is because duodenal extraction is more difficult and hazardous and also because if the object gets out of reach of the endoscope a surgical operation then becomes necessary in the event of complications.

Large foreign bodies chronically retained in the stomach should be removed endoscopically, especially those associated with symptoms of epigastric discomfort. Chronic ulcers may be found, and may not heal unless the objects are removed. Gastric bezoars should first be treated endoscopically, with the exception of trichobezoars which, unless small, usually require surgery.

If a swallowed object is first discovered beyond the pylorus, an initial wait-and-see attitude is justified. It may take up to 1 month to pass, but the average time taken is 1 week.[3] Failure of progress with development of abdominal pain, obstruction, ileus, or fever are indications of complications, and therefore surgical treatment. Only infrequently is early ileocecal impaction detected when the migration of the object has been followed carefully. Colonoscopic retrieval is indicated for these cases. Rectal impaction of foreign bodies, almost always introduced per anum, can usually be removed endoscopically before ulceration or other complications occur.

Indication for Operative Removal

Failure to remove an object in the first attempt is not necessarily an indication for surgery, since a second attempt, when both the endoscopist

Table 11-1. Radiopacity of Fishbones

Radiopaque	Faintly Radiopaque	Radiolucent
Bass	Salmon	Blue fish
Cod	Pike	Butter fish
Flounder		Mackerel
Fluke		Pompano
Gray sole		Trout
Haddock		
Halibut		
Porgie		
Red snapper		
Sea bass		
Striped bass		
Smelt		
White perch		

(Table modified from Goldman JL: Fishbones in the esophagus. Ann Otol Rhinol Laryngol 60:957, 1951.)

and the patient have been better prepared, is usually successful. The endoscopist must carefully consider the cumulative risks of repeated endoscopic procedures against the obvious disadvantage of an open surgical operation. Surgery is absolutely indicated when complications such as intestinal obstruction, fistulization, abscess formation, or perforation, have already occurred. Surgical removal is indicated as the primary treatment when the foreign body is impacted out of reach of the endoscope, when there is failure of progress over a reasonable period, or when the shape, size, or nature indicate with considerable certainty impending disaster. In general, the need to remove foreign bodies surgically is inversely proportional to the endoscopic facilities available to the patient.

FOREIGN BODIES IN THE ESOPHAGUS

Certain well-defined groups of patients swallow foreign objects. Children under age 5 swallow them accidentally or out of curiosity, alcoholics do so while inebriated, prisoners swallow objects in order to get away from the cell, and psychotic patients do so because of their psychosis. Patients with esophageal diseases present with food impaction drawing attention to the underlying disease; they do not swallow foreign objects not intended for consumption.

The nature of the objects causing impaction is different in these patient groups. Food including bones embedded therein are the usual impacted objects in adults, a significant percentage of whom have underlying esophageal lesions. Toys and a wide range of items that happen to fascinate the child may be swallowed and impacted in the small lumen. A common and dangerous item is the aluminum tab of soda or beer cans. The radiopacity of the commonly ingested objects is noteworthy. Bones are radiopaque, except for certain fishbones (Table 11-1), but thin aluminum can tabs and glass are only barely radiovisible and easily overlooked. Plastics are radiolucent unless they have been coated with a metallic paint. Thin, flat objects (such as coins and can tabs) tend to show well on anteroposterior view, as they are lodged in the cricopharyngeus, but when lodged in the larynx, they show up best on lateral view. This is because of the different anatomy: The slitlike lumen is oriented sagittally in the larynx, but is transverse in the hypopharynx and the cricopharyngeus.

The symptoms of presentation also vary widely depending on the patient. Children may not come with a history of witnessed ingestion; excessive salivation, crying, refusal to eat, or signs of pulmonary aspiration are important clues. In adults the abrupt onset of chest pain and dysphagia after heavy drinking or ingestion of food containing bones is quite characteristic; the diagnosis is usually suggested by the patient. In long-neglected cases, fortunately much rarer these days, with abscess formation or impending perforation, symptoms of mediastinal sepsis (recurrent laryngeal nerve palsy, tachycardia, pleural effusion, neck crepitus) in addition to pain and inanition may bring in a patient in an almost moribund state. Treatment is discussed under the type of object impacted.

Fish and Poultry Bones

Sharp spicules of bone become lodged after penetrating the mucosa. The patient habitually eats hastily. In the author's experience in the Far East, where fish is an important food item in a large proportion of the population, fishbones in the esophagus constitute one of the most common emergency admissions to the surgical service. Some reports suggest that patients wearing an upper denture plate may be impaired in their ability to differentiate the finer consistency of the bolus swallowed. The symptoms are pain or discomfort on swallowing and a sensation of something lodged in the pharynx; the location of lodgement usually corresponds accurately to that indicated by the patient. Three-fourths of all impactions occur at the cricopharyngeus, while impaction at the middle third (usually the aortic crossing) and the lower third (usually just above the hiatus) is about equal in fre-

quency. Plain radiographs of the neck and thorax, especially the lateral view, frequently show the foreign body, but when in doubt a contrast study such as barium-impregnated bread or marshmallow may be helpful. If still negative, the patient's symptoms may be from laceration of the mucosa, and should improve with time. If symptoms persist after 24 hours, endoscopy is indicated.

TECHNIQUE

The entire esophagus must be carefully inspected, including the pyriform sinuses and the cricopharyngeus. The author prefers using the long rigid laryngoscope first for a careful search of the pharynx, pyriform sinuses, and the cricopharyngeus under topical anesthesia. If the spicule is not found, the fiberoptic endoscope is then used to enter the cricopharyngeus under direct vision to continue the search. Most spicules are imbedded with the sharp end directed downward and are readily extractable. The best forceps for removing the bone spicules are the alligator forceps, as the serrated jaws greatly facilitate the task. The rat-toothed forceps, ideal for removing coins, are also serviceable. The bone spicules rarely fragment upon removal, leaving smaller pieces embedded in the mucosa. In any case, the site is irrigated and inspected to ensure complete removal.

Meat Bolus Impaction

Also called the steakhouse syndrome, the accident occurs when a bolus of meat, only barely masticated, is lodged at the lower end of the esophagus. The resulting intense esophageal spasm produces a boring or crushing type of chest pain quite similar to angina radiating to the back and/or to the hyoid region. In severe cases it may be associated with spontaneous rupture of the esophagus, when symptoms and signs of shock, pleural irritation, and neck crepitus, soon develop. For simple impaction, a contrast study with a very small amount of water-soluble medium confirms the diagnosis. Working with a radiologist, medical therapy[4] may first be tried by administering 0.5 to 1 mg of glucagon IV and having the patient swallow one gulp of Gastrografin after 1 or 2 minutes. Even if it only works when the impaction is not firmly lodged, it is worth a try before resorting to the more invasive endoscopic treatment. In the past enzyme instillation was advocated, but the literature is quite clear that fatal injury can result if esophagitis is present, as the unhealthy esophageal wall may be subjected to the digestive action of the proteolytic enzymes.[1,7] In any case, if glucagon alone does not work, endoscopic disimpaction must be undertaken forthwith.

TECHNIQUE

A therapeutic fiberoptic endoscope is preferred, as strong suction can be applied via its large channel if needed. A polyp retriever usually works well but, when the bolus is quite firmly lodged, multiple attempts and piecemeal removal may be possible. Glucagon may also be used as an adjunct. Strong suction on the top of the bolus has a good chance of success if the endoscope is equipped with a large channel. After suctioning the pool of saliva, the instrument is deliberately advanced to the close proximity of the bolus. Upon applying strong suction, a gray-out or red-out is experienced, indicating that the bolus has come up against the lens, a sign of success. This author prefers relinquishing suction in mid-esophagus, dislodging the bolus from the instrument channel with a closed polyp retriever and then recapturing it with the opened retriever. When suction alone is relied on, the bolus is likely to be left behind in the esophagus as the endoscope is drawn pass the cricopharyngeus, necessitating reinsertion. Alternatively, strong suction may be used with an overtube. The tube is mounted in the same manner as the sclerotherapy sheath. After endoscopic identification of the bolus, the tube is passed and positioned to the top of the bolus (Fig. 11-1). Strong suction is applied to the overtube after removal of the endoscope.

Because of the occasional association with spontaneous rupture, it is unwise to try to push the bolus into the stomach with the endoscope. Since an underlying pathology is often found (15 to 70 percent),[6,9,12] including strictures, esophageal web, Schatzki's ring, esophagitis, or even esophageal cancer, the lower esophagus should be carefully inspected after disimpaction.

Coins, Toys, and Miscellaneous Objects

Most of these occur in children but also in psychotic patients. In children the objects are lodged predominantly at the cricopharyngeus.

TECHNIQUE

Rigid endoscopy is preferred for foreign bodies lodged at the cricopharyngeus. Passage of the rigid endoscope is described in Chapter 9. There are two major advantages in using the rigid instrument for retrieval of foreign bodies in the upper esophagus. First, the rigid endoscope serves as a sheath to provide for shielding of sharp or pointed parts of the foreign body. The width of the instrument also tends to keep

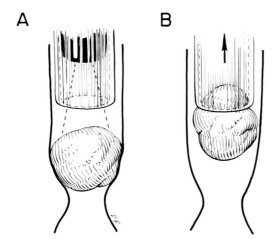

Fig. 11-1 Method to disimpact a meat bolus in the esophagus: (A) overtube is guided to the top of the meat bolus by endoscopy and (B) suction is applied.

the wall away from being scratched by the object. Second, the cricopharyngeus is entered under direct vision, and any foreign bodies lodged outside of it may be discovered before entering the sphincter. Even though the fiberoptic instrument can be passed equally well into the sphincter by direct visualization, the control is less simple and direct. General anesthesia is indicated for most patients between the ages of 2 and 5. A rigid adult or pediatric laryngoscope works well for objects impacted at the cricopharyngeus. This author prefers the fiberoptic endoscope if the site has not been localized radiographically, since its much wider angle of vision facilitates the search. The fiberoptic instrument is also preferred for extraction well below the cricopharyngeus. The techniques for removal of various foreign bodies using the rigid endoscope have been well reviewed by Tucker.[10] The principle is the same with the fiberoptic endoscope. A dry run using a duplicate of the foreign body, when identified by radiographic examination, is a major help. It is unreasonable to expect success at closing an open safety pin inside the esophagus without first trying out the technique with the pin lying on the table. Adequate exposure, as in any operation, is crucial.

There is a wide choice of forceps for the rigid endoscopes but the alligator forceps serve most extractions well. For the fiberoptic endoscope, the rat-toothed forceps are indispensable. Even though these instruments appear delicate in comparison with the rigid endoscopic accessories, the grip on foreign objects is tight enough to disengage all but the worse impaction. This is the best instrument for extraction of flat objects such as coins and watch batteries. Rubber-tipped grasping forceps for the fiberoptic endoscope have recently become commercially available and are suitable for removal of pins and wires.

Irregular objects such as open safety pins, T-shaped can openers, whistles, and small toys must be considered on their individual merits, as different solutions have to be devised for the widely different situations. If the direction of the sharp end and the location of impaction favors reduction into the stomach, this should be accomplished first, since much more room is available for maneuver. An example is the open safety pin lodged at the lower end of the esophagus with the point pointing upward. Using grasping forceps, the ring of the safety pin is grasped and the pin pushed into the stomach. Alternatively, the endoscope is maneuvered so that the instrument channel can be slipped over the sharp point. Even the 2-mm rubber cuff of some endoscopes may be enough to protect the sharp point from lacerating the mucosa as reduction into the stomach is being effected (Fig. 11-2). The pin may be closed in the stomach and left there to be passed spontaneously, or it may be removed (see Gastric Foreign Bodies). For whistles and other more bulky objects, the polypectomy snare works well. The right-angled snare (see Gastric Foreign Bodies) may be used with advantage when the conventional snare is hard to maneuver.

Chronic impaction may lead to chronic perforation, abscess or fistula formation, or mediastinal sepsis. Such patients typically give a history of chronic dysphagia, attributed variously to psychological or other nonorganic causes. The

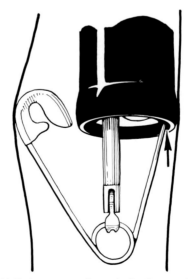

Fig. 11-2 An open safety pin in the esophagus is reduced into the stomach with the sharp point shielded by the edge of the hood.

symptoms may not be investigated until inanition, pain, and sepsis supervene. Removal of chronically impacted foreign bodies poses the additional hazard of perforation of the extremely tenuous area, and a full surgical standby must be arranged. However, when complications have already developed, surgical, rather than endoscopic removal is indicated, since the complication must be treated surgically (see Complications).

Blind retrieval with the Foley catheter may be successful in an alert patient with good cough reflexes and in no danger of aspiration of the dislodged object but, since the physician has no control of the object whatsoever, any success is attributable to chance, and cannot be recommended. Similarly, attempting to disimpact by reaching into the throat blindly with the finger tip is dangerous and can cause serious harm to both the patient and the physician.[10]

FOREIGN BODIES IN THE STOMACH

The variety of objects that have been ingested and retained in the stomach is truly amazing; most experienced endoscopists, like most fishermen, have interesting anecdotes of gastroscopic retrieval. The infinite variety of sizes and shapes provide a continuing challenge to the imagination and ingenuity of the endoscopist to improvise technique and tools for extraction. Unlike esophageal impaction, chronic gastric retention of blunt or round objects pose much less of a hazard of acute perforation, and treatment can be planned more elaborately. Both history and radiographic examination provide important information that can point to the appropriate technique and instruments. Metallic objects are identified as being in the stomach by the drastic changes in location shown in different positions on radiographic examinations. As many of these patients may have surprisingly large stomachs, a heavy object may appear to be in the pelvis on erect abdominal film, but on the supine film it may appear under the left hemidiaphragm (Fig. 11-3).

Techniques

The selection of equipment and technique are based on the following considerations:

SECURING A HOLD ON THE OBJECT

This depends on the shape of the object. The snare remains the most versatile instrument, but the following situations may be dealt with using different or modified instruments.

Round Spherical Objects

The basket principle is very useful for retrieving round objects such as light bulbs and ping-pong balls. A rubber condom has been used to retrieve ball bearings, using the trawling technique; although even sizable industrial bearings (under 2 cm in diameter) may be expected to pass uneventfully in the adult. A short condom is taped to the tip of the endoscope to serve as a basket (Fig. 11-4). Once in the stomach, the condom comes into view, and the object is maneuvered into the condom by dragging the condom over it, much like the practice of trawling in the sea. For light bulbs and ping-pong balls, a nylon net may be used in a similar manner. The stone baskets (Dormier) are suitable for lighter and smaller objects. This author once improvised a four-wire snare (by soldering the tips of two ordinary snares at right angles (Fig. 11-5) to retrieve larger plastic balls and found it to work substantially better than trawling.

Objects with Holes

Passing the biopsy forceps through the hole in objects such as keys and tubings and then opening the forceps provides a ready means of securing the key (Fig. 11-6), but in adults objects of this size rarely require endoscopic removal. The span of the fully opened jaws of

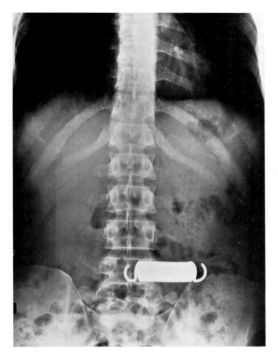 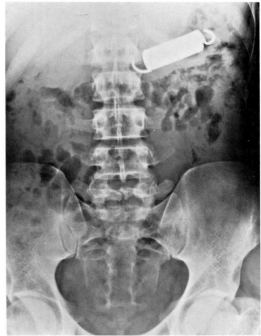

Fig. 11-3 Drastic change of position of a spring shown on supine and upright radiographs indicates that the object is in the stomach.

the forceps is 6 mm. A closed safety pin may be removed this way, but it can be expected to be passed uneventfully as well. An open safety pin, on the other hand, should be closed with a snare. The open pin is lassoed and the blunt end held against the gastric wall to counteract the tendency to slip and is closed as shown in Figure 11-7. When a double channel endoscope is used, a biopsy forceps holding the pin eliminates much frustration. A method that has wider and more flexible application than the open biopsy forcep technique is to thread a long suture, passed with the endoscope and held by the preinserted biopsy forceps (Fig. 11-8),

Fig. 11- 4 A condom taped to the tip of the endoscope to form a basket to retrieve round objects: trawling. (Chung RS: Therapeutic endoscopy, P 70. In Fromm D (ed): Gastrointestinal Surgery. Churchill Livingstone, New York, 1985.)

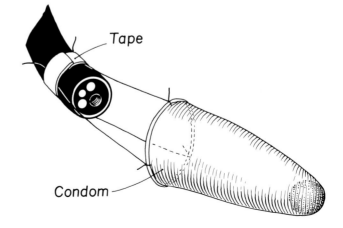

Tape

Condom

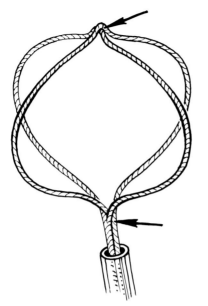

Fig. 11-5 A homemade four-wire snare to retrieve ping-pong balls.

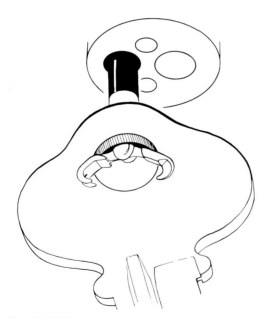

Fig. 11-6 Biopsy forceps inserted through hole in the swallowed key and opened. If hole is smaller than 6 mm, the open forceps will secure it for removal.

through the hole. By maintaining purchase on the ends of the suture, the object can be removed under visual guidance along with the endoscope.

Long Objects

A conventional polypectomy snare may be used to remove objects such as rods, toothbrush handles, and pens, but a right-angled snare designed by the author greatly simplifies the task of transporting the object into the esophagus. Tightening the conventional snare around a pen, for example, tends to make it assume a position transverse to the axis of the endoscope or the esophagus (Fig. 11-9). To clear the gastroesphageal junction, a useful tip is to ensnare the pen 1 to 2 cm toward one end and to loosen the snare slightly when the gastroesophageal junction is approached. By contrast, a right-angled snare holds the pen in the same axis as the esophagus, allowing it to negotiate the gastroesophageal junction easily. Such a snare (Fig. 11-10A) can be modified readily from commercially available polypectomy snares by blocking the Teflon sheath with a pin machined to a round tip on one end and a very steep slope on the other, the rounded tip pointing outward. A small hole is cut into the sheath at the level of the sloped end of the pin to allow the loop element to protrude. Alternatively, a 5-cm thin metal sheath can be made for the snare, rounded at one end, with a small hole drilled on the side to allow the wire elements to protrude. A right-angled snare results if the sheath is slipped on and glued securely to an ordinary polypectomy snare (Fig. 11-10B). Such a modified snare opens and closes at right angles to the catheter body. In using the snare, at least 4 cm of the sheath should extend beyond the endoscope. Since the pen is held in the same axis as the endoscope, the end of the pen may be steadied against the tip of the endoscope, facilitating its withdrawal into the esophagus (Fig. 11-11). To remove a long wire, a rubber-tipped forceps is used. The wire must be grasped on one end. It is then immaterial how it lies, as it will auto-

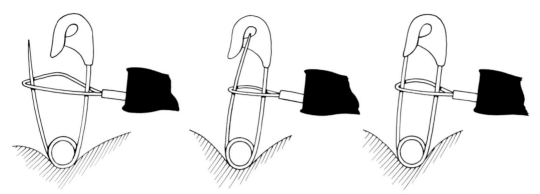

Fig. 11-7 The open safety pin may be closed with a snare, steadying the blunt end against the gastric wall. If a double-channel endoscope is used, the pin may be first steadied with the forceps. (Chung RS: Therapeutic endoscopy, P 70. In Fromm D (ed): Gastrointestinal Surgery. Churchill Livingstone, New York, 1985.)

matically align itself to the axis of the esophagus once it has been moved into the esophagus.

Flat Objects

Coins, buttons, toy soldiers, watch batteries, and other objects that can be grasped with forceps can be removed with rat-toothed forceps. It is important to remember to maintain a good grip on it while passing the last hurdle, the cricopharyngeus.

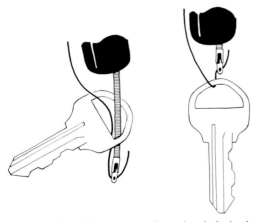

Fig. 11-8 Threading a suture through a hole in the swallowed object prior to retrieval.

Adjuncts

Glucagon, 0.5 mg bolus IV, relaxes the smooth muscles of the gut immediately, lasting for 15 minutes or more. It is a useful adjunct in removal of larger objects, such as plastic

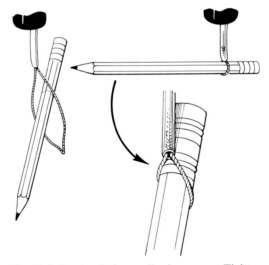

Fig. 11-9 Retrieval of a pencil using a snare. Tightening the snare causes it to swing transversely to the axis of the esophagus, rendering negotiation of the gastroesophageal junction impossible. By contrast, loosening the snare allows it to hang, assuming a more vertical position, facilitating its entry into the esophagus.

A

B

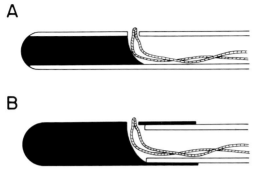

Fig. 11-10 Two methods of making a right-angled snare. (A) Blocking the tip with a metal pin and making a side hole in the sheath for the loop to exit. (B) Machining a hood with a blunt tip and a side hole, to be slipped and glued over the conventional snare.

spheres to be used when the gastroesophageal junction is being negotiated. Manipulating the position of the patient is a useful aid to expose the presenting part of the foreign body, such as the tip of a rod hidden in the gastric fundus.

Shielding of Sharp Points and Edges

A razor blade is best shielded by withdrawing it into a sheath and removing them together. One type of sheath is the overtube, such as that used for sclerotherapy. Passing a sheath is cumbersome; it has to be premounted on the shaft of the endoscope and then slid into position when needed. Once the sheath is in place, friction renders deft manipulation of the endoscope difficult. Sharp points may be shielded with the cuff or short hood built into the tip of many endoscopes (Fig. 11-2). An alternative shield, much more useful in this author's experience, is a cup-shaped Latex cuff of 3 to 4 cm mounted on the tip of the endoscope (Fig. 11-12). The mounted cuff is first everted to facilitate passage. Once the cuff is in the stomach, the eversion is undone by withdrawing it against the gastro-esophageal junction. Even wide razor blades are accommodated in the cuff. As long as the cuff shows no through-and-through cuts, the mucosa has been adequately protected. Another

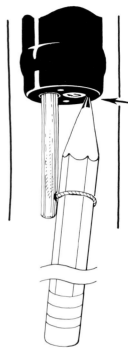

Fig. 11-11 Retrieving a pencil using a right-angled snare. The tip of the pencil is steadied by the tip of the endoscope.

method of shielding is to use a floppy balloon. A cuff with a large balloon (20 cc) may be slipped over the endoscope. When inflated it keeps the esophageal wall from being lacerated while removing a mass with jagged edges (Fig. 11-13). It may not be completely safe while passing the cricopharyngeus, however. This author has also used a nasogastric tube with the rounded tip cut off and passed alongside the endoscope to serve as a shield for a pin, the point of which is manipulated into the open end of the tube, and the entire ensemble is removed together (Fig. 11-14).

Technique

The extraction procedure for long objects such as pencils and spoons can be done under sedation alone. General anesthesia is indicated for children, for patients unable to cooperate, and for

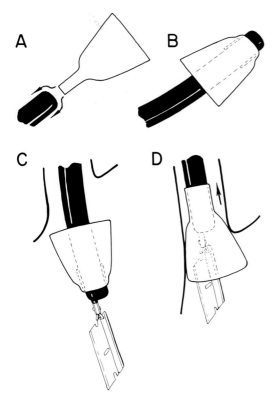

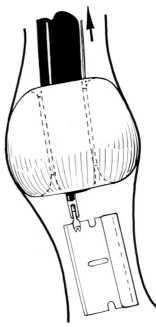

Fig. 11-13 Shielding of sharp objects by a floppy balloon cuff mounted on the endoscope. The balloon tends to hold the esophageal wall away ahead of the sharp edge, but problems may still arise at the cricopharyngeus, depending on the size and shape of the object.

Fig. 11-12 A thin rubber hood used for shielding sharp objects. (A) Elastic hood mounted on tip of endoscope. (B) Hood everted before endoscope is passed; endoscopic view is not impeded by the everted hood. (C) Foreign body secured with the forceps in the usual manner. The endoscope (but not the forceps) is withdrawn into the esophagus, a move that restores the original shape of the hood. (D) The object is now drawn into and is shielded by the hood. The ensemble is withdrawn.

those with multiple objects or when prolonged and difficult manipulations are anticipated. An operating table is advantageous but not mandatory. The therapeutic endoscope, with one or two channels, provides some convenient features but is not indispensable. The endoscope is inserted in the usual manner. The object is readily found, usually partially submerged in the fundic pool of secretions, as both are dependent. As a rule, the secretions must be removed first: If the object is heavy, one is unable to see the parts immersed in order to lasso it; if

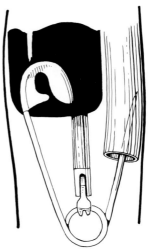

Fig. 11-14 Shielding of the sharp point by slipping a catheter over it.

it is light the flotation renders securing it impossible. The time to remove secretions is before the instrument channel has been occupied. The stomach is then distended to a moderate degree with air to flatten out the folds in order to see the ends of the object. A snare catheter is passed, and the gastric wall may be pushed away by the catheter to expose the tip, if it is not already free. The snare loop is next opened, allowing one wire of the loop to slide underneath the object, thereby ensnaring it about 1 to 2 cm from the end. The loop is tightened, and the snare catheter is advanced for about 6 cm to allow the object to swing free of the endoscope, so that one can get a better view. Before negotiating the gastroesophageal junction, a bolus of glucagon, 0.5 mg, is given intravenously. Figure 11-9 shows how a long object such as a pencil can be moved into the esophagus. Rather than tightening the loop, it is actually loosened by a small amount so that the weight of the pencil tilts it to a more vertical direction. Once the esophagus is entered, the hold is tightened, although the snare will not completely close, as it lies oblique to the axis of the esophagus. The object can be seen to move toward the lens as the snare is pulled without resistance. The endoscope and snare are removed together, with the closure of the snare continuously maintained by the assistant. It is not necessary to reintroduce the endoscope routinely, after extraction, to look for lacerations in the esophagus and gastroesophageal junction, unless there has been pulling against resistance, or unless there is a suspicious area in the stomach not adequately seen during extraction. Extraction of other objects follows a similar strategy. A double-channel endoscope permits insertion of a second instrument, but it is not of much use other than steadying a slippery object. For example, an open safety pin may be steadied by the alligator forceps down one channel while being closed by the snare inserted via the second channel (Fig. 11-15), and a round object may be steadied by a multipronged polyp retriever while being lassoed by a four-wire snare. Since both instruments occupy the same axis, they tend to be in each other's way when they con-

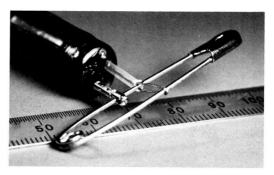

Fig. 11-15 Safety pin steadied by forceps while being closed by snare, using a double-channel endoscope.

verge for the purported concerted action. The use of accessories such as sheaths and nets often requires a dry run, if just to get acquainted with the handling characteristics of the tools one seldom gets to use.

Complications

LACERATION OF THE GASTROESOPHAGEAL JUNCTION AND THE ESOPHAGUS

Minor laceration results, as a rule, from extraction attempts rather than from swallowing. Hemorrhage is the usual manifestation. If it does not irrigate clear within a few minutes, electrocautery may be considered. Perforation must be ruled out by monitoring symptoms and signs and by immediate radiography, looking for air in the mediastinum. Mallory-Weiss type of tears usually require little treatment but rarely surgical suturing is necessary for hemostasis.

PERFORATION

Chronic impaction may lead to perforation. This usually occurs in the esophagus, although duodenal, gastric and colonic perforations are also well documented. In particular, sigmoid perforation by poultry bone with abscess formation clinically masquerades as diverticular abscess. The diagnosis is not usually made before finding the bone in the center of the abscess at laparotomy. Most of such perforations are chronic, and manifest with abscesses or fistulae rather than sudden onset of free peritonitis or mediastinitis. Surgical treatment consists of drainage of the abscess, with resection when possible, of the necrotic area and either proximal diversion or primary repair, depending on circumstances, such as location of perforation, amount of soiling, adequacy of vascular supply of the tissues, and degree of edema and inflammatory reponse.

ASPIRATION OF FOREIGN BODY INTO THE BRONCHUS

When foreign bodies are being removed from the upper GI tract, the experienced endoscopist thinks of the cricopharyngeus as a grasping hand. As the retrieved object is drawn past the sphincter, it closes and often tears the object away from a tenuous grip. This is the most common point of losing hold of the object, which is either still inside the esophagus or simply dropped at the entrance of the respiratory tract, setting the stage for aspiration. In the vigorous and healthy person, the cough reflex usually prevents this from happening. In any case, some precautionary measures may be wise, such as a head-down position, a firm hold on the object at the moment of passing the cricopharyngeus, and avoidance of oversedation. This is especially so if the patient's airway is not protected.

MIGRATION OF FOREIGN BODIES INTO THE COELOM

Long sharp needles are the most frequent offenders. The typical scenario is as follows. The unwary physician has elected to follow the progress of the swallowed needle with abdominal radiograph examinations, since it has already passed the pylorus. Soon it stops progressing and stays in the same position for days, causing much concern. Even though the patient remains asymptomatic, a decision to retrieve with open operation is made. At laparotomy no needle can be found in the gut. After much searching, aided with a metal detector, the needle is eventually identified in the mesentery. This author has encountered this twice and in neither instance can a fistulous tract or telltale scar be identified. The needle may well remain indefinitely outside the gut without causing symptoms, but the exact fate can never be known.

INTESTINAL OBSTRUCTION

Postgastrectomy patients and patients with postoperative adhesions can become obstructed, requiring surgical intervention. The most frequent site of holdup in a normal gastrointestinal tract is the ileocecal junction, and retrieval by colonoscopy is indicated (see Retrieval from Colon).

Results

The success of extraction is a measure of careful planning, patience, and skill. Failure at the first attempt is often due to lack of a suitable retrieval device and the procedure proved too long and taxing on the patience of both the endoscopist and the patient. A second attempt is usually successful, as the endoscopist will have better preparation, such as being more attuned to the specific technical problems, arming himself with better equipment. An open surgical operation is hardly ever necessary for removal of uncomplicated intragastric foreign bodies[8] unless the size of the object has substantially grown during its sojourn in the stomach, as for instance, in the case of a trichobezoar (see Gastric Bezoar). In a personal series of 46 foreign bodies (excluding bezoars) extracted from the GI tract, only two surgical operations were performed. Both were long pins that had migrated into the mesentery. As many as four metal rods were removed from the stomach at one sitting without mucosal injury (Fig. 11-16).

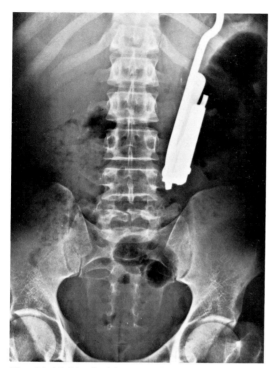

Fig. 11-16 Metal objects swallowed by a prisoner retrieved without operation. Two spoon handles, one hook (28 cm), and one iron rod (10 cm).

Similar results have also been reported in the literature.[12,14]

GASTRIC BEZOARS

Bezoars are defined as concretions of organic substances altered by digestion or chemical action of the GI secretions and retained in the gut. Concretions in the intestine are usually passed; in exceptional circumstances they cause intestinal obstruction and are then recognized as bezoars. For all practical purposes, bezoars are mostly found in the stomach. Gastric bezoars fall into three broad categories: phytobezoars, trichobezoars, and the nondescript gelatinous food residue seen mostly in patients with poor gastric emptying following gastrectomy. This last variety is not a true bezoar in the sense it is not a solid ball-like concretion, even though

it is commonly reported by radiologists as such. It is difficult to tell consistency from shadows.

The clinical presentation is vague. The major symptom is epigastric pain, but early satiety, weight loss, foul eructations, and a background history of previous gastric operations are also significant. An elderly edentulous patient, a patient with ill-fitting dentures, or one who habitually ingests hair should alert the clinician to the possibility of gastric bezoars. Sometimes a vague mass may be palpable in the upper abdomen. A plain film may show a circular soft tissue density partially silhouetted against the gastric bubble, but faint calcification may make the mass obvious, such as in trichobezoars. Contrast study is diagnostic: It first appears as a large, irregular, but movable filling defect in the stomach, but delayed films clearly show the barium-impregnated bezoar sitting in a stomach emptied of contrast. The endoscopic appearance is also striking: a huge spherical mass of dark color with interstices filled with amorphous material, and normal-appearing gastric musoca in the visible area. If the bezoar is hard or firm, the endoscope may be prevented from travelling around the mass. When most of the bezoar can be recognized as a hairball, surgical treatment is indicated. Trichobezoars are usually large when discovered. They resist enzymatic digestion and are too tough to be cut with endoscopic scissors. Piecemeal removal is possible only in exceptional circumstances, and only with infinite patience.

Phytobezoars may be treated with per-oral cellulase preparations, but dissolution is much faster by intrabezoar injections of the same enzyme, followed by repeat endoscopy a day or two later when it is found to be lavageable with pulsating water jets. The most common kind of bezoar, the gelatinous semifluid mixture of retained food usually found in the postgastrectomy stomach, is quite amenable to breaking up with jets of irrigation and suction, or other mechanical means. Follow-up endoscopy is indicated after the dissolution, since complete endoscopic examination can then be performed to rule out anastomotic strictures, stomal ulcers, and other possible causes of poor emptying. Although much has been made of the association of food bezoars with ill-fitting dentures in an elderly patient, neither it nor the eating habit has been convincingly incriminated as the major factor in the formation of bezoars.

FOREIGN BODIES IN THE SMALL INTESTINE

Except for the duodenum and the terminal ileum, foreign bodies that lodge in the small intestine are for all intents and purposes out of reach of the endoscope. The author has, however, retrieved the cutoff distal segment of a Cantor tube via the ileostomy in a patient with Crohn's disease, the tube being lodged in a narrowed segment of the ileum 45 cm proximal to the ileostomy. When the progress of sharp needles or wires is followed radiographically, one should bear in mind that the objects may migrate outside the gut, despite the paucity of symptoms. At laparotomy, certain surgical options are open: (1), milking the object onward into the cecum to avoid an enterostomy, provided the obstruction can be overcome and the cecum is close by; (2), milking it proximally to an area not affected by dilation, and making an enterostomy there to retrieve the object; and (3), if the object is in the proximal small intestine, it can almost always be milked into the stomach and be removed endoscopically. There is hardly ever justification for duodenostomy for foreign body retrieval, as suture lines on the duodenum court the risk of leakage or stenosis with the associated high morbidity. For long hooks, needles, and wire, a simple puncture of the intestinal wall, using the sharp end of the object, suffices for removal and repair can be done with a single stitch.

FOREIGN BODIES AT THE ILEOCECAL JUNCTION

Retained foreign bodies at the ileocecal junction are much less frequent than in the stomach, a tribute to the guardian function of the pylorus. Colonoscopy is indicated when (1) radiography shows failure of progress; (2) intestinal obstruc-tion is present, be it acute, intermittent, or chronic and partial; and (3) the shape of the object indicates that perforation is likely.

While fluoroscopy is hardly ever necessary for diagnostic colonoscopy, it is indispensable for retrieval of foreign bodies since only the presenting part is visible to the endoscope. There is hardly ever room for the endoscope to travel around it. This author finds fluoroscopy helpful in indicating which position the patient should assume to take full advantage of gravity, but it also indicates how much farther one has to go. As in the stomach, the snare and the forceps are the most useful instrument. The polyp retriever is usually too weak to be of much help despite an attractive design. The lack of room for maneuvering in the terminal ileum is hardly a disadvantage as objects may actually be steadied by the intestine for the snare. Theoretically displacement into the cecum suffices for relief of obstructive symptoms, but since there is a significant incidence of perforation of the sigmoid colon with long or sharp objects, it is best removed with the endoscope.

FOREIGN BODIES IN THE COLON

Long intestinal tubes cut off to be passed because it cannot be removed, may remain in the GI tract for a long period. The ileocecal valve, the splenic and the sigmoid flexures are the usual sites of arrest, unless it is held up by an intrinsic lesion elsewhere in the gut. The technique of removal does not differ from that described for the ileocecal junction. A word of caution against traction is necessary. If, after securing the end of the tube with a snare, it does not move easily in response to reasonable pulling, excessive traction must be avoided. The intestine should be distended with air, and fluoroscopy will then show the location of hold up. The snare is rotated a few times, first clockwise and then counterclockwise, and traction applied again. Glucagon may be administered. If all else fails, surgical intervention (e.g., milking) should be done before onset of necrosis. Multiple pressure necrosis of the mesenteric border of the small intestine secondary to traction have been reported. The practice of cutting off long intestinal tubes at the nose cannot be recommended.

FOREIGN BODIES IN THE RECTUM

Impaction of large objects in the rectum is almost always by introduction from the anus, but ingested spicules of bone or even toothpicks have been known to cause perforation in the sigmoid and rectum. When foreign bodies are lodged firmly in the rectum, the risk of pressure necrosis is considerable and must be relieved without delay.[2,11] The range of objects found here is completely different from those retained in the stomach. It is likely to be bulky and round, although the most slippery part tends to be directed cephalad (e.g., umbrella handles, doorknobs, vibrators, and battery-operated toys). Because of the tight impaction, the sturdy forceps and snares used with rigid sigmoidoscopes are much better suited to the task of removal, although a preliminary survey may be done with the fiberoptic instrument. The level of impaction is seldom beyond the reach of a rigid sigmoidoscope. Glucagon may facilitate the process of extraction, but to relax the anal sphincter adequately in order to carry out complicated maneuvers general or caudal anesthesia is usually necessary.

Technique

Under caudal or general anesthesia, the patient is positioned in the lithotomy position. The anus is usually patulous; if not, manual dilation to four fingers width may be necessary. The operating rigid sigmoidoscope is passed until the lower-most part of the object is seen. Depending on the shape of the presenting part, the alligator forceps or the sigmoidoscope snare are generally the most useful tools. After a good purchase of the object has been obtained, the anesthesiologist is asked to administer a bolus of glucagon, 0.5 mg IV, while air is insufflated to distend the distal sigmoid. Both the object

and the sigmoidoscope are moved together. Reinsertion of endoscopes (fiberoptic or rigid) to inspect the mucosa is usually prudent, as severe damage may require surgical intervention such as diversion colostomy.

REFERENCES

1. Andersen HA, Bernatz PE, Grindlay JH: Perforation of the esophagus after use of a digestant agent: Report of case and experimental study. Ann Otol Rhinol Laryngol 68:890, 1959
2. Barone JE, Sohn N, Nealon TF: Perforations and foreign bodies of the rectum: Report of 28 cases. Ann Surg 184:601, 1976
3. Carp L: Foreign bodies in the gastrointestinal tracts of psychotic patients. Arch Surg 60:1055, 1950
4. Ferrucci JT, Long JA: Radiologic treatment of food impaction using intravenous glucagon. Radiology 125:25, 1977
5. Goldman JL: Fishbones in the esophagus. Ann Otol Rhinol Laryngol 60:957, 1951
6. Holinger PH, Johnston KC, Greengard J: Congenital anomalies of esophagus related to esophageal foreign bodies. Am J Dis Child 78:467, 1949
7. Holsinger JW Jr, Fuson RL, Sealy WC: Esophageal perforation following meat impaction and papain ingestion. JAMA 204:734, 1968
8. Manegold BC: Fiberendoscopische fremdkoerperextraktion und intraoperative endoskopie. Langenbecks Arch Chir 345:299, 1977
9. Ray ES, Vinson PP: 584 foreign bodies removed from the esophagus; a statistical study. Va Med 85:61, 1958
10. Tucker GF Jr: Management of foreign bodies in the esophagus. Mod Treatm 7:1301, 1970
11. Viceconte G, Viceconte GW, Bagliolo G, et al: Endoscopic removal of foreign bodies in large bowel. Endoscopy 14:176, 1982
12. Vizcarrondo FJ, Brady PG, Nord JH: Foreign bodies of the upper gastrointestinal tract. Gastrointest Endosc 29:208, 1983
13. Votteler TP, Nash JC, Rutledge JC: The hazard of ingested alkaline disc batteries in children. JAMA 249:2504, 1983
14. Waye JD: Removal of foreign bodies from the upper intestinal tract with fiberoptic instruments. Am J Gastroenterol 65:557, 1976

12

Intubations

ENDOSCOPIC INTUBATIONS: RATIONALE

Tubes are inserted into the GI tract for two general therapeutic indications: for decompression/diversion of gas and liquid and for enteral nutrition when oral intake is not feasible. Stents (endoprostheses) inserted for palliation of malignant obstruction are discussed in Chapters 10 (endoprosthesis for esophageal tumors) and in Chapter 6 (biliary tumors). Surgical insertions of tubes and drains are usually ancillary procedures to major operations, although some of these techniques have been adapted for the percutaneous route. For most clinical occasions, however, simple decompression of the gut with tubes via the nose or rectum, without the use of radiology or endoscopy, may suffice. Even intubations into the small intestines or colon are possible with long tubes with weighted tips passed via the nose, relying on the gut's own peristalsis. However, unaided passage of long tubes is an uncertain and time-consuming process that frequently fails because of obstruction or ileus. At times decompression is urgently needed and it is not prudent to wait for the tube to pass. Endoscopic or radiologic guidance overcomes many of these difficulties when performed properly. Since the chance of success of either method is dependent on the skill of the operator as well as the adequacy of the facili-

ties, the selection should be based on this consideration as well as the patient's condition.

Specific Indications

1. Postgastrectomy gastric dysfunction (gastric atony), is a temporary failure to empty, attributed to poor contractility rather than outlet obstruction, but edema at the anastomosis cannot be ruled out. Since this condition is self-limiting, maintenance of nutrition in the interim is an important therapeutic objective. Although total parental nutrition may be employed, a less invasive modality is by endoscopic or radiologic placement of a feeding tube into the jejunum.

2. Failure of progression of a Cantor tube into the duodenum may occur in attempting intestinal decompression. The clinical setting is usually subacute intestinal obstruction from multiple adhesions, where a long intestinal tube is indicated. Through endoscopy the tube can be placed into the duodenum in a few minutes.

3. A small feeding tube may be passed across an esophageal stricture for nutritional management, while leaving enough room for saliva to pass.

4. Percutaneous endoscopic gastrostomy and jejunostomy are indicated for prolonged enteral feeding when the patient cannot be fed by mouth. In addition, gastrostomy may also be used for prolonged gastric drainage. When such

243

needs are anticipated at the time of a major operation, feeding jejunostomy or gastrostomy drainage tubes should be placed as an adjunctive procedure rather than relying on endoscopic placement at a later date, since surgical adhesions may increase the hazards of the endoscopic procedure. The complications associated with longstanding indwelling nasogastric intubations are well known. These include erosion of the nose and pharynx, ear and sinus infections, gastroesophageal reflux and aspiration, esophageal stricture, and esophagotracheal fistula. Short-term enteric feeding by means of nasojejunal tube is safe when the fine soft tubes are used.

5. Decompression of pseudo-obstruction of the colon can be achieved by the passage of a tube into the descending colon or high sigmoid colon. For the lower gut, intubation of the descending colon for colonic ileus has been shown to be effective.[1,3,7,8,13] However, the safety of prolonged intubation is unproven and on general principles is ill advised. If needed, such intubation may be repeated but an indwelling colonic tube is hazardous since pressure points are likely to be multiple when many curves have to be spanned.

ENDOSCOPIC PERORAL AND PERANAL INTUBATIONS

Equipment

TUBES AND GUIDEWIRES

The gastrostomy tubes are short and wide (up to 32 Fr. may be placed endoscopically). Jejunostomy tubes are longer and thinner (40 to 50 cm long and typically 7–12 Fr.), usually equipped with a weighted tip containing either mercury or metallic pellets. As red rubber tubes are too irritating by modern standards and the rubber deteriorates quickly; they are unsuitable for long-term use. Latex tubes are softer, last longer in the body, and are quite well tolerated by the tissues. Silastic tubes are the least reactive, do not deteriorate significantly with im-

plantation in the GI tract, and stay soft and pliable for long periods of time. However, both Latex and Silastic tubes offer considerable friction and do not slide well over surfaces. Polyvinylchloride or polyurethane tubes are soft, nonreactive, but offer much less friction in passing through endoscopes. A guidewire coated with Teflon or other low-friction material slides well over a polyvinylchloride surface, less well over polyurethane, and least easily over Silastic. A disadvantage of polyvinylchloride tubing is that it hardens with prolonged exposure to the digestive juices of the gut, becomes brittle, and cracks. The time taken for this to occur is variable but is generally over 2 weeks for the upper GI tract and is said to be due to leaching out of the plasticizer.[4] Neither polyurethane nor Silastic would harden appreciably, even with prolonged use. If a guidewire is not needed, the Silastic or polyurethane tubes are preferred for prolonged intubations. Generally speaking, when intubation is needed solely for feeding, the smallest diameters (e.g., 7 Fr.) are selected, as risks and discomfort of intubation increase with the size of the tube; but when used for decompression, a larger diameter is necessary in order to avoid clogging. For colonic decompression, even the largest tubes become clogged, frequent irrigation notwithstanding.

The guidewire may be used as a stiffening device, but it is also useful for changing a tube already in position. Guidewires must be flexible and slippery. The friction between the guidewire and tube depends on the length and number of curves as well as the material it is made of, and so a satisfactory "dry run" before intubation does not necessarily guarantee that the wire can be removed easily without disturbing the position of the tube. Guidewires are definitely less popular with endoscopists than with radiologists.

Techniques

Tubes may be passed by mouth paraendoscopically, via a channel in the endoscope, or over the endoscope which acts as an introducer. The proximal end may be rerouted through the nose for security and comfort.

PARAENDOSCOPIC METHOD

A 7 Fr. polyurethane feeding tube is preferred. It is prepared by tying several ligatures at 3 to 5 cm intervals from the tip, with each ligature left about 3 cm long (see Fig. 12-1). The biopsy forceps are first preinserted into the instrument channel, and the ligature nearest the tip is held by the forceps, which are then withdrawn into the channel. As long as the assistant maintains a hold of the forceps on the ligature, the tube is secured to the endoscope. The entire assembly (endoscope plus tube) is passed. The gastrojejunostomy anastomosis (or the pylorus, as the case may be) is negotiated, and the forceps, carrying the suture tied to the feeding tube, is extended as far as can be seen, usually 10 cm. The grip on the ligature is now released, and the forceps are withdrawn to catch a more proximal ligature; the tube is advanced again by advancing the forceps. While maintaining the hold on the last ligature, the endoscope is slowly withdrawn while the forceps are advanced at about the same rate so as to keep the tip stationary and to prevent dislodgement. Soon a point is reached at which the last ligature will have to be relinquished, but the position of the tube can still be monitored through the endoscope. As the endoscope comes out of the cricopharyngeus, the friction on the tube is greatly diminished and the risk of dislodgement thereafter is minimal. The endoscopist reaches into the back of the patient's mouth and steadies the tube during the last phase of withdrawal of the endoscope.

Another variant of the paraendoscopic method is to pass the tube by itself first. An example is guiding the Cantor tube into the duodenum endoscopically. Endoscopy is performed with the patient in the right lateral position. A suitable length of the Cantor tube is fed and allowed to coil in the fundus. The mercury bag is identified and picked up with the biopsy forceps, and the endoscope is then advanced to the pylorus. The bag is then delivered by the forceps and dropped into the pylorus much like dropping mail into the mailbox. The weight of the mercury makes advance easier with the duodenum in the dependent position. More tube is fed to reaccumulate a coil in the fundus. Should friction in the esophagus cause some length of the Cantor tube to be pulled out as the endoscope is withdrawn, it would only affect the excess coiled in the fundus. After completion of endoscopic placement, the head of the bed is raised, and the patient is instructed to lie on the right side for another hour. The position of the mercury bag is checked by radiography.

Yet a third variant of this technique is to use an add-on temporary channel to the endoscope (Fig. 12-2), a useful trick in passing a fine feeding tube across an edematous gastrojejunostomy.[2] The add-on channel overcomes the most common obstacle, namely, dislodgement of the tube at the time the endoscope is withdrawn. This author uses a polyethelene tube, PEG 360, internal diameter 3.8 mm and external diameter 4.7 mm, taped to the side of the pediatric endoscope with Parafilm, just behind the bending section, to serve as a temporary large channel (Fig. 12-2). The feeding tube,

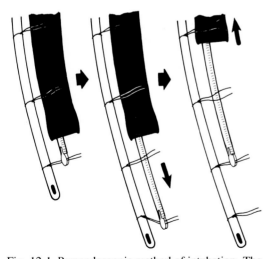

Fig. 12-1 Paraendoscopic method of intubation. The tube is carried into the small intestine with the biopsy forceps holding onto a ligature tied near the tip. (Fromm D (ed): Gastrointestinal Surgery. Churchill Livingstone, New York, 1985.)

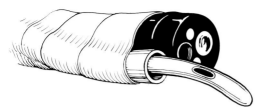

Fig. 12-2 A large add-on channel for passing an intestinal tube, created by taping PE tubing to a pediatric endoscope.

prepared with multiple ligatures, is preinserted into this large channel. The entire assembly is passed and tube placement carried out as described above. While the endoscope is more difficult to pass and the controls somewhat stiffer to use, it avoids the frustrating experience of pulling out the tube as the endoscope is removed.

Still another variant of the paraendoscopic method, suitable for intubation of the sigmoid or descending colon, is to utilize a thread guide.[3] For colonic decompression, a large tube is required since clogging is common despite diligent irrigation and nursing care. A 1-meter-long No. 1 silk suture is tied to the tip of a rectal tube, and the free end of the suture is passed retrograde through the instrument channel of the 60-cm fiberoptic sigmoidoscope, emerging from the proximal port (Fig. 12-3). The sigmoidoscope is first inserted, followed by insertion of the rectal tube alongside it, and both are advanced a few centimeters at a time; the tip of the sigmoidoscope is never more than 10 to 15 cm ahead of the tube (Fig. 12-4). The standard colonoscopy technique is utilized to reduce the sigmoid loop (frequent withdrawals until a straight luminal view is attained before further insertion) so that the endoscope is in a relatively straight configuration. When the lumen of the

descending colon is in sight, traction on the suture just outside of the biopsy port combined with manual advancement of the rectal tube will bring the tip into view. The hold on the suture is released and the endoscope withdrawn, keeping the tube and the suture in view on the way out. The suture is cut short at the anus and the tube taped to the buttocks.

INSERTION THROUGH THE INSTRUMENT CHANNEL

When a therapeutic endoscope is used, a large channel is available for insertion of a small feeding tube. To overcome the considerable friction inside the channel, lubrication with silicone lubricants is essential. The only success this author has had was to use a somewhat stiff polyethylene tubing, such as PE 240 (internal diameter 1.6 mm, external diameter 2.4 mm), which is preinserted into the channel after the channel valve had been removed. The friction is minimal, and the endoscope can be removed easily without disturbing the tube's position but the material is not as durable as the commercial feeding tubes made with polyurethane. Some advocate the use of a guidewire inserted inside a polyurethane feeding tube to make it passable. One must be aware however, that the guidewire may be hard to remove once the tube is in place.

INSERTION OVER THE ENDOSCOPE

When a large tube is to be inserted, such as for colonic decompression, the overtube principle may be used. A rectal tube with an inside

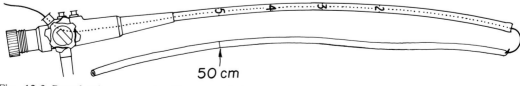

Fig. 12-3 Rectal tube prepared with suture tied to tip; suture is then passed through biopsy channel. (Chung RS: Therapeutic endoscopy. p. 73. In Fromm D (ed): Gastrointestinal Surgery. Churchill Livingstone, New York, 1985.)

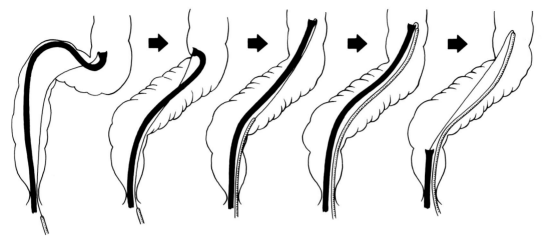

Fig. 12-4 Guiding a rectal tube into the sigmoid or left colon by traction of the ligature. (Chung RS: Therapeutic endoscopy. p. 73. In Fromm D (ed): Gastrointestinal Surgery. Churchill Livingstone, New York, 1985.)

diameter just larger than the endoscope (e.g., a 44 Fr. tube used with the 10-mm diameter sigmoidoscope), with the round end cut off and the sharp edges sanded smooth, is slipped over the free end of the endoscope after liberal application of lubricant. Sigmoidoscopy is performed, reducing the loops as the endoscope is advanced. In this position the endoscope assumes a straight form, or at most a gentle curve. The rectal tube is advanced with a gentle twisting motion. Whenever any resistance is met, the tube must be withdrawn a few centimeters and more air insufflated (to keep the wall away) and then advanced again. This is because there is a risk of catching the mucosa between the tube and the endoscope. When it is in position, the shiny inside wall of the tube will become visible. The sigmoidoscope is removed while pressure is maintained on the tube to prevent dislodgement.

All rectal tubes carry considerable risk of erosion and perforation, since they are bulky, are inserted retrograde, and have to be maintained in place against the induced peristalsis. To counter being expelled, some form of external anchoring is necessary. Such anchorage is likely to produce multiple pressure areas at the curves. Rectal tubes must never be indwelling

for more than 24 hours. Repeated intubations of the sigmoid are preferred to indwelling tubes.

Complications

No statistics are available in the literature, but clinical experience indicates that the following complications are quite common:

DISPLACEMENT

Displacement is the usual cause of failure. Regurgitation of the tube into the stomach from the duodenum may be attributed to reverse peristalsis but displacement during withdrawal of the endoscope is also common. Feeding tubes anchored to the nose are at risk from being coughed out during a bout of pharyngeal irritation.

BLOCKAGE

Blockage may be due to the physical nature of the feeding. When the tube has been weakened by cutting too many holes, blockage occurs by acute kinking in the weakened areas. Sometimes this can be corrected by putting hydrostatic pressure in the system with a syringe and at the same time slowly withdrawing the tube to undo the kink. All rectal tubes will be blocked by virtue of the nature of the contents and must be irrigated conscientiously in order to keep it patent even if it were used just for evacuation of gas, by far and away the main function of rectal tubes.

EROSION

Tube erosion of the small bowel is unusual unless traction is put on it (see knotting). However, when the tubes with weighted tips have been indwelling for a long time in the small intestine, hemorrhage may occasionally be seen due to mucosal erosion.

DETERIORATION AND LEAKAGE

Polyvinylchloride tubes tend to lose their elasticity and crack when implanted in the gut lumen for several days. This is due to leaching out of the plasticizer. Leakage of feeding into the stomach through the cracks may cause the patient to regurgitate tube feedings despite the radiographic evidence showing the tip of the tube in the small bowel. The tube should then be changed.

KNOTTING

Knotting is seen mostly in passing long intestinal tubes. Excessive coiling in the stomach may predispose to knotting. Sometimes what appears to be knotting in the stomach on radiography is not found on endoscopy, an optical illusion due to lack of three-dimensional perception. The diagnosis is made by withdrawal under fluoroscopy: A true knot will offer resistance and will retain its shape. If the knot is reducible into the stomach but not into the esophagus, it can be untied endoscopically. If it is found far

down into the small intestine and the tube cannot be withdrawn, all exterior anchoring should be removed. The attempt to dislodge the tube can be repeated every hour or so until it is removed; usually patience and persistence are rewarded. Constant traction should never be exerted on the tube to overcome resistance. The intestinal loops proximal to the knotting become gathered, creating multiple pressure sores where the folds impinge on the tube. This author once operated on a patient with this complication and found 23 perforations in one segment of intestine, all on the mesenteric side. Cutting the tube off at the nose after pulling back as much as it would come in order to allow it to pass is an option to be taken only when all else has failed. Like most foreign bodies it would pass spontaneously but it may take a long time. Impaction with symptoms of obstruction, when within reach of the colonoscope, may be treated endoscopically, but failure of progress above the colon means surgical intervention.

Results

Even though endoscopy may enable successful placement of the tube into the duodenum close to 100 percent, progress further into the small intestine still depends on the integrity of the motor function. Regurgitation of the tube into the stomach is frequent if ileus is not resolved.

RADIOLOGIC PLACEMENT

Gastrointestinal intubations can be accomplished under fluoroscopy, borrowing the technology of angiography. A useful device is the steerable tip catheter with the control attachment developed by the Medi-Tech Corporation, used in conjunction with a special decompression tube. The Medi-Tech intestinal decompression tube is a 16 Fr. polyvinylchloride tube equipped with a fine spring in the first 20 cm to reduce friction in steering, and a balloon at the tip. It is usable as a sump suction tube (Fig. 12-5).

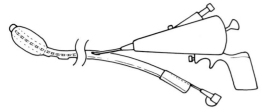

Fig. 12-5 Steerable-tip catheter inserted into a double-lumen intestinal tube equipped with a balloon for duodenal intubation under fluoroscopy. Steerable catheter is removed when tube is in duodenum. Balloon is then inflated for further progress.

At its proximal end is a slit through which a 7 Fr. Medi-Tech steerable catheter can be inserted for directable intubation under fluoroscopy. Combined with instillation of small amounts of thin barium suspension to illuminate strategic locations, only a small dose of irradiation is required (less than that used in the upper GI series). In expert hands, even difficult intubation can be accomplished in minutes.[5] Radiologic methods should be used when the patient objects to the discomfort of endoscopy. A distinct advantage over the endoscopic method is that the tube can be threaded quite far into the small intestine under fluoroscopy, as compared to only 10 to 15 cm attainable with endoscopy.

PERCUTANEOUS ENDOSCOPIC GASTROSTOMY

Operative gastrostomy, like the operation of polypectomy through colotomy, is being replaced by equivalent procedures performed through the endoscope, and for similar reasons. It is much less invasive, carries a lower mortality and morbidity, and accomplishes the same objective without an open operation. With the exception of a few clinical situations, any kind of gastrostomy tube can be placed endoscopically. The notable exceptions are as follows: (1) the gastrostomy placed for retrograde dilation of long and difficult esophageal strictures; (2) for feeding in patients with advanced esophageal malignancy that cannot be dilated enough to admit an endoscope; and (3) a small gastric

remnant of a previous high subtotal gastrectomy, inaccessible from the abdomen as it resides under the dome of the diaphragm well protected by the left lower ribs. Operative gastrostomy is expeditious when done as part of another operative procedure, and should not be deferred simply because it can be done later endoscopically.

Indications

Gastrostomy is indicated for long-term feeding or decompression; the vast majority of the demand is in the long-term nursing care of patients unable to feed themselves. The side effects of an indwelling nasogastric tube must be balanced against the invasiveness of a gastrostomy. Chronic nasogastric intubation promotes reflux, aspiration, esophagitis, stricture, and even tracheoesophageal fistula when the patient is chronically ventilator dependent. Many patients are referred for gastrostomy to facilitate nursing care, while recovering from complicated craniofacial trauma, maxillofacial reconstructions, certain neurologic diseases. Gastronomy is indicated as a permanent method of feeding in certain patients with stroke, cervical spinal fractures, and so forth. Gastrostomy for decompression is indicated where prolonged ileus is expected or when prolonged diversion of gastric secretions may be beneficial, such as in pancreatitis or in leakage from duodenal suture lines.

Contraindications

A stricture of the upper GI tract preventing passage of the endoscope is the major contraindication for endoscopic placement. Major gastric resection that leaves no stomach accessible below the costal margin is another contraindication. If drainage tubes (e.g., sump drains placed after pancreatic or hepatic resection) interpose between the abdominal wall and the stomach, an endoscopic gastrostomy in the vicinity of the drainage tubes may be complicated by leakage, since the gastric wall is separated from the abdominal wall by the drains. Patients with ventriculoperitoneal shunts should not undergo this procedure because of the risk of contamination of the shunt, particularly when the peritoneal component has been implanted to the left upper quadrant. Massive ascites is a contraindication: Sealing of the gastrostomy to the abdominal wall is likely to be impaired in the presence of ascitic fluid. Leakage of ascites may lead to infection. Prolonged steroid administration, multiple abdominal scars, and adhesions in the upper abdomen, especially around the stomach, are conditions in which complications of the percutaneous methods are expected to be high. These are considered relative contraindications in the present state of the art.

Endoscopic Techniques

The original technique was described by Gauderer and Ponsky.[6] The simplicity of the equipment needed is a measure of its ingenuity. The principle is to insert percutaneously a fine cannula into the stomach so that a thread can be passed via the cannula into the stomach. The thread is retrieved endoscopically and brought out through the mouth by removing the endoscope. A tapered gastrostomy tube (the other end being the mushroomed expansion) is tied to it and by pulling on the thread the tube is guided from the mouth into the stomach, tapered end first, and out through the abdominal wall. When seated correctly, the mushroom head should rest snugly against the gastric mucosa. A modified method, often called the push technique, as contrasted with the original pull technique of Gauderer and Ponsky, uses a long guidewire instead of the thread. After the guidewire has been retrieved from the mouth, a long gastrostomy tube with a relatively rigid plastic taper is inserted over the guidewire and pushed through the anterior gastric wall and out onto the abdominal wall. A different approach is to introduce the tube percutaneously from the abdomen into the stomach. A trocar and cannula is inserted percutaneously over a guidewire into

the stomach under endoscopic guidance, followed by insertion of the tube via the cannula which is then removed.[6]

THE GAUDERER-PONSKY PULL TECHNIQUE

Equipment

A Fr. 16 latex mushroom-tipped catheter is modified by cutting off and discarding the trumpet end and wedging the cut end into the cone-shaped intravenous catheter (Medicut). The wedging is performed by pulling a suture passed through the latex catheter near the edge (Fig. 12-6) and threaded through the intravenous catheter. A 3-cm crossbar made of latex tubing is mounted onto the modified catheter and slid over to the mushroom tip. A 150-cm (60-inch) No. 2 silk is also needed. These items are now available commercially as a kit.

Procedure

With the patient in the supine position, the anterior abdominal wall is prepared with scrubbing and sterile drapping as for an operation (see Fig. 12-7). The endoscope is passed in the usual manner, anesthetization of the pharynx

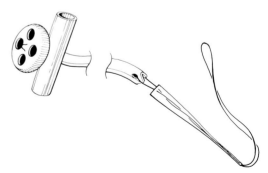

Fig. 12-6 Preparing the gastrostomy catheter. The trumpet end of the de Pezza catheter (16 Fr.) is cut off. The resulting squared end is tapered by two cuts. A silk suture is passed through this tapered tip and brought through the plastic catheter of a No. 16 Medicut.

A   B

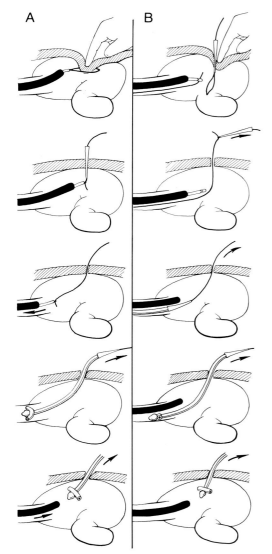

Fig. 12-7 (A) Steps in endoscopic gastrostomy: the Gauderer-Ponsky pull method. (B) Steps in endoscopic gastrostomy: the simplified pull method.

should be thorough, since the endoscope is to be passed twice. Some prefer adding atropine 0.4 mg SC to the premedication, if there are no contraindications, to prevent the troublesome coughing spells from aspiration of saliva when the patient is supine. In any case, frequent oral suction must be maintained throughout the procedure.

After a quick examination of the upper GI tract, the stomach is distended with air and the room is darkened. The tip of the endoscope is directed towards the anterior abdominal wall for transillumination. This is an important step in order to select the portion of the stomach closest to the abdominal wall. The abdominal operator then firmly pushes with one finger on the abdominal wall onto the distended stomach in the region of maximum transillumination, which usually correspond to an area 4 cm to the left of the midline and 2 to 4 cm below the left costal margin. The endoscopist should see a well defined indentation of the gastric wall produced by this maneuver, not just a diffuse movement. If this is not seen, the abdominal finger should be repositioned until this is beyond doubt. A polypectomy snare is passed down the instrument channel and opened directly under this indentation. After topical anesthetization with 5 ml of 1 percent lidocaine, the abdominal operator makes a 0.5-cm incision at this site of finger pressure, deepened through the subcutaneous fat. Through this incision a Medicut i.v. cannula (No. 16, 10 cm long) is used to puncture into the stomach. The endoscopist verifies the entry of the needle and cannula, which should be within the opened snare. The needle is removed and the end of the 150-cm-long No. 2 silk ligature passed via the cannula into the stomach. The ligature is retrieved with the snare, and the endoscope and snare withdrawn, bringing the ligature out through the mouth. The tapered tip of the prepared mushroom-tip catheter is now tied to the ligature.

The abdominal operator then removes the plastic cannula, and by steady traction on the silk ligature, pulls the mushroom-tipped catheter into the mouth, tapered end first. Continuous steady traction will bring the tapered end into the abdominal incision, until the body of the catheter is clearly visible. The endoscope is now reintroduced, and the progress of the mushroom-tipped catheter is monitored closely. Traction should continue until the crossbar of the catheter is seated correctly without undue pressure on the gastric mucosa. Since the fascia is only punctured, the latex catheter is held snugly by friction and the approximation of the abdominal and gastric wall will be maintained even when traction is stopped. It is well to remember that while it is simple to pull the gastrostomy catheter further out, it is hard to push it back in and must be snared through the endoscope. Traction must therefore be applied judiciously under close endoscopic scrutiny during the last 1 to 2 cm of travel.

The gastrostomy tube is anchored securely to the skin by friction sutures. Ponsky uses another latex tubing crossbar for anchoring the tube to the skin. The gastrostomy tube should be fitted with an adaptor and connected to a bag and may be used for feeding after 18 to 24 hours. For decompression, it may be connected to drain by gravity. No suction is applied to gastrostomy tubes inserted for drainage. As a final step, it is always wise to deflate the stomach by opening the gastrostomy tube and to endoscopically verify that no excessive tenting is created by the gastrostomy in the deflated state, prior to removal of the endoscope.

THE SIMPLIFIED PULL TECHNIQUE

The major objection to the technique described above is the need to insert the endoscope twice. By simple modification of the equipment supplied with the commercially available Gauderer-Ponsky gastrostomy kit (American Endoscopy Inc, Mentor, OH), the author has further streamlined the procedure.

Equipment

The gastrostomy kit comes with a disposal snare, a 150-cm No. 2 silk ligature, a 16-gauge Medicut, and the ready-to-insert tapered-end gastrostomy tube (16 Fr. mushroom-tipped catheter). The first modification is to remove the plastic sheath of the disposal snare, using only the bare wire element. The second modification is preinsertion of the biopsy forceps into the instrument channel of the endoscope, with the forceps securing the No. 2 silk ligature for passage into the stomach.

Technique

The abdomen is prepared and draped (see Fig. 12-7B). The endoscope is passed with ligature held paraendoscopically. Transillumination, location of the gastrostomy site, local anesthetic infiltration, and incision are all done as the original method. The 16-gauge plastic intravenous cannula is inserted into the stomach at the point of maximum finger indentation. The bare wire element of the snare is introduced into the stomach through the plastic cannula, which acts as its sheath. The long ligature is threaded into the snare loop by means of the biopsy forceps. It is unnecessary to thread the end of the ligature; any loop of the thread can be snared. The loop is closed against the plastic cannula, its temporary sheath, thereby securing the ligature, which is brought through to the outside of the abdominal wall by withdrawing both the medicut and the wire loop together. It should be remembered that the trumpet portion of the medicut cannula would not hold the ligature, and so the loop must not be withdrawn too far into it. The oral end of the ligature is then tied to the tapered end of the gastrostomy tube. The tube is thinly coated with povidone-iodine ointment and then with a coat of lubricating gel. By traction on the abdominal end of the ligature, the gastrostomy tube is pulled into position, monitored by the endoscope, which stays in the stomach throughout the procedure. The gastrostomy tube is finally anchored with sutures when it has seated correctly. Under no circumstance should this anchorage be too tight.

This streamlining of the Gauderer-Ponsky technique eliminates not only the repeated insertion of the endoscope but the unnecessary up-and-down travel of the silk and snare in the esophagus as well. Another advantage is that multiple tubes (such as a draining gastrostomy tube and a feeding jejunostomy tube) can be placed with a single pass of the endoscope. The only possible disadvantage of this technique is that the gastrostomy tube has to pass the esophagus where the endoscope has taken up some space, a more than theoretical consideration in the pediatric patient. In more than 50 procedures, this author has not encountered any difficulty in adult patients without preexisting esophageal narrowing. Lubrication of the tube is a useful precaution since it reduces the friction with the endoscope while passing through the esophageal sphincters.

THE PUSH TECHNIQUE

Equipment

The equipment is commercially available as the Sachs-Vine percutaneous gastrostomy kit (Microvasive Inc., Milford, MA). It consists of a tapered catheter, 80 cm long, and 14 Fr. in diameter. A flexible guidewire, 160 cm long, and an 18-gauge needle, 2¾ inches long mounted on a syringe, are also supplied.

Technique

Gastroscopy and transillumination are performed as in the pull technique and the ideal location determined with finger indentation of the gastric wall. Under sterile conditions and infiltration anesthesia, an 0.5-cm stab incision is made in the skin at the selected location. The 18-gauge needle is inserted percutaneously into the stomach followed by insertion of a guidewire via the lumen of the needle. The tip of the guidewire is snared endoscopically inside the stomach and brought out from the mouth, as the endoscope is removed. The long feeding tube, tapered end first, is next threaded over the guidewire into the mouth. Advancing the tube into the stomach will cause the tapered end to appear at the abdominal wall. Traction of the tapered end until the mushroom tip is seated snugly against the gastric wall, monitored by reinsertion of the endoscope, completes the procedure.

It is possible for the operator to run out of catheter, which has disappeared into the mouth, and yet the tip has not penetrated to the outside. This usually happens when the tip is prevented from penetrating the abdominal wall because of a kink in the guidewire at that location, causing coiling of the catheter in the stomach. The catheter must be retrieved from the mouth, the catheter uncoiled and reinserted after reducing the kink in the guidewire.

Another cause of difficulty is low-grade esophageal stenosis, which prevents the passage of the crossbar and the mushroom end. The crossbar should be reduced in length, or be eliminated altogether. To further reduce the bulk of the mushroom, a 150-cm-long ligature may be looped through the mushroom, and countertraction used as the catheter is pulled from the abdominal aspect.

MODIFIED SELDINGER TECHNIQUE

The only special equipment is a plastic cannula that can be removed by peeling into two halves (Russell gastrostomy kit, Wilson Cooke, Inc., Winston-Salem, NC).[11] In this technique, needle puncture of the stomach is again monitored endoscopically. A guidewire is next inserted into the stomach through the needle. After removal of the needle, the trocar (with a central lumen) and cannula are inserted over the guidewire into the stomach by the Seldinger technique. For this to be possible, the skin, fascia, and rectus muscle must be first incised with the blade and the gastric wall must be pushed against the anterior abdominal wall by gaseous distention and also by the tip of the endoscope, which is rammed against the mucosa next to the site of entry of the guidewire. A rotary motion of the trocar facilitates entry. When the cannula is in place, the trocar is removed. A 14 Fr. Foley catheter is inserted via the cannula into the stomach and the balloon inflated. The catheter is pulled back until the balloon is seated correctly, as observed endoscopically. The cannula is then removed by peeling away and separating into halves without disturbing its content, the Foley catheter.

If the peel-away cannula is not used, a regular steel cannula and trocar (16 Fr.) can be substituted. The Foley catheter (14 Fr.) is then inserted after the trocar is removed and the balloon inflated. To remove the cannula, the funnel end of the Foley catheter is amputated obliquely, saving the balloon channel so that the cannula can slide out easily. An adaptor can be fitted to the amputated catheter for attachment to either a drainage bag or an infusion set.

The advantage claimed for the Seldinger technique is that the tube is introduced sterilely from outside into the stomach, as contrasted with the pull method, in which the tube is contaminated by oral organisms. Also, the endoscope is passed only once in this technique. The disadvantage is that the gastric wall tends to be pushed away from the abdominal wall in executing this technique, as Preshaw has noted[10] in a radiologic percutaneous method utilizing only air distension of the stomach. The Seldinger technique was originally described for puncture of arteries, which are well supported by surrounding tissues; it is hard to see how the freely moving stomach can be anchored well enough for this to be done consistently and safely. In all other methods described, the freely moving gastric wall tends to be approximated to the abdominal wall when the tube makes its way to the outside, the single most important safety factor. In the original report of 28 cases,[11] there were no complications related to failure of puncturing the stomach, such as multiple attempts causing multiple holes. One dislodgement of tube occurred due to a ruptured Foley balloon shortly after insertion, requiring operation. The gastrostomy tube requires redesigning since the Foley balloon cannot be depended upon for any amount of traction, as any seasoned house officer knows only too well.

REMOVAL OF GASTROSTOMY TUBE

When the tube has served its purpose, it can be simply removed by firm, steady traction. The procedure causes transient pain but premedication is not necessary if the patient has been reassured. With traction, the pliable mushroom tip slips through the transverse bar and out through the tract. The bar is left in the stomach to be passed later. The tract must be well-formed and removal is therefore contraindicated any sooner than two weeks after placement. The gastrostomy tube may also be removed by endosopy after cutting short at the skin level; but leaving the combined crossbar and intragastric segment to be passed is not recommended as the T-shaped structure is quite large. Straightening the mushroom tip by traction against an internal introducer may not work since the introducer may slip out of the tube through one of the holes in the mushroom head. The posterior gastric wall may be injured instead.

Complications

Although the technique is simple in principle, a number of what appear to be trivial details must be attended to. Thus the following complications are all avoidable if these are heeded.

CANNULA IN THE SUBCUTANEOUS SPACE

Loss of the plastic cannula in the subcutaneous tissue may occur when the procedure is done in obese patients. While the space between the stomach and the skin may be reduced with depression of the abdominal wall and the stomach successfully penetrated, the cannula may disappear on release of pressure and become buried in the subcutaneous fat. Worse, the cannula may be lifted up and dislodge from stomach. Another puncture is then required. Usually the original puncture seals without sequelae. A 20 cm No. 14 or 16 cannula should be used in obese patients. A plastic cannula lost in the fat requires cutting down for retrieval.

INABILITY TO PENETRATE THE STOMACH

When transmitted movement is misinterpreted as indentation of the gastric wall, percutaneous puncture in the selected location with the 10-cm cannula may not penetrate the stomach. This may also happen if the puncture is not vertical to the gastric wall. When multiple punctures are required, the chance of puncturing the transverse colon or small intestine is increased. If the first puncture did not enter the stomach, the operator must desist. He or she must then explore carefully with finger pressure to produce the well-defined indentation as verified by the endoscopist, before puncturing again.

CONE SEPARATION

Separation of the plastic cone from the gastrostomy mushroom catheter occurs when traction is applied to the cone instead of the suture, which is attached to the gastrostomy catheter itself. If the cone separates, the square end of the catheter will meet with much resistance, and the suture may break or cut through the latex rubber. Rather than keep on pulling, the catheter end must be exposed by dissection in the subcutaneous tissue. The holdup is usually at the level of the dermis.

HOLDUP

A situation may arise when the gastrostomy is performed for palliation of carcinoma of the gastroesophageal junction in which the gastrostomy catheter is held up in the esophagus. While no difficulty has occurred in the initial endoscopy, resistance may be encountered when the gastrostomy tube was being pulled through the vicinity of the neoplasm, possibly because the line of traction was substantially different from the available lumen (Fig. 12-8). The bowstringing of the long silk cuts into the tumor, which holds up the catheter. Disimpaction is easily achieved endoscopically, although there may be embarrassing bleeding.

The cross bar may slip off the mushroom end at locations of hold up such as the gastroesophageal junction. The gastrostomy tube may function without the bar but it risks dislodgement and peritonitis. It is safer to change the tube by bringing it back into the mouth with a snare and tying a new tube to the end of the long silk.

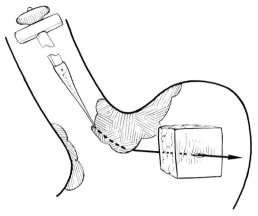

Fig. 12-8 Even when a tumor at the gastroesophageal junction is nonobstructing, it may lead to difficulty in placing an endoscopic gastrostomy tube due to alteration of the line of traction, such that the string may cut into the tumor.

LEAKAGE

Leakage around the gastrostomy is usually due to too much traction on the catheter, resulting in major pressure necrosis of the gastric and/or the abdominal wall. The hole may become large and the catheter may be extruded. This is a disastrous complication resulting in a large hole in the abdominal wall with excoriation of surrounding skin. Fortunately a fibrous track usually has formed so that no peritonitis results. Management involves removal of the original catheter and replacement with a smaller (not larger) catheter, so that the tract can contract around it. Protection of the skin with stoma adhesive in the interim is mandatory. The care must be supervised by a skilled stomal therapist.

Leakage into the peritoneal cavity is due to dislodgement before the fibrous tract is formed.

LOCAL INFECTION

If the catheter is too large or the fascial opening too tight local infection around the catheter may occur. Fasciitis has been reported. This author believes that the condition can be avoided if pressure necrosis of the fascia has not occurred around the catheter. Ponsky[9] advocates prophylactic antibiotics administered in the perioperative period in three doses. Strodel et al.[14,15] believe that good oral hygienic care as a method of preoperative preparation will reduce such infection.

PNEUMOPERITONEUM

Early pneumoperitoneum, if asymptomatic, may be disregarded, as some escape of air from the stomach around the puncture site is common. Overinflation of the stomach during the procedure is the usual cause. However, if it is persistent (over several days), leakage around the tube should be suspected. This can be confirmed with a contrast radiologic study. If the leakage is significant or if peritoneal signs are present, operative repair should be undertaken without delay to prevent continuous peritoneal soilage.

GASTROCOLIC FISTULA

Injury of the transverse colon may lead to abscess formation adjacent to the gastrostomy. A fistula forms with spontaneous drainage into the stomach.

TUBE BLOCKAGE

Blockage by tube feeding is rare unless improperly cared for. Blenderized feeding is the usual offender, but since this has been largely replaced by commercial liquid diets, clogging is uncommon. When it has become hopelessly clogged, the tube should be removed and replaced. This is possible without endoscopy, provided a tract has formed around the tube. Following removal of the clogged tube, a new No. 16 mushroom catheter, without modification, is then inserted with an introducer stretching the mushroom tip to reduce the diameter. Alternatively, a Foley catheter may be used with the balloon for internal anchorage. Even a simple catheter may suffice if it is sutured to the skin. Blockage in the early post-insertion period is best treated by judicious guidewire probing combined with irrigation.

DISLODGEMENT

The tube is rarely dislodged after endoscopic insertion using the mushroom-tipped catheter with crossbar unless pulled on intentionally. In this author's experience in surgical gastrostomy, the dislodgement commonly occurs from a deflated Foley balloon, a notoriously unreliable device for anchoring gastrostomy tubes. The consequences of early dislodgement are disastrous, as the ensuing generalized peritonitis requires prompt operative intervention.

FAILURE OF RETURN WHEN ASPIRATED

All gastrostomy tubes exhibit this characteristic. The mucosa immediately blocks off the tube as soon as suction is applied. It is important to recognize this so as to avoid unnecessary replacement of a perfectly good gastrostomy tube. By the same token, the tube should never be connected to suction for the purpose of drainage.

Results

The popularity of the endoscopic technique is attested to by a proliferation of reports in the endoscopic literature in the short interval since introduction. A success rate of more than 95 percent can be expected, as judged from more than 1,000 cases reported to date from many centers. Most of the complications described above occurred early in the experience. No procedure-related mortality has been found in the results published so far. When used as the feeding route, aspiration occurred in 15 to 20 percent of patients with neurologic disorders where swallowing had been impaired, a complication not of the technique itself, but of the choice of procedure. An overall complication rate of 5 to 10 percent is a representative figure.[15] This is compared with the open operation of gastrostomy, where mortality is 5 to 33 percent and an overall complication rate of 20 percent in the same type of patient population.[16] Even though no study has addressed specifically the reason for the difference, the cumulative hazards of wounds in the stomach and abdomen, the possibility of contamination, and the effects of anesthesia in the compromised host are all probable contributory factors. A wound communicating with the gut a few centimeters from the main incision is certainly an important concern for infection of the main wound.

PERCUTANEOUS ENDOSCOPIC FEEDING JEJUNOSTOMY

A feeding jejunostomy may be performed endoscopically by a technique identical to that of gastrostomy. Compared with the clinical success of percutaneous gastrostomy, however, feeding jejunostomy is at best a mediocre performer.

The primary indication is for long-term feeding when the patient has significant gastroesophageal reflux. Jejunostomy is not the preferred feeding route, it should be noted, as it bypasses the gastric regulation of temperature and osmolarity, and is more prone to the production of diarrhea, nausea, and electrolyte imbalance. One advantage of the jejunostomy tube inserted via the stomach is that it can be replaced easily through an established tract, unlike the jejunostomy created by the Weitzel technique.

When there is a previously established gastrostomy, a jejunostomy tube may simply be inserted through the gastrostomy tract after removing the gastrostomy tube. Some jejunostomy kits are designed to fit into the previously placed gastrostomy tube (e.g., Microvasive Inc, Milford, MA). If the holes in the mushroom tip are not large enough, one connecting bridge of rubber between the holes can be cut with endoscopic scissors at endoscopy. The jejunal tube is fed through the gastrostomy tract or tube into the stomach. The endoscopist catches the

tip intragastrically with a snare and brings it into the second or third portion of the duodenum. The endoscopist then lets go of the weighted end and, while keeping the tube in full view, inflates the intestine to a moderate extent and withdraws the endoscope, trying not to dislodge the tube.

To establish a feeding jejunostomy de novo, special tubes are necessary. These are available commercially (American Endoscopy, Mentor, OH) but they can be prepared simply from ordinary hospital supplies. A 7 Fr. Silastic feeding tube with weighted tip (e.g., Keofeed tube, Ivac Corporation, San Diego, CA) is threaded through the mushroom tip and cross bar of the endoscopic gastrostomy tube (Fig. 12-9). The adaptor end of the feeding tube is excised, and together with the proximal end of the gastrostomy tube, are wedged into the plastic cone of a No. 16 Medicut intravenous catheter after anchoring both with a suture (Fig. 12-9). Percutaneous puncture of the stomach is then performed using a 16-gauge IV cannula as described for gastrostomy. A snare wire loop is inserted through the cannula into the stomach, to catch the string introduced paraendoscopi-

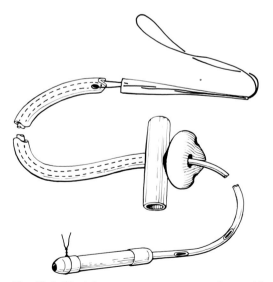

Fig. 12-9 The jejunostomy–gastrostomy tube combination. Both tubes are to be wedged into the plastic cone, aided by a suture. A short tie at the weighted tip serves as a "handle" for the grasping forceps.

cally as the endoscope is inserted. The string is pulled from the abdominal aspect, the oral end of the string being attached to the gastrostomy–jejunostomy tube combination. After seating the gastrostomy tube correctly, the rest of the feeding tube can be brought down the esophagus endoscopically. This is accomplished by withdrawing the endoscope to the esophagus to 30 cm from the incisor, catching the tube with endoscopic forceps, and then advancing into the stomach. The weighted tip should now be visible in the stomach and should be caught with the forceps. The endoscope is next advanced to the second portion of the duodenum, where the feeding tube is relinquished.

The gastrostomy tube is no longer usable for decompression, as most of the lumen is occupied by the feeding tube. Leakage of gastric juice can be a nuisance, however, and must be prevented by slipping a rubber hood, (an IV tubing connecting rubber hood serves well), over the junction of the feeding and gastrostomy tube.

Where both drainage gastrostomy and feeding jejunostomy are required, a separate gastrostomy tube must be placed. The endoscope needs to be passed only once if two long silk sutures are carried into the stomach paraendoscopically held by the biopsy forceps in the instrument channel. Upon reaching the stomach, only one suture is picked up and delivered to the snare introduced percutaneously, as described for placement of gastrostomy, under the simplified pull method. At a second puncture, the second suture is picked up and used for placement of the second tube.

Most of the jejunal feeding tubes do not have enough weight on the tip, particularly those using metallic pellets rather than mercury. When combined with a rather stiff polyvinyl body, lack of progress is predictable. This author has the best experience with the Anderson pediatric long intestinal sump tube with the air vent tubing removed, passing it through a dilated track of a preexisting gastrostomy. The tube is suitably soft and the mercury compartment substantial; once delivered beyond the pylorus, self-propagation can be relied on every time.

The placement of the jejunostomy tube is subject to the same complications as the gastrostomy tube, but aspiration of feeding is less common. However, regurgitation of feedings should alert the clinician to the possibility of either a leak in the feeding tube so that the feedings are delivered into the stomach or of displacement of the tip, so that it now lies in the stomach. If leakage is not the problem and the tip is weighted, it usually corrects itself. It can be replaced easily endoscopically. Since the progress of the tip into the jejunum is dependent on the motor function of the small bowel, the tube may not be usable for a long time if ileus is not resolved. It is therefore inferior to feeding jejunostomy placed at operation.

ENDOSCOPIC VERSUS SURGICAL INTUBATIONS

For gastrostomy placement, the published data as well as clinical experience of surgeons who are experienced in both procedures clearly favor the endoscopic method, mostly because of the vastly reduced complications. An important difference is in infection and other complications of the main wound. The incision into the stomach for insertion of the gastrostomy tube, repaired by a pursestring suture, is apparently subject to healing problems depending on the soundness of the technique. Junior surgeons, often given this operative task, tend to encounter more problems in leakage around the tube, tube dislodgement, hematoma, and infection. A lower complication rate is seen in community hospitals for the same type of gastrostomy operations.

By contrast, endoscopic jejunostomy performs only fairly, although it carries a lower complication rate. Surgical jejunostomy remains the more effective, mainly because of the uncertainty and the time required for the feeding tube to travel to the jejunum. Until a safe, direct percutaneous technique is perfected, operative jejunostomy will remain the procedure of choice.

REFERENCES

1. Bernton E, Myers R, Reyna T: Pseudoobstruction of the colon: Case report including a new endoscopic treatment. Gastrointest Endosc 28:90, 1982
2. Chung RS, Denbesten L: Improved technique for placement of intestinal feeding tube with the fiberoptic endoscope. Gut 17:264, 1976
3. Chung RS: A technique for rapid intubation of the sigmoid and left colon. Surg Gynecol Obstet 157:279, 1983
4. Duke HN, Vane JR: An adverse effect of polyvinylchloride tubing used in extracorporeal circulation. Lancet 2:21, 1968
5. Edlich RF, Gedgaudus E, Leonard AS, et al: New long intestinal tube for rapid nonoperative intubation. Arch Surg 95:443, 1968
6. Gauderer MWL, Ponsky JL: A simplified technique for constructing a tube feeding gastrostomy. Surg Gynecol Obstet 152:82, 1981
7. Ghazi A, Shinya H, Wolff W: Treatment of volvulus of the colon by colonoscopy. Ann Surg 183:263, 1976
8. Groff W: Colonoscopic decompression and intubation of the cecum for Ogilvie's syndrome. Dis Colon Rectum 26:503, 1983
9. Ponsky JL, Gauderer MWL, Stellato TA: Percutaneous endoscopic gastrostomy: Review of 150 cases. Arch Surg 118:913, 1983
10. Preshaw RM: A percutaneous method for inserting a feeding gastrostomy tube. Surg Gynecol Obstet 152:659, 1981
11. Russell TR, Brotman M, Norris F: Percutaneous gastrostomy; a new simplified and cost-effective technique. Am J Surg 148:132, 1984
12. Sachs BA, Glotzer DJ: Percutaneous reestablishment of feeding gastrostomies. Surgery 85:575, 1979
13. Starling JR: Initial treatment of sigmoid volvulus by colonoscopy. Ann Surg 190:36, 1979
14. Strodel WE, Lemmer J, Eckhauser F, et al: Early experience with endoscopic percutaneous gastrostomy. Arch Surg 118:449, 1983
15. Strodel WE, Ponsky JL, Knol JA, et al: Percutaneous endoscopic gastrostomy. P. 113. In Dent TL, Strodel WE, Turcotte JG (eds): Surgical Endoscopy. Year Book, Chicago, 1985
16. Wasiljew BK, Vjiki GT, Beal JM: Feeding gastrostomy: Complications and mortality. Am J Surg 143:194, 1982

Index

Page numbers followed by t denote tables; those followed by f denote figures

261

Portoazygous disconnection, operative sclerotherapy and, 60f, 61
Poultry bones, removal from esophagus, 229
Power, in electrosurgery, 9–10
Precut technique, for endoscopic sphincterotomy, 101
Premedication, colonic polypectomy and, 159–160
Prophylactic sclerotherapy, 59
Propranolol, effect on variceal hemorrhage, 59
Pseudodiverticulum, endoscopic sphincterotomy and, 104
Pseudomonas
   following nasobiliary drainage and endoprosthesis placement, 123
   in primary biliary infection, 116
Pseudostalk, formation of, in colonic polypectomy, 163–164, 164f
Pull technique
   Gauderer-Ponsky, 250f, 250–252, 251f
   simplified, 251f, 252–253
"Pulsating pseudoaneurism," in diagnostic endoscopy, 19–20
Push technique, 253
   equipment for, 253
Pyloric stenosis, 205
Pyrexia, as sclerotherapy complication, 53–54

Radiofrequency (RF) currents, 8–9
Radiology
   combined with endoscopy, in placement of biliary endoprosthesis, 122
   in intestinal bleeding treatment, 78–79
   intubation placement by, 248–249
   for retrieval of retained stone, 146–147
      complications in, 148–149
      technique for, 147f, 147–148
   in upper GI bleeding treatment, 31–32
   use in nonsurgical drainage of obstructed biliary tract, 126–129
Radiopacity, of fishbones, 228t
Razor blade, shielding of, during removal from stomach, 237f
Rectal carcinoma, 222
   cryotherapy for, 223–224
   electrocoagulation for, 222–223
   photoablation for, 224–225
Rectal tube, 246, 246f, 247f
   insertion over endoscope, 246–247
Rectum
   anastomotic stricture of, 206
   carcinoma of. *See* Rectal carcinoma
   foreign body removal from, 242
   intubation of. *See* Rectal tube
   polypoid lesions of, 155t
Reflux, of duodenal content into biliary tree, endoscopic sphincterotomy and, 108
Reflux esophagitis, advanced esophageal carcinoma and, 214

Restenosis
   endoscopic sphincterotomy for, 94
   with or without recurrent stones, endoscopic sphincterotomy and, 108
Retained common duct stone
   defined, 137
   operative endoscopy for, 137–138. *See also* Operative choledochoscopy
   radiologic retrieval of, 146–149, 147f
   therapeutic options for, 150–151
Retrograde dilation, of strictures, 192–193, 193f
RF. *See* Radiofrequency (RF) currents
Rigid endoscope technique, in sclerotherapy, 51–52
Rigid esophagoscope, 185–188, 186f
Rigid esophagoscopy, for stricture dilation, 185–188, 186f
Round objects, in stomach, endoscopic removal of, 232, 233f, 234f

Safety-pin
   in esophagus, extraction of, 231, 231f
   shielding of point, 237f
   in stomach, endoscopic removal of, 233, 235f
   technique for, 238, 238f
Savary dilator, 183, 185
Sclerosants. *See also* Sclerotherapy
   angiodysplastic lesion and, 73–74
   biology of, 16
   cardiovascular action of, 43, 44t–46t, 45–46
   results with, 31
   upper GI bleeding and, 7, 25–26, 26f
Sclerosis, esophageal wall, 45–46
Sclerotherapy. *See also* Sclerosants
   acute effect hypothesis of, 43, 43f
   for acute hemorrhage, results of, 57
   chronic, results of, 57–59
   complications from, 53–56
   contraindications for, 41–42
   equipment for, 46–47
   indications for, 40–41
   injection frequency in, 53
   in integrated approach to variceal hemorrhage, 61–63, 62f
   mechanisms of action of, 42–46
   operative, 60f, 61
   patient preparation for, 47–48
   postinjection management and, 52–53
   prophylactic, results of, 59
   with propranolol, results of, 59
   surgery versus, 59–61
   techniques in
      critique of, 52
      free-hand, 48–51, 49f
      rigid endoscope, 51–52
      sheath, 51
   variceal pressure changes due to, 42–43, 43f
Sedation, in diagnostic endoscopy, 18
Seldinger technique, modified, 253–254